OXFORD MEDICAL PUBLICATIONS

Oxford Handbook of
Obstetrics and Gynaecology

Oxford Handbooks

Oxford Handbook of
Obstetrics and Gynaecology

Edited by

S. Arulkumaran

Professor of Obstetrics & Gynaecology
St. George's Hospital Medical School,
University of London, UK

I. Symonds

Senior Lecturer and Honorary Consultant in
Obstetrics and Gynaecology
Derby City General Hospital, Derby, UK

A. Fowlie

Consultant in Obstetrics & Gynaecology
Derby City General Hospital, Derby, UK

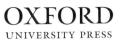

OXFORD
UNIVERSITY PRESS

OXFORD
UNIVERSITY PRESS

Great Clarendon Street, Oxford OX2 6DP

Oxford University Press is a department of the University of Oxford.
It furthers the University's objective of excellence in research, scholarship,
and education by publishing worldwide in

Oxford   New York

Auckland   Bangkok   Buenos Aires   Cape Town   Chennai
Dar es Salaam   Delhi   Hong Kong   Istanbul   Karachi   Kolkata
Kuala Lumpur   Madrid   Melbourne   Mexico City   Mumbai   Nairobi
São Paulo   Shanghai   Taipei   Tokyo   Toronto

Oxford is a registered trade mark of Oxford University Press
in the UK and in certain other countries

Published in the United States
by Oxford University Press Inc., New York

A catalogue record for this title is available from the British Library

ISBN 0 19 263181 0

10 9 8 7 6 5 4 3 2 1

Typeset by Cepha Imaging Pvt Ltd
Printed in Italy
on acid-free paper by Legoprint S.p.A

Contents

Part 2 **Gynaecology**

Contributors

Mandy Abbett
Breastfeeding Counsellor,
Sure Start Chesterfield Infant
Feeding Specialist, South Lodge,
Boythorpe Ave, Chesterfield
S40 2LD
Chapter 39

Mrs. R. A. Adekunle, MB BS
MRCOG
Consultant Obstetrician &
Gynaecologist,
Dewsbury and District Hospital,
Halifax Road, Dewsbury
WF13 4HS
Chapters 50, 51

Dr. S. Ahuja
Specialist Registrar in Obstetrics &
Gynaecology,
Luton & Dunstable Hospital,
Lewsey Road, Luton,
Bedfordshire LU4 ODZ
Chapter 1

Professor S. Arulkumaran
Dept of Clinical Developmental
Sciences – Obstetrics &
Gynaecology,
St. George's Hospital Medical
School, Cranmer Terrace,
London SW17 0RE
Chapters 3–5, 7, 12, 15, 16, 19,
26, 27, 31–4, 37, 40, 43, 48, 49, 63,
87, 93

J. Ashworth, MD MRCOG
Sub-speciality Trainee in
Feto-maternal Medicine,
Birmingham Women's Hospital,
Metchley Park Road,
Birmingham B15 2TG
Chapters 22–5, 30

Dr. A. Bali, MD MRCOG
Gynaecology Oncology Fellow,
Women's Services, Gynaecology
Oncology Unit,
2nd Floor, KG V Building,
St. Bartholomew's Hospital,
West Smithfield, London EC1A 7BE
Chapter 29

Mr. A. Bunkheila, MBChB BSc
M (ART) MD MRCOG
Specialist Registrar,
Dept of Obstetrics & Gynaecology,
University Hospital, Queen's
Medical Centre,
Nottingham NG7 2UH
Chapter 52

Mr. Roger Chapman, FRCS, FRCOG
Consultant Obstetrician &
Gynaecologist,
Derby City General Hospital,
Uttoxeter Road, Derby DE22 3NE
Chapter 35

Mr. M. Cust
Consultant Obstetrician &
Gynaecologist,
Derby City General Hospital,
Uttoxeter Road, Derby DE22 3NE
Chapters 60, 66, 75, 78,
80, 81, 94

Mr. F. J. Darné, MD MRCOG
Consultant Obstetrician &
Gynaecologist,
Derby City General Hospital,
Uttoxeter Road, Derby DE22 3NE
Chapters 53–5, 61, 62, 67–72

Dr. Soo Downe
Director,
Midwifery Studies Research Unit,
University of Central Lancashire,
Preston, Lancs PR1 2HE
Chapter 41

Miss Alison Fowlie, FRCOG
Consultant Obstetrician &
Gynaecologist,
Derby City General Hospital,
Uttoxeter Road, Derby DE22 3NE
Chapters 6, 8, 9, 14, 18, 22–5, 30,
44, 57

Dr. David Guthrie Ph.D, FRCOG,
FRCR
Consultant Clinical Oncologist,
Derbyshire Royal Infirmary,
London Road, Derby DE1 2QY
Chapters 90, 91

Mrs. Hasiba Hamoud, MRCOG
Consultant in Obstetrics &
Gynaecology,
East Kent Hospitals NHS Trust,
William Harvey Hospital,
Kennington Road, Willesborough,
Ashford, Kent TN24 0LZ
Chapters 20, 21, 56, 65, 79

Mr. R. Hayman, MRCOG
Lecturer in Obstetrics &
Gynaecology,
The City Hospital,
Hucknall Road,
Nottingham NG5 1PB
Chapters 14, 18, 44

M. Jackson
Dept of Midwifery,
Derby City General Hospital,
Uttoxeter Road, Derby DE22 3NE
Chapter 39

Mr. H. M. L. Jenkins, DM FRCOG
Consultant Obstetrician &
Gynaecologist,
Derby City General Hospital,
Uttoxeter Road, Derby DE22 3NE
Chapters 82, 89, 95

Mr. Olujimi Jibodu, MRCOG
Specialist Registrar in Obstetrics &
Gynaecology,
Mid Trent Rotation, Derby City
Hospital, Derby DE22 3NE
Chapters 6, 8, 11, 17, 46, 57

Dr. Devendra Kanagalingam
Honorary Clinical Lecturer,
Dept of Clinical Developmental
Sciences—Obstetrics &
Gynaecology, St. George's Hospital
Medical School,
Cranmer Terrace,
London SW17 0RE
Chapters Introduction Part 1,
Introduction Part 2

Dr. V. L. Keeley, MA, MB, BS, PhD,
DRCOG, MRCGP
Consultant in Palliative Medicine,
Derbyshire Royal Infirmary,
Nightingale Macmillan Unit,
117A London Road, Derby DE1 2QS
Chapter 92

Mrs. Anne Meadows
Risk Coordinator,
Dept of Midwifery,
Derby City General Hospital,
Uttoxeter Road, Derby DE22 3NE
Chapter 96

Dr. John McIntyre
Senior Lecturer in Child Health,
Academic Division of Child Health,
Derbyshire Childrens Hospital,
Uttoxeter Road, Derby DE22 3NE
Chapter 36

Mr. S. Mitra, MD DNB MRCOG
Specialist Registrar,
Oxford Deanery, Oxford PGMDE,
Headington, Oxford OX3 7XP
Chapters 85, 88

Dr. M. P. Mohajer, FRCOG MD
Consultant Obstetrician and
Gynaecologist,
Royal Shrewsbury Hospital,
Mytton Oak Road,
Shrewsbury SY3 8XQ
Chapters 13, 28

Contributors

Mr. George E. Morgan, MB ChB
MRCOG
Consultant Obstetrician
Gynaecologist & College Tutor,
University Hospital of North
Durham, North Road,
Durham DH1 5TW
Chapters 3–5, 7, 12, 19, 27, 31–3,
40, 43, 63

Mrs. Andrea Morris, RGN RM
RHV BScHons
Primary Care Midwife,
Amber Valley North Primary Care
Midwifery Team,
Alfreton Community Clinic,
Grange Street, Alfreton,
Derbyshire D55 7JA
Chapter 41

E. P. Morris, MD MRCOG
Consultant Obstetrician &
Gynaecologist,
Norfolk & Norwich University
Hospital, Colney lane,
Norwich NR4 7UZ
Chapter 2

Mr. S. Mukhopadhyay, MD DNB
MRCOG
Specialist Registrar,
Department of Obstetrics &
Gynaecology, Norfolk & Norwich
University Hospital, Colney lane,
Norwich NR4 7UZ
Chapters 1, 2, 26, 29, 82, 89

Karen Payne, RGN RM DPSM
Infant Feeding Support Midwife,
Dept of Midwifery,
Derby City General Hospital,
Uttoxeter Road, Derby DE22 3NE
Chapter 39

Dr. S. Peatman
Specialist Registrar,
Dept of Obstetrics & Gynaecology,
University Hospital, Queen's Medical
Centre, Nottingham NG7 2UH
Chapter 54

Mrs. Lesley Roulstone, RM RGN
DPPM (Nottingham University)
Clinical Lead Midwife,
Derby Central Primary Care
Midwifery Team, Southern
Derbyshire Acute Hospitals NHS
Trust, Ward 22,
Derby City General Hospital,
Uttoxeter Road, Derby DE22 3NE
Chapter 41

Dr. W. Scott
Consultant Anaesthetist,
Derby City General Hospital,
Uttoxeter Road, Derby DE22 3NE
Chapter 35

Mr. I. Symonds, MD BMedSci
MRCOG ILTM
Senior Lecturer,
Dept of Obstetrics & Gynaecology,
Derby City General Hospital,
Uttoxeter Road, Derby DE22 3NE
Chapters 20, 21, 38, 42, 47,
56, 58, 59, 64, 65, 74, 76, 79,
83, 86, 94

Mr. Onnig Tamizian, BMBS
BMedSci MRCOG
Specialist Registrar in Obstetrics &
Gynaecology,
Derby City General Hospital,
Uttoxeter Road, Derby DE22 3NE
Chapters 4, 9, 12, 15, 16, 27,
31–4, 37, 40, 43, 46, 48, 49, 73,
87, 93

Dr. S. Wallace, BA BM BCh
Specialist Registrar in Obstetrics &
Gynaecology,
King's Mill Hospital, Mansfield
Road, Sutton in Ashfield,
Notts NG17 4JL
Chapter 10

Preface

Obstetrics and gynaecology have seen major advances in knowledge and a rapid growth of technology. Evidence based medicine and clinical governance are the themes of the day and are here to stay. The field of obstetrics and gynaecology is expanding into reproductive health because women are expected to bear offspring and to lead a healthy life, bringing up children who will be useful and productive citizens. Each nation has a responsibility to uphold the sexual and reproductive rights of women. The medical curriculum and the care provided should respect human rights—this aspect has not been covered as it is beyond the scope of this Handbook.

This Oxford Handbook is designed to provide the breadth and depth of knowledge needed in obstetrics and gynaecology that is necessary for one to identify, investigate, diagnose, and manage the more common clinical problems. This is a good revision book for examinations and will be a quick reference guide for family practitioners and house officers. The editors have considered the vast number of topics that need to be covered, and placed more emphasis on the core knowledge that is needed for practitioners. In order to make this book useful for both the student and the senior clinician, most chapters have been designed and written by a multidisciplinary group of authors of varying seniority.

It is our hope that this book will serve the purpose of a handbook for every student, doctor, and nurse in the field of reproductive health. Special attention has been paid to incorporate the latest evidence, and to follow a uniform style to make navigation easy for the reader. The editors and the publishers would be keen to receive any comments and criticism that will help to improve future editions of the Handbook. We hope it will help you on a daily basis in the clinics and wards to diagnose and manage the simple, as well as complex, problems and emergencies in obstetrics and gynaecology.

S.A.
I.S.
A.F.

Acknowledgements

The editors would like to acknowledge the authors of chapters for their valuable contribution. To conform to style and to avoid repetition, the original contributions have been considerably edited and we thank the authors for their understanding. We are grateful to Professor A. Biswas of the National University of Singapore for researching possible cover pictures and Dr. Leonie Penna for some pictures in some chapters. Our sincere and greatest thanks to Mrs. Sue Cunningham of St. George's for organizing and helping us with the manuscripts and Miss Catherine Barnes of OUP for her patience, understanding, and editorial advice. We acknowledge the tremendous help from every member of the publishing team at OUP, especially that of Dr. Kate Smith.

S.A.
I.S.
A.F.

5-FU	5-fluorouracil
5HIAA	5-hydroxyindoleacetic acid
5-HT	5-hydroxytryptamine (serotonin)
ABC	airway, breathing, and circulation (resuscitation protocol)
AC	abdominal circumference (of fetus)
ACE	angiotensin-converting enzyme
aCL	anticardiolipin antibody
ACTH	adrenocorticotrophic hormone (adrenocorticotrophin)
ADH	antidiuretic hormone
AFE	amniotic fluid embolism
AFI	amniotic fluid index
AFLP	acute fatty liver of pregnancy
AFP	alpha-fetoprotein
AFS	American Fertility Society
AIS	adenocarcinoma *in situ*
ALT	alanine aminotransferase
ANA	antinuclear antibodies
AP	anteroposterior
APCR	activated protein C resistance
APH	antepartum haemorrhage
APS	antiphospholipid syndrome
APTT	activated partial thromboplastin time
ARDS	adult respiratory distress syndrome
ART	assisted reproduction techniques
ASD	atrial septal defect
ATP	adenosine triphosphate
AUC	area under the curve
BCG	bacille Calmette–Guérin
bd	*bis die* (twice daily)
BMI	body mass index
BNA	borderline nuclear abnormalities
BP	blood pressure
BPD	biparietal diameter
BSO	bilateral salpingo-oophorectomy

DMT	dimethyltryptamine
DR	detection rate
DS	Down's syndrome
dsDNA	double-stranded DNA
DUB	dysfunctional uterine bleeding
DVT	deep vein thrombosis
DZ	dizygous
E3	oestriol
ECG	electrocardiography
ECT	electroconvulsive therapy
ECV	external cephalic version
EDC	estimated date of confinement
EDD	estimated date of delivery
EE	ethinyloestradiol
EFM	electronic fetal monitoring
EOC	epithelial ovarian cancer
ELISA	enzyme-linked immunosorbent assay
ESR	erythrocyte sedimentation rate
ET	embryo transfer
ETT	endotracheal tube
EUA	examination under anaesthetic
FAS	fetal alcohol syndrome
FAST	fetal acoustic stimulation test
FBC	full blood count
FBS	fetal blood sampling
FDPs	fibrinogen degradation products
FFP	fresh frozen plasma
FHR	fetal heart rate
FIGO	International Federation of Gynaecologist and Obstetricians
FISH	fluorescent *in situ* hybridization
FL	femur length (of fetus)
FPR	false-positive rate
FS	fundal–symphyseal (height)
FSH	follicle-stimulating hormone
fT_3	free tri-iodothyronine
fT_4	free thyroxine
FTA	fluorescent treponemal antibody (test)
FTA-ABS	fluorescent treponemal antibody absorption (test)
G&S	group and save serum

GBS	group B streptococcal infection
GCSF	granulocyte colony-stimulating factor
GDM	gestational diabetes mellitus
GFR	glomerular filtration rate
GH	growth hormone
GIFT	gamete intrafallopian transfer
GnRH	gonadotrophin-releasing hormone
GP	general practitioner
GTT	glucose tolerance test
HAART	highly active anti-retroviral therapy
Hb	haemoglobin
HbA_{1c}	haemoglobin A_{1c}
HBeAg	hepatitis B core antigen
HBIg	hepatitis B immune globulin
HbAS	sickle cell trait
HBsAg	hepatitis B surface antigen
HbS B thal	sickle cell β thalassaemia
HbSC	sickle cell haemoglobin C disease
HbSS	sickle cell anaemia
HBV	hepatitis B virus
HC	head circumference (of fetus)
hCG	human chorionic gonadotrophin
HCT	haematocrit
HDL	high-density lipid
HDL-C	high-density lipoprotein cholesterol
HDU	high-dependency unit
HELLP	haemolysis, elevated liver enzymes, and low platelet count (syndrome)
HIV	human immunodeficiency virus
HNIG	human normal immunoglobulin
HOCM	hypertrophic obstructive cardiomyopathy
hPL	human placental lactogen
HPO axis	hypothalamo-pituitary-ovarian axis
HPV	human papillomavirus
HRT	hormone replacement therapy
HSG	hysterosalpingogram
HSV	herpes simplex virus (HSV1 and HSV2)
IBD	inflammatory bowel disease
IBS	irritable bowel syndrome
IC	interstitial cystitis
ICSI	intracytoplasmic sperm injection
ICU	intensive care unit

IDDM	insulin-dependent diabetes mellitus
IGF	insulin-like growth factors
IH	idiopathic (familial) hirsuitism
IM	intramuscular
INR	international normalized ratio
IOL	induction of labour
ITP	idiopathic thrombocytopenia
ITU	intensive therapy unit
IU	international units
IUCD	intrauterine contraceptive device
IUD	intrauterine death
IUGR	intrauterine growth restriction
IUI	intrauterine insemination
IUI + OI	intrauterine insemination plus ovulation induction
IUS	intrauterine system
IV	intravenous
IVD	instrumental vaginal delivery
IVF	*in vitro* fertilization
IVF-HIC	IVF with a high insemination concentration
IVU	intravenous urogram
JVP	jugular venous pressure
L	litre
LA	lupus anticoagulant
LATS	long-acting thyroid stimulator
LBW	low birth weight
LDL	low-density lipid
LDL-C	low-density lipoprotein cholesterol
LFTs	liver function tests
LH	luteinizing hormone
LLETZ	large loop excision of the transformation zone
LMP	last menstrual period
LMWH	low-molecular-weight heparin
LOA	left occipitoanterior
LOT	left occipitotransverse
LSCS	lower segment Caesarean section
LSD	lysergic acid diethylamine
MAC	minimum alveolar concentration
MAOIs	monoamine oxidase inhibitors
MAP	mean arterial pressure

MAS	meconium aspiration syndrome
MBL	menstrual blood loss
MCH	mean corpuscular haemoglobin
MCHC	mean corpuscular haemoglobin concentration
MCV	mean corpuscular volume
MDMA	3,4-methylenedioxymethamphetamine (Ecstasy)
MG	myasthenia gravis
MIBG	metaiodobenzylguanidine
MoM	multiples of the median
MPA	medroxyprogesterone acetate
MRI	magnetic resonance imaging
MS	maternal serum (as in MSAFP) or multiple sclerosis
MSU	midstream urine
MZ	monozygous
NET-EN	norethisterone oenanthate
NFP	natural family planning
NFT	nuchal fold translucency
NHS	National Health Service (UK)
NHSLA	NHS Litigation Authority
NICE	National Institute of Clinical Excellence (UK)
NIDDM	non-insulin-dependent diabetes mellitus
NSAIDs	nonsteroidal anti-inflammatory drugs
NTDs	neural tube defects
NYHA	New York Heart Association
od	*omni die* (once daily)
OD_{450}	optical density at 450 nm
OHSS	ovarian hyperstimulation syndrome
PAPP-A	pregnancy-associated plasma protein A
PB	placental biopsy
PCO	polycystic ovary
pCO_2	partial pressure of carbon dioxide
PCOS	polycystic ovary syndrome
PCP	*Pneumocystis carinii* pneumonia or phencyclidine
PCR	polymerase chain reaction
PCT	postcoital test
PCV	packed cell volume
PDA	patent ductus arteriosus
PE	pulmonary embolism
PESA	percutaneous epididymal sperm aspiration
PG	prostaglandin (PGE_2, $PGF_{2\alpha}$)
PID	pelvic inflammatory disease
PMS	premenstrual syndrome

PMT	premenstrual tension (same as PMS)	
po	*per os* (by mouth)	
POP	progestogen-only (contraceptive) pill	
PP	placenta praevia	
PPH	postpartum haemorrhage	
PPROM	preterm pre-labour rupture of membranes	
p.r.n.	*pro re nata* (whenever needed)	
PROM	pre-labour rupture of membranes	
PTU	propylthiouracil	
PUPP	pruritic urticarial papules and placques of pregnancy	
PV	*per vaginam*	
PZD	partial zona dissection	
qds	*quater die sumendum* (to be taken four times a day)	
RA	rheumatoid arthritis	
RCOG	Royal College of Obstetricians and Gynaecologists	
Rh	rhesus	
Rh (D)	rhesus D (antigen)	
RPR	rapid plasma reagin (test for syphilis)	
SAH	subarachnoid haemorrhage	
SC	subcutaneous	
SCJ	squamo-columnar junction	
SFH	symphyseal–fundal height	
SGA	small for gestational age	
SHBG	sex-hormone-binding globulin	
SLE	systemic lupus erythematosus	
SOL	space-occupying lesion	
SP-1	pregnancy-specific beta-1 glycoprotein	
SRY	sex-related Y (gene)	
SSRIs	selective serotonin reuptake inhibitors	
stat	immediately	
STD	sexually transmitted disease	
STIs	sexually transmitted infections	
SUZI	subzonal insemination	
SVD	spontaneous vaginal delivery	
SVT	supraventricular tachycardia	
T_3	triiodothryonine	
T_4	thyroxine	
TAH	total abdominal hysterectomy	

TAH + BSO	total abdominal hysterectomy and bilateral salpingo-oophorectomy
TAMBA	Twins and Multiple Births Association
TAT	thrombin–antithrombin III (complexes)
TB	tuberculosis
TBG	thyroid-binding globulin
tds	*ter die sumendum* (to be taken three times a day)
TENS	transcutaneous electrical nerve stimulation
TESA	testicular/epididymal sperm aspiration
TFT	thyroid function tests
TIBC	total iron-binding capacity
TOP	termination of pregnancy
TORCH	toxoplasma, rubella, cytomegalovirus, and herpes
TPHA	*Treponema pallidum* haemagglutination (test)
TPI	*Treponema pallidum* immobilization (test)
TPR	temperature, pulse, respiration
TSH	thyroid-stimulating hormone
TSIg	thyroid-stimulating immunoglobulin
TV	transverse (presentation at birth)
TZ	transformation zone
U&Es	urea and electrolytes (test)
UC	ulcerative colitis
uE_3	unconjugated oestriol
UR-NAP	urea-resistant neutrophil alkaline phosphatase
U/S	ultrasound
UTI	urinary tract infection
UV_{max}	maximum umbilical vein velocity
VDRL	Venereal Disease Research Laboratory (test for syphilis)
VIN	vulval intraepithelial neoplasia
VMA	vanillymandelic acid
VSD	ventricular septal defects
VT	ventricular tachycardia
VTE	venous thromboembolism
VZIG	varicella zoster immune globulin
VZV	varicella zoster virus
ZIFT	zygote intrafallopian transfer

Part 1

Obstetrics

Introduction

Obstetric history and physical examination

History-taking and physical examination are essential skills for good clinical practice. Competence in this area requires a sound clinical knowledge in order to direct questions that will help to shape the presentation appropriately. The basic framework to history-taking and physical examination can be readily acquired but the best result can only be achieved by improving these skills by practice and better knowledge.

The obstetric history

The obstetric history is both a synopsis of a woman's background risk as well as an account of the progress of her index pregnancy. A carefully taken history provides a clinical guide to the physical examination to follow. Further physical signs which are not routinely elicited in a pregnant woman may become necessary if the history warrants it. It is useful to have a template for taking the obstetric history. This allows the history to be taken and presented in a logical sequence and avoids inadvertent omission of important details. The following is a guide to taking an obstetric history.

Current pregnancy

In presenting an obstetric case, it is appropriate to begin with a summary of the details to follow. This is especially so if the history that is to follow is complicated. It allows the listener to focus on the clinical issues in the pregnancy. The summary is best constructed by having some organisation in history taking and is given below;

- *Personal and pregnancy details.*

A polite introduction of you followed by permission to take the history and examination is vital. Start with the enquiry of her name, age, gravidity (i.e. number of pregnancies including the current one) and parity (i.e. number of births beyond 24 weeks gestation). The expected date of delivery (EDD) can be calculated from the last menstrual period (LMP) by Naegele's rule (add one year and seven days to the LMP and subtract 3 months).

Inquire about her health and that of her fetus (e.g. after 20 weeks inquire about fetal movements). This should be followed by details of the current problems if there are any.

A chronological and concise account of the events in pregnancy is best obtained by enquiring about her pregnancy in the first, second and third trimester. If she was in the postnatal period details of labour and delivery are relevant.

This inquiry should include details of laboratory tests and ultrasound scans. The date pregnancy was confirmed by a pregnancy test, results of the routine antenatal blood tests and the date and details of the first scan (dating or nuchal translucency scan) are important. Subsequent antenatal check ups and tests done including subsequent scans should be noted. The details of the results may be asked from the woman and if necessary can be cross checked against the notes.

There should be an organisational logic of history taking. At times it may be necessary to revisit an area of the history as the story unfolds further or during or after clinical examination.

Obstetric history and physical examination

- *Menstrual history* – State the last menstrual period (LMP) and any details that may influence the validity of her EDD as calculated from the LMP, such as long cycles irregular periods or recent use of the combined oral contraceptive pill.
- *Past obstetric history* – Outcome of previous pregnancies and any significant antenatal, intra or postpartum events may have influence in the management of the current pregnancy. Previous maternal complications, mode of delivery, birth weights and the life and health of babies may be relevant.
- *Past gynaecological history* – Details of contraceptive history, previous surgical procedures and cervical smears should be noted.
- *Past medical/surgical history* – Some medical conditions may have a significant impact on the course of the pregnancy. Heart disease, epilepsy, bronchial asthma, thyroid disorders, insulin-dependent diabetes mellitus and other medical conditions or the medications they take for these conditions may have significant impact on the pregnancy. Alternatively pregnancy may have an impact on the medical condition. The condition may remain the same or get better or worse. These may be incorporated under "current pregnancy" if it is of concern in this pregnancy. Outcome of joint consultations should be known and if it has not been done, arrangements need to be made for looking after the mother in a multidisciplinary clinic or with the relevant physician.
- *Drug history* – *History of allergies* should be highlighted and any use/abuse of drugs during pregnancy should be noted. Arrangements may have to be made to wean off the drug.
- *Family/social history* – History of hereditary illnesses or congenital defects is important and may be of concern to the couple. Appropriate counselling and investigations may have to be organised. This will be a good opportunity to discuss about stopping to smoke or to reduce excessive alcohol intake. Relevant social aspects such as childcare arrangements and plans for breastfeeding and contraception can be discussed at this point.
- *Final summary* – This should include the salient details that will impact on the investigations to be carried out and the proposed plan of management.

It may be necessary to vary this template to suit different clinical situations. In a woman who has experienced many problems during her pregnancy, it may be better to provide details of each problem separately rather than a chronological account of the pregnancy.

Physical examination

Many aspects of the obstetric physical examination are unique. There are several necessary techniques and skills, which are not required in other specialities.

General examination

The assessment should begin with a general examination. This is intended to provide the clinician with an overview of the woman's condition upon which more specific examinations can be directed. The general examination should include the woman's height and weight. From these, the body mass index (BMI) can be calculated as follows:

$$BMI = \frac{weight\ (kg)}{Height^2\ (m)}$$

Some antenatal and perinatal complications are associated with a BMI < 20 or > 25. The thyroid gland and breasts should be examined at a booking visit and auscultation of the heart sounds and lungs is essential. For many women, the obstetric booking visit will be their first visit to a doctor in many years. Hence, it is not unusual for asymptomatic conditions such as a cardiac murmur from valvular heart disease, breast lumps or goitre to be detected at these visits. These conditions may have significant implications on the course of her pregnancy and, indeed, subsequent health. More detailed examinations are indicated when a sign is detected (e.g. multinodular of the goitre, bruit over the mass, ophthalmic signs, tremors etc.) or in specific situations, for example examination of the eyes with an ophthalmoscope to look for retinopathy in a diabetic or hypertensive woman.

The measurement of maternal blood pressure is of great importance in pregnancy. It is not appropriate to measure this in the supine position as pressure from a gravid uterus on the inferior vena cava impedes venous return resulting in a falsely low blood pressure. This is often referred to as the supine hypotension syndrome. The correct position is 'semi recumbent' – a 45° tilt. When auscultating the brachial artery in measuring the diastolic blood pressure, the value at which the sounds disappear (Korotkoff V) is currently accepted as it gives the closest reading to the direct arterial blood pressure measurement. An appropriate size cuff should be utilised with a larger cuff for those with a larger upper arm circumference – the smaller cuff in these women would give a falsely high reading.

Abdominal examination

The fundamental steps in abdominal examination, namely inspection, palpation and auscultation apply to the pregnant woman and occasionally the art of percussion to elicit fluid thrill when polyhydramnios is suspected. The specific manoeuvres and techniques vary in an obstetric examination. The clinician may be guided by the preceding history and general examination to conduct this more specific part of the physical examination. For instance, a history of abdominal pain should prompt a careful palpation for uterine contractions (suggestive of labour) or localised tenderness (associated with red degeneration of a fibroid, accident of an adnexal mass, dehiscence of a previous scar or rarely placental abruption).

Obstetric history and physical examination

Inspection

- Note the distension of the abdomen that may indirectly indicate the shape and size of the uterus. Any asymmetry of the abdomen and fetal movements should be recorded.
- It is important to note any surgical scars, particularly a low transverse Pfannenstiel incision that may be obscured by pubic hair and a laparoscopic scar within the umbilicus. The scars observed should be correlated to previous surgical and gynaecological history.
- Cutaneous signs of pregnancy such as linea nigra (dark pigmented line stretching from just below the xiphi sternum through the umbilicus to the supra-pubic area) or striae gravidarum (recent striae are purplish in colour) are often present though they are of no clinical significance. Old striae (striae albicans) are silvery-white and are evidence of previous parity. The umbilicus may be flat with the surface or everted due to increased intra-abdominal pressure. Superficial veins may be seen denoting alternate paths of venous drainage due to pressure on the inferior venacava by the gravid uterus.

Palpation

- Uterine size – The uterine size is objectively measured and expressed as fundo-symphyseal height. First the highest point of the fundus of the uterus should be palpated. One should bear in mind that the uterus may be displaced to the left or right of the midline. Use the ulnar border of the left hand and move it downwards from below the xiphi sternum and from below each subcostal margin until the fundus is located. Once the highest point of the uterine fundus is identified the fundo-symphysial height (SFH) can be measured with a tape measure. The upper margin of the bony pubic symphysis is located by palpating downwards in the midline starting from few centimetres above the pubic hair margin. The SFH in centimetres ± 2 cm should approximate the gestation of the pregnancy in weeks from 20 until 36 weeks gestation. From 36 to 40 weeks this could be +/− 3 cm and at 40 weeks it is +/− 4 cm. The decrease in height is due to reduction in the amniotic fluid volume and descent of the fetal head. On the contrary the increase in size may be due to further growth of the fetus, increase of amniotic fluid and non descent of the fetal head.

  It is important at this stage that the number of fetuses is determined. Palpation of a larger uterus than that expected for that gestation, two heads, three poles, multiple fetal parts, excessive amniotic fluid, and auscultation of two fetal heart rates with a difference of greater than 10 beats per minute suggests the presence of multiple pregnancies.
- Presentation – Presentation is the part of the fetus that overlies the pelvic brim and is of importance especially after 37 weeks gestation when the majority of women go into labour. This is determined by placing both hands on either side of the lower pole of the uterus while facing the woman's feet. Approximate the hands firmly but gently towards the midline to ascertain the presenting part. A hard rounded presenting part suggests a cephalic presentation while a broader, soft object suggests breech presentation. In cephalic presentation, it is usual to report the number of fifths of the head palpable. This is a rough approximation of how many finger breadths are necessary to cover the head above the pelvic brim. As this step is performed it is important to look at the woman's face as

Physical examination (*continued*)

palpation of the fetal head may be tender. The clinician should detect any signs of discomfort from her facial expression and be gentle with the palpation. Paulik's grip is a one-handed technique to feel for the presenting part. The cupped right hand is used to grasp the lower pole of the uterus and it is possible to feel the hard rounded fetal head in nearly 95% of pregnancies at term. It can cause discomfort and is not a necessary part of the examination if the head can be palpated with ease by the two hands. If the hands on the sides of the head converge above the pelvic brim then the head is not engaged as more of the head is above whilst if the hands diverge then it is suggestive of engagement i.e. more than half the head has descended below the pelvic brim.

- Lie of the fetus and location of the fetal back – Lie of the fetus describes the relationship of the longitudinal axis of the fetus to the longitudinal axis of the uterus. This is best done by facing the woman and placing one hand on each side of the uterus and applying gentle pressure when one should be able to perceive the resistance of the firm fetal back and on the opposite side it may be possible to feel the fetal limbs. This can be confirmed by alternately palpating with one hand while using the opposite hand to steady the fetus. If the presentation is cephalic or breech (the buttocks of the fetus) it has to be a longitudinal lie as the lower pole of the longitudinal lie of the uterus is occupied by one pole of the longitudinal axis of the fetus. If no presenting part was palpable in the lower pole and if the head or a breech was in one of the iliac fossa it is an oblique lie and if the longitudinal axis of the fetus straddles right across the horizontal axis of the uterus then it is a transverse lie. Once the fetal lie is determined the anterior shoulder should be palpated as the fetal heart sounds are best heard over this area. A shallow groove palpable between the presenting part and the rest of the fetus helps to identify the prominent anterior shoulder in most cases.

- Estimation of fetal weight and quantity of amniotic fluid – Assessing fetal weight can be difficult but it is important to determine whether the fetus is small, average or big. It is usually assessed by placing one hand over each pole of the fetus and by guessing the approximate weight. With experience and by checking the guessed weight to the actual weight after delivery the clinician is able to improve his/her performance although many a times the error would exceed more than 10% especially with the very small and the very large fetuses. The ease with which the fetal parts are palpable, ballotment of the fetal parts and the 'cystic' feeling for the fluid in the uterus should give some idea of the amniotic fluid.

Auscultation

The fetal stethoscope or an electronic device like the Doptone can be placed over the anterior shoulder and the fetal heart can be heard. The rate can be determined by auscultation over one minute.

Percussion

Percussion is generally not used in an obstetric examination. If the quantity of amniotic fluid is felt to be excessive (shining, stretched abdomen with difficulty in feeling fetal parts) then the sign of ballotment is useful to identify the head. Fluid thrill may be elicited by tapping in the mid point of the uterus on one side and trying to feel it with the hand placed on the opposite side at the same level. The passage of surface vibrations should be damped by an assistant or patient keeping the ulnar border of the hand firmly in the midline on the abdominal wall.

Vaginal examination

Vaginal speculum and digital examinations are not a routine part of the obstetric physical examination but are performed when indicated e.g. A speculum examination to confirm leaking amniotic fluid in cases of pre-labour rupture of membranes, or to carry out inspection and take swabs in cases with abnormal vaginal discharge.

Reporting your history and examination findings

A concise, clear and logical sequence of reporting the history and examination findings is essential to ensure that that the rest of the medical team and the patient can understand the clinical condition. It should form the basis for further investigations if needed and to help plan effective management.

A summary of the history should be followed by a summary of the examination findings. The general examination findings should be reported first, emphasising any aspects that may influence management. Abdominal findings should be reported in the order that they were elicited using the appropriate terminology (e.g. lie, presentation, engagement).

Chapter 1

Anatomy of the female pelvis and the fetal head

The bony pelvis

The pelvis is made up three bones—the two innominate bones and the sacrum. When articulated they enclose a cavity. The sacrum is wedged between the two innominate bones. Each innominate bone is made up of three parts:

- Ilium.
- Ischium.
- Pubis.

The innomimate bones are joined anteriorly at the symphysis pubis.

Pelvic brim

The pelvic brim is formed by the pubic crest, the pectineal line of the pubis, the arcuate line of the ilium, the alae of the sacrum, and the promontory of the sacrum. The brim separates the false pelvis above from the true pelvis below. Inferiorly it is separated from the perineum by the urogenital diaphragm. The plane of the pelvis is at an angle of 55° with the horizontal. In an anatomical position the pelvic cavity projects backward from the pelvic brim. The upper border of the symphysis pubis, the ischial spines, the tip of the coccyx, the head of the femur, and the greater trochanter lie in the same plane.

The female pelvis

The female pelvis differs from the male pelvis. The basic differences are:

- The female pelvis is broader than the male pelvis and the female pelvic bones, including the neck of the femur, are more slender than those of the male.
- The outline of the male pelvic brim is heart-shaped and the brim is widest towards the back, whereas the female pelvic brim is transversely oval (widest further forwards) due to less prominence of the sacral promontory.
- The female pelvis has evolutionally developed for giving birth. Therefore it is roomier. The outlet is also wider than that of the male pelvis.
- The subpubic angle is acute like a Gothic arch in the male pelvis, whereas it is rounded like a Roman arch in a female pelvis.

The major obstetric interest in the bony pelvis is that it is not distensible. Only minor degrees of movements are possible at the symphysis pubis and sacroiliac joints. Its dimensions are therefore critical at childbirth. The diameters of the pelvis vary at different parts of the pelvis.

In addition, the shape of the pelvis determines the availability of pelvic diameters. There are four basic shapes.

- *Gynaecoid type* (Fig. 1.1). The classical female pelvis with the inlet transversely oval and a roomier pelvic cavity.
- *Android type*. The inlet is heart-shaped. The cavity is funnel-shaped with contracted outlet.
- *Anthropoid type*. This results from high assimilation, i.e. the sacral body assimilated to the fifth lumbar vertebra. It is long, narrow, and oval in shape.
- *Platypelloid type*. This is a wide pelvis flattened at the brim with the promontory of the sacrum pushed forward.

Pelvic walls

The inner aspect (cavity) of the pelvic bones is covered by muscles. Above the brim it is covered by iliacus and psoas. The sidewalls are clad with obturator internus and its fascia. The curved posterior wall is covered by the pyriformis, which courses laterally to the greater sciatic foramen. The levator ani and coccygeus with their opposite counterparts constitute the pelvic floor.

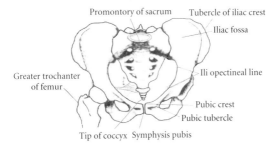

Fig. 1.1 A gynaecoid pelvis. (Reproduced from *Last's anatomy, regional and applied*, ninth edition (ed. R.M.H. McMinn), p.395, © 1994 by permission of the publisher, Mosby.)

Adequacy of the pelvis to achieve vaginal delivery

This is best demonstrated using a model of a pelvis and a fetal head but a description useful in understanding the mechanism of labour is given here.

The true pelvis is bounded anteriorly by the symphysis pubis (3.5 cm long) and posteriorly by the sacrum (12 cm long) (Fig. 1.2).

- The *zone of inlet* is made anteriorly by the upper border of the pubis, posteriorly by the sacral promontory, and laterally by the iliopectineal line. The transverse diameter is 13.5 cm and the anteroposterior (AP) diameter is 11.5 cm.

- The *zone of cavity* is most roomy just below the inlet zone and appears almost round with a transverse diameter of 13.5 cm and an AP diameter of 12.5 cm.

- The *zone of midpelvis* that follows is bounded by the apex of the pubic arch anteriorly, the tip of the sacrum posteriorly, and the ischial spines laterally (the interspinous distance should be > 10 cm). This area is ovoid in shape and is the narrowest part of the pelvis.

- The *zone of outlet* has the pubic arch (desirable angle > 85°) as its anterior border, whilst the sacrotuberous ligaments and ischial tuberosities delineate the posterolateral margins leading to the coccyx posteriorly.

The ideal female pelvis should be able to accommodate the head of a fetus at term. It has an oval brim, a shallow cavity, non-prominent ischial spines, a curved sacrum with large sciatic notches (> 90°), and a sacrospinous ligament more than 3.5 cm long. The angle of the pelvic brim is 55° to the horizontal. The anterior posterior diameter of the inlet is at least 12 cm and the transverse diameter is about 13.5 cm. The subpubic arch is rounded and is > 90° and the ischial intertuberous distance is at least 10 cm. The pelvis is said to be clinically favourable if:

- The sacral promontory cannot be felt.
- The ischial spines are not prominent.
- The subpubic arch and base of the sacrospinous ligaments both accept 2 fingers and the intertuberous diameter accepts 4 knuckles on pelvic examination.

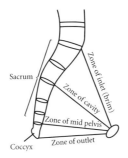

Fig. 1.2 Different zones of the pelvis. (Reproduced from *Oxford handbook of clinical specialties*, 5th edn (ed. J. Collier, M. Longmore, and T.D. Brown), p. 87, © 1997 by permission of the publisher, Oxford University Press.)

The fetal head

The fetal head is described using identifiable anatomical features.
- The *bregma* is the anterior fontanelle.
- The *brow* lies between the bregma and the root of the nose.
- The *face* lies below the root of the nose and the supraorbital ridges.
- The *occiput* is the bony prominence that lies behind the posterior fontanelle.
- The *vertex* is the diamond-shaped area between the anterior and posterior fontanelles and the parietal eminences.

Identification of the sutures and the fontanelles of the skull (Fig. 1.3) helps us to identify the position of the head in labour. The two frontal bones, two parietal bones, two temporal bones, the wings of the sphenoid, and the occipital bone form the skull. The area where the bones unite is not bony but is membranous and is called a *suture*.
- The *frontal suture* is situated between the frontal bones.
- The *sagittal suture* is situated between the parietal bones.
- The *coronal sutures* are between the parietal and frontal bones.
- The *lambdoid sutures* are between the parietal and occipital bones.
- The *temporal sutures* lie between the inferior margins of the parietal bones and the temporal bones. They cannot be felt due to soft tissue covering them.

When two or more sutures meet there is an irregular membranous area between them and this is called a *fontanelle*.
- The *anterior fontanelle* or the *bregma* is a diamond-shaped space between the coronal and the sagittal suture. This measures about 3 cm in the AP and the transverse diameters and usually ossifies about 18 months after birth.
- The *posterior fontanelle* or the *lambda* is a smaller triangle-shaped space that lies between the sagittal and the lambdoid sutures.
- The *temporal* or the *casserian fontanelles* lie at the intersection of the lambdoid and the temporal sutures. They cannot be felt.

The position of the sutures and fontanelles in labour plays a very important role in determining the position of the fetal head in labour.

The important diameters of the fetal head (Fig. 1.4) are:
- *Biparietal* diameter (9.5 cm). The greatest transverse diameter of the head. It extends from one parietal eminence to the other.
- *Bitemporal* diameter (8.0 cm). The greatest distance between the two temporal sutures.
- *Bimastoid* diameter (7.5 cm). The distance between the tips of the mastoid processes. It is impossible to decrease this diameter by any obstetrical operation.
- *Suboccipitobregmatic* diameter (9.5 cm). The well flexed vertex presents with this diameter, which extends from the middle of the bregma to the undersurface of the occipital bone where it joins the neck. The circumference of the fetal head at this plane is the smallest and measures 32 cm.
- *Suboccipitofrontal* diameter (10.5 cm). The partially flexed vertex presents with this diameter, which extends from a point just above the root of the nose to the undersurface of the occipital bone where it joins the neck.
- *Occipitofrontal* diameter (11.5 cm). A deflexed head presents with this diameter, which extends from a point just above the root of the nose to the most prominent point on the occipital bone. The circumference of the fetal head at this plane measures 34.5 cm.

- *Mentovertical diameter* (13.0 cm). A brow presentation has the largest AP diameter and it extends from the chin to the most prominent point of the occiput.
- *Submentobregmatic* diameter (9.5 cm) A face presentation has a small diameter and it extends from the chin to the middle of the bregma.

Moulding of the head

With the descent of the head into the pelvis, the frontal bones slip under the parietal bones. In addition, one parietal bone can override the other parietal bone and they in turn slip under the occipital bone, thereby reducing the head circumference. The degree of moulding is assessed vaginally.
- Usually the suture lines are separate (moulding = 0).
- If the suture lines meet the degree of moulding is 1+.
- If they overlap but can be reduced with gentle digital pressure, the degree of moulding is 2+.
- If the overlap is irreducible with gentle digital pressure, the degree of moulding is 3+.

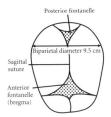

Fig. 1.3 Fontanelles, sagittal suture, and biparietal diameter. (Reproduced from *Oxford handbook of clinical specialties*, 5th edn (ed. J. Collier, M. Longmore, and T.D. Brown), p. 87, © 1999 by permission of the publisher, Oxford University Press).

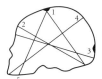

1 Suboccipitobregmatic 9.5 cm
  flexed vertex presentation
2 Suboccipitofrontal 10.5 cm
  partially deflexed vertex
3 Occipitofrontal 11.5 cm deflexed vertex
4 Mentovertical 13 cm brow
5 Submentobregmatic 9.5 cm face

Fig. 1.4 Different presenting diameters of the head. (Reproduced from Oxford handbook of clinical specialties, 5th edn (ed. J. Collier, M. Longmore, and T.D. Brown), p. 87, © 1999 by permission of the publisher, Oxford University Press.)

Chapter 2

The placenta

The human placenta is discoid in shape, haemochorial, and deciduate. It is called haemochorial as chorion is in direct contact with the maternal blood and deciduate as some of the maternal decidual tissue is shed at parturition. The placenta is attached to the uterine wall and is connected to the fetus via the umbilical cord. Placental tissue is fetal in origin and the fact that maternal and fetal tissues come in direct contact with each other without rejection suggests some complex immunological mechanisms favouring acceptance of the fetus as a graft by the mother.

Development

- Implantation occurs at blastocyst stage. It usually starts at day 7 and is completed on the 11th day. The inner cell mass within the blastocyst forms the embryo, yolk sac, and amniotic cavity while the trophoblast will form the future placenta, chorion, and extraembryonic mesoderm.
- When the blastocyst embeds into the decidua, trophoblastic cells differentiate and syncytiotrophoblast and cytotrophoblast are defined. This is followed by appearance of lacunar spaces in the syncytium. These cells advance into the surrounding tissues as early or primitive villi, each of which consists of cytotrophoblast surrounded by the syncytium. The lacunar spaces soon become filled with maternal blood.
- The villi subsequently mature to secondary and tertiary villi with the appearance of first the mesodermal core and then fetal blood vessels in the mesodermal core of the villi, respectively. This process is completed by day 21.
- At 16 to17 days the surface of the blastocyst is covered by branching villi, which are best developed at the embryonic pole. The chorion here is known as chorionic frondosum and the future placenta is developed from this area.
- Simultaneously, lacunar spaces become confluent with one another and by weeks 3 to 4, form a multilocular receptacle lined by syncytium and filled with maternal blood. This space becomes the future intervillous space.
- With the growth of the embryo the decidua capsularis becomes thinner and both villi and the lacunar spaces in the decidua get obliterated, converting the chorion into chorionic laeve.
- The villi in the chorionic frondosum show exuberant division and subdivision and, with the accompanying proliferation of the decidua basalis, the future placenta is formed (Fig. 2.1). The process starts at 6 weeks and the definitive number of stem villi are established by 12 weeks.
- Thereafter, placental growth continues up to term and possibly beyond. Until the 16th week the placenta grows both in thickness and circumference due to the growth of the chorionic villi with accompanying expansion of the intervillous space. Thereafter, growth occurs mainly circumferentially till term or beyond.

Stem villi and the placental barrier (Fig. 2.2)

Stem villi arise from the chorionic plate and extend to the basal plate. A major stem villus with its branching villi forms the fetal cotyledon or placentome. There are approximately 60 stem villi in human placenta. Thus each cotyledon contains 3–4 major stem villi. The villi are the functional units of the placenta. Some of them anchor the placenta to the decidua but the majority of them float in the intervillous space.

In the early placenta, the following structures are present from outside inward.
- Outer syncytiotrophoblast.
- Cytotrophoblast.
- Basement membrane.

- Stroma-containing mesenchymal cells and the endothelium and basement membrane of the fetal blood vessel.

This also constitutes the placental barrier (Fig. 2.2(b)). In spite of close proximity, there is no mixing of the maternal and fetal blood. The barrier is about 0.025 mm thick. Near term with the attenuation of the syncytial layer and sparse cytotrophoblast with marked distension of fetal capillaries, the placental membrane becomes very much thinner to the extent of 0.002 mm in places. However, all the constituents forming the layer in early pregnancy can be identified microscopically.

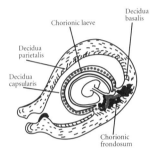

Fig. 2.1 Early development. Chorionic frondosum forms the future placenta.

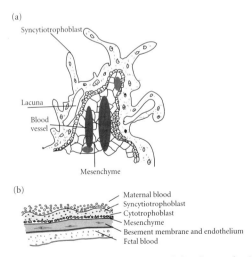

Fig. 2.2 (a) Structure of chorionic villi. (b) Simple line diagram showing cell layers of placental barrier.

The placenta at term

The placenta at term is circular in shape and has a diameter of 15–20 cm. It is about 2.5 cm thick at the centre and weighs approximately 500 g. The ratio of fetal and placental weight at term is about 6:1. Normally at term the placenta occupies 30% of the uterine wall. It presents two surfaces.

- The *fetal surface* is covered by smooth glistening amnion with the umbilical cord attached at or near to its centre. The branches of umbilical blood vessels are visible beneath the amnion as they radiate from the insertion of the cord. The amnion can be peeled off from the underlying chorion except at the insertion of the cord.
- The *maternal surface* has a rough and spongy appearance. A shaggy layer may be visible on the maternal surface. This is the remnant of decidua basalis. The maternal surface is divided into several cotyledons (15–20) by septa arising from the maternal tissues. Each cotyledon may be supplied by its own spiral artery. Numerous small greyish spots are also visible on the maternal surface. These are due to calcium deposition in the degenerated areas.

Placental circulation

The placental circulation consist of two distinctly different systems—the utero-placental circulation and the fetoplacental circulation.

Uteroplacental circulation

This involves circulation of maternal blood through the intervillous space (Table 2.1). The intervillous blood flow at term is estimated to be 500–600 mL/minute and the blood in the intervillous space is replaced 3–4 times per minute. The pressure gradient between the fetal capillaries and the intervillous space favours placental transfer of oxygen and other nutrients.

Arterial system
The spiral arteries respond to the increased demand of blood supply to the placental bed. They become more tortuous and less elastic by trophoblastic invasion. Trophoblastic invasion starts early in the pregnancy. It appears to occur in two stages.

- The decidual segments of the spiral arterioles are structurally modified during the first trimester.
- The second wave of trophoblastic invasion, occurring in the second trimester, begins to invade the myometrial segments of the spiral arteries.

These morphological changes in the blood vessels create a low-pressure high-flow system in the placenta. The blood vessels become dilated, tortuous, and possibly less capable of responding to vasoactive amines. Sometimes these physiological changes, particularly the second wave of trophoblastic invasion of myometrial segments of spiral arteries of the placental bed, fail to occur in pregnancies complicated by pre-eclampsia and intrauterine growth restriction.

Venous system
The venous blood through the intervillous space drains into the uterine veins. The blood from the spiral artery enters the intervillous space. Lateral dispersion occurs after the entering blood jet reaches the chorionic plate. Losing the original momentum, the blood then gradually flows towards the basal plate. This is

facilitated by mild movement of the villi and uterine contraction. From the basal plate the uterine veins drain the deoxygenated blood. Shunting of blood from the arterial circulation to the neighbouring venous channel is prevented by the increased pressure of the endometrial spiral arteries driving the blood in jets towards the chorionic plate. Venous drainage only takes place during uterine relaxation and arterial flow is reduced during contraction. Spiral arteries are perpendicular and veins are parallel to the uterine wall. Therefore, larger volumes of blood are available for exchange at the intervillous space even though the rate of flow is decreased during contraction.

Fetoplacental circulation

The two umbilical arteries carry blood from the fetus and enter the chorionic plate underneath the amnion. Each of them supplies to one-half of the placenta. The arteries divide into small branches and enter the stem of the chorionic villi. Further division of vessels to arterioles and then to capillaries takes place within the villi. The blood then flows to the corresponding venous channel and subsequently to umbilical vein. Maternal and fetal bloodstreams flow side by side, in an opposite direction. This counter current flow facilitates exchange between mother and fetus. The haemodynamics of fetoplacental circulation are shown in Table 2.2.

Table 2.1 Haemodynamics of uteroplacental circulation

Volume of blood in the intervillous space	150 mL
Blood flow in the intervillous space	500–600 mL/min
Pressure changes in the intervillous space	
Height of uterine contraction	30–50 mm Hg
Uterine relaxation	10–15 mm Hg
Pressure in the spiral artery	70–80 mm Hg
Pressure in the uterine veins	8–10 mm Hg

Table 2.2 Haemodynamics in the fetoplacental circulation

Fetal blood flow through the placenta	400 mL/min
Pressure	
in the umbilical artery	60–70 mm Hg
in the umbilical vein	10 mm Hg
Oxygen saturation	
in the umbilical artery	60%
in the umbilical vein	70–80%
Partial pressure of O_2	
in the umbilical artery	20–25 mm Hg
in the umbilical vein	30–40 mm Hg

Functions of the placenta

The placenta functions primarily as an organ responsible for the transfer of substances to and from the fetus. Far from acting as a simple filtering mechanism, it has many other important roles some of which are not fully understood.

Placental transfer

The placenta acts as a relative barrier to most substances, but the speed of exchange and concentration of substance exchanged depends upon the concentration on each side of the placenta, the molecular size, lipid solubility, ionization, placental surface area, and maternofetal blood flow (Table 2.3). For example a fast transfer to the fetus would be achieved by a low-molecular-weight, lipid-soluble substance with a high concentration gradient across the placenta.

The placenta as a barrier

Infection

The placenta forms an effective barrier against most maternal-blood-borne bacterial infection to the fetus. Other organisms such as syphilis, parvovirus, hepatitis B and C, rubella, human immunodeficiency virus (HIV), and cytomegalovirus (CMV) are able to infect the fetus during pregnancy.

Drugs

Almost all drugs administered to the pregnant woman can pass across the placenta into the fetus. They may have little effect on the fetus (e.g. paracetamol) and be considered 'safe', but other drugs (e.g. warfarin and thalidomide) may significantly affect the development, structure, and function of the fetus—a process known as *teratogenesis*. Before giving any drug to a pregnant woman it is the prescriber's obligation to ensure that it is considered safe for that stage of the pregnancy.

The placenta as an endocrine organ

The placenta has been shown to be capable of producing most peptide and steroid hormones. The production of human chorionic gonadotrophin (hCG), oestrogens, and progesterone by the placenta is vital for the maintenance of pregnancy.

- hCG levels are detected from 6 days after fertilization and form the basis of modern pregnancy testing, being reliably measurable in urine and blood from at least 2 weeks post-fertilization. Concentrations of hCG reach a peak at 10–12 weeks gestation and then plateau at a lower level for the remainder of the pregnancy.
- Progesterone and oestrogen increase in concentration throughout pregnancy, with peaks reached prior to the onset of labour. Progesterone appears to antagonize uterine contractility but the role of oestrogen is unclear—possibly improving uterine blood flow, encouraging breast growth, and priming myometrial receptors to oxytocin.
- Human placental lactogen antagonizes the effects of insulin and enhances the passage of amino acids across the placenta. Prolactin concentrations also increase during pregnancy from both the placenta and pituitary, promoting breast development.

Table 2.3 Transfer mechanisms across the placenta for common anabolites and catabolites

Substance	Transfer mechanism(s)	Direction of transfer
Oxygen	Simple diffusion	To fetus
Carbon dioxide	Simple diffusion	From fetus
Glucose	Simple and facilitated diffusion	To fetus
Amino acids	Facilitated diffusion	To fetus
Iron	Endocytosis	To fetus
Fatty acids	Facilitated diffusion	To fetus
Water	Simple diffusion	To and from fetus
Electrolytes	Counter-transport mechanisms	To and from fetus
Urea and creatinine	Simple diffusion	From fetus

Chapter 3

Pre-pregnancy counselling

Attention to reproductive health should start before conception, but expectations must be realistic. Not all poor obstetric outcomes can be anticipated or avoided. For general health education, a pre-pregnancy counsellor needs to be informed, enthusiastic, dedicated, and skilful, but not necessarily medically qualified. Where specific risks and diseases are identified, specialists in those areas have to be involved as part of the multidisciplinary team required to provide adequate information for appropriate decision-making. The family physician is in an ideal position to identify obstetric risk pre-conception.

Couples preparing for pregnancy will probably need some time to develop a relationship by living together and to learn more about each other. On the other hand, once a woman is over 35 years old, her fertility starts to decline and by 40 years of age it drops very quickly. Age also carries with it an increased risk of chromosomal abnormalities in the baby—the most common abnormality being Down syndrome. Older mothers are also more likely to suffer from age-related illnesses, e.g. high blood pressure, diabetes mellitus, and uterine fibroids—all of which may affect the outcome of the pregnancy.

Preparing for pregnancy

Preparation for a baby should begin before conception because the development of the fetus begins from the third week after the last menstrual period (LMP). Any damaging effect, e.g. exposure to drugs, would have occurred even before the woman was aware she was pregnant.

The intended mother should keep herself healthy by eating sensibly as well as exercising moderately to improve her cardiovascular and muscular fitness in readiness for the challenging task of pregnancy and delivery. The best exercises are low impact aerobics, swimming, brisk walking, and jogging.

Nutritional preparation for pregnancy

Women who are extremely underweight or obese are likely to have menstrual problems that may affect their fertility. These women are also more likely to have problems during pregnancy. Obesity is the most common nutritional disorder in the affluent industrialized world, with its attendant risks of gestational diabetes, hypertension, and monitoring/assessment difficulties for the mother during pregnancy, whereas malnutrition is a major life hazard for mother, fetus, and infant in the developing world. Malnutrition is a cause of anaemia with its own attendant problems for the mother and with intrauterine growth restriction a sequela for the fetus.

Undernutrition in pregnant women of low socio-economic status is associated with the delivery of low-birthweight (less than 2500 g) infants. An improvement in nutritional status and maternal weight may therefore have a positive effect on birth outcome.
- The intending mother should be made aware of the fact that a pregnant woman should consume an extra 350 kilocalories a day. This might comprise, for example:
  —Two slices of wholemeal bread and butter/margarine.
  —One carton (150 g/5 oz) yoghurt.
  —One apple.

- Food delicacies such as undercooked meats and eggs, pates, soft cheeses, shellfish and raw fish, and unpasteurized milk should be avoided as they are all potential sources of *Listeria*. Listeriosis in pregnancy is known to cause a poor obstetric outcome with death of the fetus.
- Periconceptional multivitamin supplementation, including folic acid, has been shown to reduce the occurrence of neural tube defects (NTDs), not just for those at risk of recurrence but also for the first occurrence of NTD.
- Ingestion of preformed vitamin A in excess of 25 000 to 150 000 international units (IU) has been found to be associated with an increased incidence of fetal growth restriction and urinary tract abnormalities but ingestion of vitamin A precursors, carotenoids, is not.
- Women with low serum zinc levels have been found to be at increased risk of pre- and post-term labour and intrauterine growth restriction. Vegetarians should increase non-meat zinc sources such as leafy and root vegetables, whole grains, and nuts. Those who are able to take milk and dairy products will usually have an adequate zinc intake from their diet alone.
- Calcium metabolism may be adversely affected by smoking and alcohol consumption and these should be avoided. Supplementation of calcium may be necessary if intake of calcium is low, but the ideal is increased calcium from dietary sources.
- Routine iron supplementation may not be necessary for all pregnant mothers. Iron should be prescribed only when medically indicated and iron supplementation should be considered as a routine in areas where the incidence of iron deficiency anaemia is high.
- Iodine deficiency is endemic in some parts of the world, resulting in cretinism and neonatal hypothyroidism. Where iodized salt is not available, iodized oil should be used. The maximum benefit will be achieved when iodized oil is given before conception.

Alcohol

Regular drinking of small amounts of alcohol has not been shown to be harmful but excessive alcohol intake has been shown conclusively to be a cause of fetal malformations. The exact threshold of alcohol that will cause malformation in the fetus has not been established, but mothers to be should try to avoid alcohol whenever possible.

Medication

Most drugs carry warnings about use in pregnancy. The pharmacist or a doctor should be consulted before using any over-the-counter drugs. Some conditions may not really need medication, e.g. tetracycline is sometimes used for the treatment of acne and long-term use may cause staining of baby's teeth and weakening of bones, even when tetracyclines were taken months before conception.

Relaxation and exercise

Relaxation is probably the most difficult and yet the most important guideline to follow whilst planning for pregnancy. The standard medical advice to men and women almost regardless of age and complaint is to exercise more since cardiorespiratory function will be improved, weight reduced, and blood pressure lowered. Exercise is associated with higher self-esteem and confidence. The intending mother should be encouraged to exercise.

Preparing for pregnancy (*continued*)

Work
Some workplaces are more likely to present hazards for the pregnant woman, e.g. chemical factories, operating theatres, and X-ray departments. Health-care workers are at higher risk as they are exposed to anaesthetic gases in the operating theatre and come into contact with toxic drugs, particularly those used in the treatment of cancer, ionizing agents in the diagnostic X-ray department, and infections such as hepatitis and AIDS. The intending mother must continually take precautions when coming into contact with these potential hazardous situations.

The computer terminal (video display unit or VDU) has been intensely scrutinized since the early 1980s when reports linked it to pregnancy problems. So far, no study has been able to prove a definite link between the low-level radiation emitted by VDUs and miscarriage.

Routine examination
- General examination including blood pressure, heart, and lungs.
- Family history of inherited disorders or congenital abnormalities.
- Routine urine examination for protein, sugar, and white blood cells.
- Blood tests for thalassaemia, sickle cell disease, toxoplasma, and syphilis may be offered if at risk.
- The presence or absence of immunity against hepatitis and rubella should be ascertained and vaccination given pre-conception if not immune.
- HIV screening if at risk—may be advised to avoid pregnancy if infected.
- Dental examination.

Existing medical problems

Pre-existing illnesses may be made worse by pregnancy. The pregnancy effect may be transient and the condition may return to pre-pregnancy state after the delivery, e.g. diabetes mellitus. Unfortunately, the deterioration may sometimes be permanent and progressive and may eventually result in death (e.g. severe kidney impairment). Where the risk is high, the intending mother may be advised not to attempt pregnancy at all. The advice of a specialist should be sought in cases of severe chronic illnesses, e.g. chronic renal failure and severe cardiac disease.

Pregnancy undertaken when the illness is in remission, stable, or cured will ensure a better outcome. For instance, a good control of diabetes would prevent congenital malformation in the baby.

Avoidance of pregnancy

Women should be advised about an effective method of contraception if they are not ready for parenthood or have just been given a vaccination. It is advisable to wait at least 3 months before conception after immunization with rubella.

Chapter 4

Normal pregnancy

Physiological changes

Physiological changes occur in pregnancy to provide a suitable environment for the nutrition, growth, and development of the fetus and to prepare the mother for the process of parturition and subsequent support for the newborn infant.

Hormonal changes

- Progesterone is synthesized by the corpus luteum until 35 days post-conception and mainly by the placenta thereafter. It decreases smooth muscle excitability (gut, ureters, uterus) and raises body temperature.

- Oestrogens, mainly oestradiol (90%), increase breast and nipple growth and pigmentation of the areolar. With the progress of pregnancy, they make the uterus more sensitive to oxytocin by making uterine muscles more active and excitable by increasing the frequency of action potential of individual fibres. They also increase water retention and protein synthesis.

- Human placental lactogen (hPL), also called chorionic growth hormone or human somatomammotropin, is lactogenic and has some growth-stimulating activity. It promotes growth and insulin secretion, but decreases insulin's peripheral effect, liberating maternal fatty acids (hence sparing maternal glucose use). These actions divert glucose to the fetus. It also stimulates mammary growth and maternal casein, lactalbumin, and lactoglobulin production.

- The maternal thyroid enlarges in 70% of all pregnant women due to increased colloid production. Increased urinary excretion of iodine leads to a relative plasma iodide deficiency. The thyroid gland responds by tripling its iodide uptake from the blood hence the hypertrophy. Thyroid-binding globulin (TBG) is doubled by the end of the first trimester. As a result total T_3 (triiodothryonine) and T_4 (thyroxine) rise early in pregnancy and then fall to remain within the normal non-pregnant range. Thyroid-stimulating hormone (TSH) may decrease slightly in early pregnancy but tends to remain within the normal range. T_3 and T_4 do not cross the placental barrier and there is therefore no relationship between maternal and fetal thyroid function. Iodine, anti-thyroid drugs, and long-acting thyroid stimulator (LATS), however, do cross the placenta.

- The pituitary gland enlarges in normal pregnancy mainly due to changes in the anterior lobe. Prolactin levels increase substantially probably due to oestrogen stimulation of the lactotrophes. Gonadotrophin secretion is inhibited whilst plasma adrenocorticotrophic hormone (ACTH) levels increase. Maternal plasma cortisone output increases but the unbound levels remain constant. The posterior pituitary releases oxytocin principally during the first stage of labour and during suckling.

Haemodynamic changes

The average weight gain for a nullipara throughout the whole pregnancy is 12.5 kg and is probably 0.9 kg less for multiparas. From 10 weeks the plasma volume rises until 32 weeks when it is about 3.8 litres (about 50% increase from non-pregnant state). Acute excessive weight gain is commonly associated with abnormal fluid retention. Failure to gain weight and sometimes slight weight loss may occur during the last 2 weeks of pregnancy.

- Red cell volume (sometimes called red cell mass) rises from 1.4 litres (L) in the non-pregnant state to 1.64 L at term if iron supplements are not taken (an increase of 18%). An increase of 30% has been reported with iron and folate supplements. The discrepancy between the rate of increase of plasma volume and that of red cell mass results in a decline in haemoglobin concentration, haematocrit, and red cell count during pregnancy and, in particular, in the second trimester—leading to 'physiological anaemia'. Mean corpuscular haemoglobin concentration remains constant.

- Total white cell count rises during pregnancy, mainly due to the increase in neutrophil polymorphonuclear leucocytes, which reaches its peak at 32 weeks. A further massive neutrophilia occurs during labour. Eosinophils, basophils, and monocytes remain relatively constant during pregnancy, but there is a profound fall in eosinophils during labour and they are virtually absent at delivery. Although the lymphocyte count and the number of B and T cells remain constant, lymphocyte function and cell-mediated immunity are profoundly depressed by a factor in maternal serum giving rise to a lowered resistance to viral infection.
- Platelets, erythrocyte sedimentation rate (ESR; up to fourfold), cholesterol, β-globulin, and fibrinogen are also raised.
- Albumin and gamma-globulin levels fall due to the dilution effect caused by the increase in plasma volume.

Cardiovascular changes

Major cardiovascular changes occur in pregnancy, the most significant changes taking place within the first 12 weeks.

- Cardiac output rises from 5 to 6.5 L/min by increasing stroke volume (10%) and pulse rate (by about 15 beats/min). During labour, contractions may increase cardiac output by 2 L/min probably due to injection of blood from the distended intervillous space. Pregnancy proceeds normally even when the mother has an artificial cardiac pacemaker—compensation occurring mainly from increased stroke volume.
- Secondary to hormonal changes peripheral resistance falls. Blood pressure (BP), particularly diastolic, falls during the first and second trimesters by 10–20 mm Hg rising to non-pregnant levels by term. The fall of peripheral resistance to nearly 50% of the non-pregnant values is probably due to production of vasodilator prostaglandins. The balance between vasodilator and vasoconstrictor factors regulating peripheral resistance may be the basis of blood pressure regulation in pregnancy and the development of pregnancy-induced hypertension. Vasodilatation and hypotension also stimulate renin angiotensin release, which also plays a part in blood pressure regulation in pregnancy.
- The supine hypotension syndrome is due to compression of the inferior vena cava leading to reduced venous return and hence the reduced cardiac output. Aortic compression may result in a conspicuous difference between brachial and femoral blood pressures giving a pressure difference of 10–15% from the supine to the lateral position.
- Progressive enlargement of the uterus results in upward displacement of the heart and the diaphragm.
- The heart enlarges during pregnancy by 70–80 mL in volume as a result of increased diastolic filling and muscle hypertrophy.

Physiological changes (*continued*)

Respiratory system changes

In pregnancy the level of the diaphragm rises and the intercostal angle increases from 68° in early pregnancy to 103° in late pregnancy. Breathing therefore tends to be more diaphragmatic rather than costal.

- Tidal volume rises from 500 to 700 mL (increase of 40%), the increased depth of breathing being a progesterone effect. Inspiratory capacity (tidal volume plus inspiratory reserve volume) increases in late pregnancy.
- The respiratory rate changes slightly during pregnancy. Breathlessness is common as maternal pCO_2 (partial pressure of carbon dioxide) is set lower to allow the fetus to offload CO_2.

Renal function changes

Renal size increases by about 1 cm in length during pregnancy. There is a marked dilatation of the calyces and renal pelvis and of the ureters. These changes appear in the first trimester and therefore are unlikely to be due to back pressure. Vesicoureteric reflux occurs sporadically. These changes are associated with a high incidence of urinary stasis and increased tendency to urinary tract infection (UTI).

- The bladder muscle relaxes but residual urine after micturition is not normally present.
- Renal blood flow increases by 30–50% in the first trimester and remains elevated throughout pregnancy. Effective renal plasma flow and glomerular filtration rate (GFR) increase. Creatinine and urea production remain the same and plasma levels therefore fall during pregnancy. Uric acid clearance increases from 12 to 20 mmol/mL with a consequent reduction in plasma uric acid levels. With progression of pregnancy, the filtered load of uric acid increases while excretion remains constant, and plasma levels therefore return to non-pregnant values.
- The increased GFR plays an important role in the variable glycosuria and urinary frequency that occur in pregnancy.

Changes in the alimentary system

Decreased oesophageal sphincteric tone is responsible for the reflux oesophagitis (heartburn) that occurs in pregnancy. An additional factor may be displacement of the oesophageal sphincter through the diaphragm due to increased abdominal pressure.

- Gastric mobility is low and gastric secretion is reduced resulting in delayed gastric emptying. Gut motility is generally reduced resulting in constipation.

Changes in the uterus

The non-pregnant uterus weighs 100 g. It undergoes a 10-fold increase in weight to weigh 1000 g at term. Muscle hypertrophy occurs up to 20 weeks with stretching after that.

- The uterus is divided functionally and morphologically into three sections, namely, the cervix, the isthmus (later to develop into the lower uterine segment, becoming more clearly defined from 18 weeks), and the main body of the uterus (corpus uteri).
- Reduction in cervical collagen later in pregnancy enables its dilatation. Hypertrophy of cervical glands leads to the production of profuse cervical mucus and to the formation of a thick mucous plug or operculum that acts as a barrier to infection.

- Vaginal discharge increases due to cervical ectopy and cell desquamation.
- The uterine body increases in size, shape, position, and consistency. The uterine cavity expands from 4 to 4000 mL.
- Uterine blood flow has been shown to increase from approximately 50 mL/min at 10 weeks gestation to 500–700 mL/min at term. The vessels that supply the uterus, the uterine and ovarian arteries, and branches of the superior vesical arteries undergo massive hypertrophy.

Changes in the vagina

In pregnancy the rich venous vascular network in the connective tissue surrounds the vaginal walls with blood and gives rise to the slightly bluish appearance of the vagina.

- High oestrogen levels stimulate glycogen synthesis and deposition, and the action of lactobacilli on glycogen in vaginal cells produces lactic acid, which in turn lowers the vaginal pH to keep the vagina relatively free from any bacterial pathogens.

Skin changes

Pigmentations in linear nigra, nipple, and areola or as chloasma (brown patches of pigmentation seen especially on the face) are seen in pregnancy.

- Palmar erythema, spider naevi, and striae are also common. These changes vary in different women and in different populations. They represent the effect of disruption of collagen fibres in the subcuticular zone. They are probably related to the effect of increased production of adrenocortical hormones in pregnancy as well as to the actual stress in the skin folds associated with expansion of the abdomen.

Diagnosis and dating of pregnancy

The most common presenting symptom of pregnancy is cessation of periods, i.e. a period of amenorrhoea in a woman having regular menstruation.

Other common symptoms of early pregnancy are:
- *Nausea and vomiting* (morning sickness). This is common in the first 3 months of pregnancy. Thereafter it tends to disappear although it may sometimes persist throughout pregnancy.
- *Frequency of micturition.* This is probably due to increased plasma volume and increased urine production and the pressure effect of the uterus on the bladder.
- Many women experience *excessive lassitude* in early pregnancy. This tends to disappear after 12 weeks gestation.
- *Breast tenderness* and 'heaviness' are common and are particularly noticeable in the month after the first period is missed.
- *Fetal movements* or quickening are not usually noticed until 20 weeks gestation in the nullipara and 18 weeks in the multipara. However, many women may experience fetal movements earlier than this or some may not be aware of them till term.
- *Pica.* An abnormal desire for a particular food may occur.

Clinical examination
The vagina and cervix have a bluish tinge due to blood congestion. Estimation of uterine size by vaginal examination is reasonably accurate in early pregnancy compared with later than 12 weeks gestation.

Pregnancy test
The hormone β-hCG is secreted by the trophoblastic tissue or placenta. This increases in pregnancy and peaks at 10 weeks. The levels of this hormone can be measured by blood or urine. Test kits are available commercially to carry out the pregnancy test. Monoclonal antibodies have been raised against β-hCG and tagged with latex or red cells to carry out agglutination tests. The commercial kits can show a positive reaction with colour change when the urinary hCG levels are > 50 or with some kits > 25 IU/L. The woman would be able to know about her pregnancy within 1 week of missing her period using this test.

Dating of pregnancy
Menstrual history
It is important to ascertain the date of the first day of the last menstrual period. This information may not be accurate because many women do not record the day on which they menstruate. In special circumstances such as IVF (*in vitro* fertilization) pregnancies, dating can be accurate as a record is always made of the day of embryo transfer. Gestational age is calculated from the first day of the last period. The length of the menstrual cycle is important. Ovulation usually occurs on the 14th day before the first day of menstruation but the proliferative phase may vary considerably.
- The length of the cycle, i.e. the interval from the first day of the period to the first day of the subsequent period, may vary from 21 to 42 days in normal women although menstruation usually occurs every 28 days in most women.

- It is also important to ascertain the method of contraception employed prior to conception.
- The estimated date of confinement or delivery (EDC or EDD, respectively) can be calculated from the first day of the last period especially if the cycle is 28 days. This can be obtained from Naegele's formula: add 1 year and 7 days and subtract 3 months from the date of the last menstrual period (LMP). Adjustments have to be made for long cycle lengths. This assumes a pregnancy age of 40 weeks (280 days) with conception occurring 2 weeks after the first day of the last menstrual period. For example, if LMP = 7.9.02, EDD = LMP + 9 months + 7 days = 14.6.03. About 40% of women will deliver within 5 days of the estimated date of confinement and about two-thirds within 10 days.

Ultrasound verification of dates

- *Gestation sac.* The visualization of an intrauterine sac provides the first evidence of an intrauterine pregnancy. Vaginal ultrasonography can detect a gestation sac as early as 4 weeks from the last menstrual period.
- *Crown–rump length* (CRL). This is most useful in the first trimester. Fetal flexion in the second trimester renders this of less value. It measures a straight line from one fetal pole to the other along its longitudinal axis.
- *Biparietal diameter* (BPD). This measurement is useful from 14 weeks onwards. The ultrasound probe images the fetus longitudinally and then it is rotated 90° to obtain the transverse plane through the fetal head. Specific structures such as the cavum, septum pellucidum, and the lateral ventricles with their anterior and posterior horns should be identified to make measurements valid. The BPD is measured between the leading edge of the echoes from the proximal and distal skull bones.
- *Head circumference* (HC; Fig. 4.1). The measurements are made from the same section as for BPD. Electronic callipers measure the circumference around the head. The transcerebellar diameter in millimetres gives the gestational age in weeks. It remains constant in growth restriction.

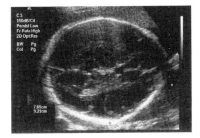

Fig. 4.1 Ultrasound measurement of the head circumference (HC).

Diagnosis and dating
of pregnancy (*continued*)

- *Abdominal circumference* (AC; Fig. 4.2). Abdominal circumference is a sensitive indicator of fetal growth. It is measured at a level where the image of the stomach and intrahepatic portion of the umbilical vein is seen.
- *Femur length* (FL; Fig. 4.3). The fetal thigh is identified and the femur measured in the plane where the buttocks and the knee are included in the view. The femur image should be parallel to the transducer. FL can be underestimated if the correct plane is not obtained.

BPD and FL give assessment of gestational age. If this differs from the menstrual date by more than 2 weeks at an early gestation of less than 20 weeks, the ultrasound measurement should be accepted as the gestational age and the date of delivery should be adjusted accordingly.

Charts of measurements and normograms are available for different population groups and should be used to get the best results (Fig. 4.4). Computer programs are incorporated into the ultrasound machines to provide the gestation once a measurement is made.

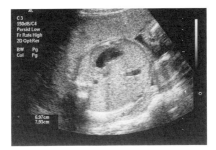

Fig. 4.2 Ultrasound measurement of abdominal circumference (AC).

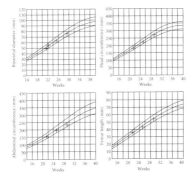

Fig. 4.3 Ultrasound measurement of femur length (FL).

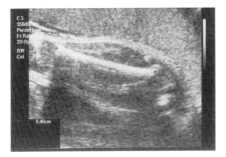

Fig. 4.4 Charts showing normograms of various indices measured by ultrasound.

Booking visit

The purpose of the booking visit is to assess the mother and make a plan for her care in pregnancy. This should include the plan for confinement. Most women in the UK have 'shared obstetric care' whereby the woman's general practitioner (GP) and community midwife undertake most of her obstetric care with a limited number of visits to the hospital (1, 2, or more) to see the consultant under whose care she is delivered. Many women elect to return home 6–72 hours after delivery. Recent recommendations[1] recommend that at least 30% of mothers should be looked after by the midwife and that in 70% of cases the mothers should know which midwife will deliver her. Increasingly therefore, 'low-risk' women are cared for by their community midwives and GPs with medical staff involvement only if complications occur. Certain risk factors, however, make specialist visits necessary.

Only 1% of women deliver at home with a 5% chance of adverse maternal and fetal outcome in low-risk pregnancy. Hence, there is the need for any domiciliary service to have good equipment available and good emergency back-up. The birthing room concept probably is a good compromise as it offers a homely birth with congenial surroundings with labour ward facilities nearby if needed. In this case, the mother is attended by her GP and a midwife in a hospital setting in a home environment.

Booking should normally be in the first trimester in order to take full advantage of antenatal care, but many women are seen the first time in hospital in the second trimester. Children born to very late bookers or especially to unbooked women run the risk of higher perinatal mortality (4–5-fold) and morbidity with an attendant increase in maternal morbidity and mortality.

History

A comprehensive history should include the following headings: personal history, family history, and previous obstetric and medical/surgical history along with the history of the present pregnancy to the time of that visit. In many institutions in the UK there are comprehensive structured sections in the clinical notes (or computer screens) to facilitate history-taking by midwives and clinical staff.

- High-risk markers from past obstetric performance or from medical, surgical, and family history should be highlighted.
- An effort should be made to obtain past obstetric notes from institutions where the women delivered before if it is thought that this information will change the course of management.
- History of inheritable diseases in close relatives of the woman and her partner should be sought as well as the history of migration and intercontinental travel. This may help to identify risk groups for diseases such as haemoglobinopathies, some forms of hepatitis, and HIV infection. With particular reference to HIV infection, intravenous (IV) drug injection and any high-risk sexual practices of the woman or her partner(s) are important.
- Histories of alcohol abuse, smoking, and/or addictive drug use are useful behavioural markers of other potential risks (e.g. fetal abnormalities, impaired growth, preterm labour).

- Recommendations from the last Confidential Enquiry into Maternal Deaths[2] emphasize the need for early identification of women at risk of postnatal depressive illness or self-harm. History should therefore be taken of maternal psychiatric disorder, severe social problems, and previous self-harm. Patients at risk should have appropriate psychiatric care and social support.
- Advice and support should be given on healthy lifestyles, including diet and exercise. Women should be told about the correct use of seat belts during pregnancy.
- Women should be made aware of symptoms and consequences associated with antepartum haemorrhage, pre-eclampsia, preterm labour, and pre-labour rupture of membranes.

Examination

A complete physical examination of the pregnant woman must be undertaken. This should include:

- Height (very small stature may indicate a small pelvis), weight, and blood pressure in the supine lateral position to avoid compression of the inferior vena cava.
- Inspection of the mucosal surfaces (mouth, conjunctiva) for pallor and the general state of dentition (caries should be treated and appropriate advice given on dental hygiene).
- The thyroid gland tends to enlarge slightly in pregnancy but any abnormal enlargement, especially if associated with tachycardia and/or thyrotoxic symptoms or signs, should be investigated.
- The heart should be examined to exclude organic murmurs and, if needed, appropriate referral to the cardiologist should be made. Flow murmurs and mammary souffles are common in pregnancy. When in doubt refer.
- The breasts are examined to exclude the presence of any lumps noting also the condition of the nipples.
- The limbs are examined for varicose veins and the presence of any shortening and the vertebral column is examined for skeletal abnormalities such as kyphosis or lordosis.

Pelvic examination

This is not routinely done in many centres. It is argued that ultrasound gives more accurate information about the pregnancy and more certain detection of adnexal masses. It does not, however, provide information on the state of the vagina or appearance of the cervix. It would therefore be advisable to do a pelvic examination including a speculum examination if the patient has never been examined, has not had a recent smear, or in cases of unusual vaginal discharge or bleeding.

If the woman has become pregnant with an intrauterine contraceptive device (IUCD) *in situ* (which is extremely rare), it is best to remove the IUCD if the threads are visible. Retention of the device may lead to septic abortion.

Abdominal examination in pregnancy

The routine of inspection, palpation, percussion (in cases of polyhydramnios), and auscultation is used to examine the abdomen in pregnancy.

Inspection
Describe the enlarged abdomen giving suggestions as to the approximate gestational age. Describe signs of pregnancy such as linear nigra, striae gravidarum, and the presence of fetal movements. Note any superficial distended veins or scars: Pfannenstiel scars (i.e. transverse low abdominal scars usually used for Caesarean sections) and laparoscopy, appendicectomy, and cholecystectomy scars.

Fundal height measurements
Although the numbers were too small in one study looked at in the Cochrane Library to draw any conclusions, the use of measurement of the fundal height from the top of the symphysis pubis to the fundus of the uterus (highest part of the uterus) is more objective than eye-balling. Measure this in centimetres. The mean fundal–symphyseal (FS) height measures approximately 20 cm at 20 weeks gestation (up to the umbilicus) and increases to approximately 36 cm by 36 weeks gestation (a centimetre per week roughly). Thereafter, the distance tends to plateau until term. Two centimetres either way of the gestation is acceptable up to 35 weeks, which becomes ± 3 cm at 36 weeks and ± 4 cm at 40 weeks due to such factors as increase in size of the baby, reduction of amniotic fluid volume, and engagement of the head.

- Using this technique, approximately 40–60% of all small-for-dates babies can be detected. The accuracy is considerably less if the measurement is made after 36 weeks gestation.

The predictive value of this method is less for large-for-dates infants. Pregnancy factors such as large baby, polyhydramnios, and twins and uterine factors such as fibroids and pelvic tumours lead to FS height greater than dates.

Oligohydramnios, leakage of amniotic fluid, intrauterine growth restriction (IUGR), presenting part deep in the pelvis, and abnormal lies may give rise to uterus smaller than dates. The clinical diagnosis of uterus larger or smaller than dates needs to be investigated further by ultrasound examination.

Palpation for fetal parts
Fetal parts are not usually palpable before 24 weeks gestation. The purpose of palpation is to describe the relationship of the fetus to the maternal trunk and pelvis.

- The lie describes the relationship of the long axis of the fetus to the long axis of the uterus. Palpate along the anterolateral sides of the abdomen and towards the midline to reveal either the firm resistance of the fetal back or the irregular projection of the fetal limbs.
  —The lie is longitudinal if the head or breech is palpable over the pelvic inlet.
  —The lie is oblique if the head or breech is in the iliac fossa.
  —The lie is transverse if the fetus lies at right angles to the uterine longitudinal axis and the poles of the fetus are palpable in the flanks.

- Feel for the head or breech by firm pressure with the two hands starting in the lower pole of the uterus as it is likely to be cephalic or breech in 96% of cases at term. The head is round, hard, and discrete. It can be 'bounced' or ballotted between the examining hands. The buttocks are softer, more diffuse, and broad and the breech is not ballottable.

Presentation

Presentation is the part of the fetus nearest to the pelvic inlet or in the lower uterine segment. Palpate with the two hands over the lower uterine pole for presentation and degree of engagement. Powlik's grip (examining the lower pole of the uterus between the thumb and the index finger of the right hand) can also be used for assessing the engagement of the head. Pressure over the head causes tenderness. This has to be observed as it allows you to stop causing the pain. The presenting part may be the head (cephalic) or the breech (podalic) in a longitudinal lie.

Engagement

This refers to the passage of maximal diameter of the presentation beyond the pelvic inlet. The level of the head is assessed as engaged or in terms of the number of 'fifths' palpable abdominally above the pelvic brim (Fig. 4.5).

When the head is engaged only two-fifths of the head can be felt abdominally. Conventionally, the palm width of the five fingers of the hand is used for this estimation. If five fingers are needed to cover the head above the pelvic brim, it is five-fifths palpable, and, if no head is palpable, it is zero-fifths. Palpation of the occiput (most prominent lateral part of the head on the same side of the fetal back) and the sinciput or forehead (most lateral part on the opposite side of the occiput) would give the degree of flexion of the fetal head.

The baby normally engages in an attitude of flexion in the transverse diameter of the pelvic inlet unless the pelvis is very roomy where it could engage in any diameter. Being able to palpate the sinciput and not the occiput (which is always ahead of the sinciput in a well-flexed head) suggests engagement. On palpating the head, if it is two-fifths palpable and if the hands are diverging on palpating the lateral border of the head it is engaged.

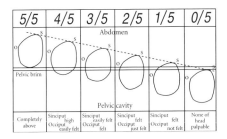

Fig. 4.5 Clinical estimation of descent of head.

Abdominal examination in pregnancy (*continued*)

In a nullipara, the head usually enters the pelvis by 37 weeks. However, non-engagement is not that uncommon at this gestation. Rare causes of non-engagement must be excluded, especially if the head is high (e.g. placenta praevia or fetal abnormality). In multiparous women, the head may not engage until the onset of labour. Due to the exaggerated lordosis in the Black population, engagement even in a primigravida takes place at the onset or during the course of labour.

Position

This describes the relationship of the denominator of the presenting part to fixed points of the maternal pelvis. These points are sacral promontory (posterior), symphysis pubis (anterior), sacroiliac joint (posterior lateral and may be right or left), and iliopectineal eminence (anterolateral and may be right or left). If the saggital suture is lying in the transverse axis of the pelvis, then the denominator is in the right or left lateral position. The denominator is the most definable peripheral prominence in the presenting part. In a vertex presentation, it is the occiput. In face presentation, it is the chin (mentum), and in breech it is the sacrum. This is illustrated in Fig. 4.5 for a vertex presentation.

Finally, note the amount of liquor present. Fetal parts are more easily palpable when the liquor is reduced (oligohydramnios) and are hardly palpable when the liquor is excessive (polyhydramnios). If there is clinical suspicion of polyhydramnios (shiny abdomen on inspection, tense to touch, FS height greater than expected for period of gestation, and difficulty in feeling fetal parts) then fluid thrill should be demonstrated. Women could help by pressing the ulnar border of their hand on the midline of the abdomen along the linea nigra to avoid feeling the surface vibrations, whilst the fluid thrill is illustrated by the clinician.

Auscultation

The fetal heart may be heard by Doppler ultrasound (Sonicaid) from about 12 weeks gestation and with a Pinard stethoscope from about 24 weeks.

- The Sonicaid or stethoscope is placed over the anterior shoulder detected by palpation. It can also be heard over the chest in the midline when the fetus is in the occipito-posterior position.
- With a cephalic presentation, when the vertex is in the occipito-anterior position, the fetal heart is best heard in the midpoint between the maternal umbilicus and the anterior superior iliac spine, where the fetal anterior shoulder could be palpated.
- In a breech presentation, the fetal heart is heard over the back of the baby and is at or above the level of the umbilicus of the mother.

The rate and rhythm of the heartbeat should be noted.

Plan for antenatal care

The aims of antenatal care can be defined as:
- Provision of education, reassurance, and support to the woman and her partner.
- Advice on minor problems and symptoms of pregnancy.
- Assessment of maternal and fetal risk factors at onset of pregnancy and as they develop throughout pregnancy.
- Provision of prenatal screening and management of abnormalities detected.
- Determination of timing and mode of delivery where complications arise.

Effective antenatal care needs to focus on what should be achieved at each key stage of the pregnancy rather than regularity of visits. Antenatal care needs to be provided as part of a broadly agreed and implemented programme but 'fine-tuned' to the individual requirements of the mother and fetus as assessed at booking and as these requirements evolve during the course of the pregnancy. The current emphasis is on provision of as much of the antenatal care as possible in the community and primary-care team setting and this is partly in response to what the patients would prefer themselves.

Pre-conception
In an ideal world antenatal care would commence at the pre-conception stage where health education (general advice about nutrition, lifestyle, avoidance of teratogens, folic acid supplementation, etc.) and risk assessment can be focused towards a planned pregnancy. Pre-conception counselling is of much greater importance where there are underlying medical conditions that may be affected by or may influence the outcome of a pregnancy.

First trimester
Antenatal care in the first trimester starts with a visit to the GP after a missed period and confirmation of pregnancy. This visit is followed by a booking visit with the community midwife. The purpose of this visit is to obtain a comprehensive history, establish gestational age, and identify any maternal or fetal risk factors. It also provides an ideal opportunity for the woman to discuss any anxieties she may have.
- During this visit routine blood tests are performed—full blood count (FBC); blood grouping and antibody screen; rubella, syphilis, hepatitis B, and HIV serology; and haemoglobin electrophoresis if appropriate. Urine is tested for glucose and protein and a midstream specimen is sent for culture and sensitivity to detect asymptomatic bacteruria.
- The hospital booking visit may be any time between 12 and 20 weeks of gestation and varies from hospital to hospital but there is an increasing tendency for earlier referral especially in older women who may wish screening tests for chromosomal abnormalities in the first trimester.
- Many hospitals offer a first trimester ultrasound scan for pregnancy dating and measurement of nuchal translucency at the 10–14 weeks stage. Nuchal translucency measurements may be combined with measurements of serum markers such as β-hCG and PAPP-A (pregnancy-associated plasma protein A) as a sensitive screening test for trisomy 21. Towards the end of the first trimester (11–12 weeks) is the time when prenatal diagnostic testing such as chorionic villus sampling (CVS) may be performed in selected groups of patients.

Second trimester

Early in the second trimester, at around 16 weeks, serum screening tests are performed for assessment of risk of open neural tube defect and Down syndrome. Prenatal diagnostic testing in the form of amniocentesis may be performed at around 16 weeks and a detailed ultrasound scan to assess fetal anatomy is usually performed at the 19–20 week stage by which time the results of serum screening should have been available and reviewed. Where fetal cardiac anomalies are suspected, a further ultrasound scan may be required at the 22–24 week stage. After this stage of pregnancy the patient is seen at 4-weekly intervals and at each visit BP, urinalysis, and fundal height as well as maternal well-being are checked and fetal activity enquired about.

Third trimester

Monthly visits to the community midwife continue in the third trimester (> 28 weeks). FBC is checked and antibody screen is repeated at 28 and 34 weeks in rhesus-negative women who are given anti-D prophylaxis at these times. In addition to BP, urinalysis, fundal height, maternal well-being, and fetal activity, from 36 weeks onwards fetal presentation is also assessed and, if not, cephalic referral to the hospital antenatal clinic is organized for appropriate investigations and counselling. During the third trimester the mother and her partner need to be prepared for what to expect regarding onset and process of labour and delivery. The final routine antenatal visit often is in hospital and is timed between 40 and 41 weeks where discussion takes place regarding induction of labour after 41 weeks. If the woman wishes to avoid induction after discussion of the rationale for induction and the risks involved in prolongation of pregnancy, then a plan of increased surveillance with cardiotocograph (CTG) and ultrasound assessment of fetal growth and liquor volume can be individualized.

Routine blood tests

A series of blood tests is performed in pregnancy. These tests are in general screening tests for potential maternal and fetal problems that, if identified, can either affect the outcome of the pregnancy or give an opportunity by adjusting antenatal care appropriately to make a difference in pregnancy outcome.

Full blood count (FBC)

This is the most commonly performed haematological investigation in pregnancy. Pregnancy is associated with a physiological dilutional anaemia due to a greater increase in plasma volume than red cell mass and therefore the lower limit for a 'normal' haemoglobin (Hb) is 10.5 g/dL in pregnancy as opposed to 11.5 g/dL in the non-pregnant individual. Many women enter pregnancy with a low iron reserve and, therefore, if anaemia is detected in pregnancy it should be investigated by assessment of haematinic indices such as ferritin, total iron-binding capacity (TIBC), serum and red cell folate, and serum B_{12} levels. The most common cause of anaemia in pregnancy is iron deficiency anaemia. FBC estimation is performed every 4 to 8 weeks in the second half of pregnancy and a low haemoglobin on admission in labour is an indication for sending a specimen to the lab for 'group and save' in case of intrapartum or postpartum bleeding.

Blood grouping and screening for antibodies

Determining the blood group at booking makes it possible to identify those women who are rhesus-negative and therefore at risk of rhesus isoimmunization. The incidence of rhesus disease has dramatically fallen over the last 30 years following the introduction of anti-D administration. Despite administration of prophylactic anti-D after screening at 28 and 34 weeks and after any potential sensitizing event, a small number of rhesus D-negative women still develop anti-D antibodies because of small silent haemorrhages predominantly in the third trimester or because of failure of timely administration of anti-D. Screening for red cell antibodies should be repeated in all women early in subsequent pregnancies even if rhesus positive as there may be other clinically significant antibodies as a consequence of previous pregnancy or blood transfusion.

Infection screening

- All booking bloods are screened for evidence of immunity to rubella due to the devastating implications on the fetus of rubella in early pregnancy. The present data show that around 2% of primigravida and 1% of multigravida are non-immune to rubella, and it is recommended that these women receive postpartum rubella vaccination. Vaccination in pregnancy is not recommended but there have been no reports of adverse outcome where this has been performed inadvertently in pregnancy.
- Screening for syphilis is also routinely performed with around 250 cases detected annually in the UK. The rationale for screening for syphilis lies in the fact that early treatment of the disease can prevent congenital syphilis in the neonate.
- Hepatitis B screening is also universally performed on all antenatal booking bloods. A combined course of active and passive immunization can then be undertaken in the neonate at risk after birth. The importance of preventing hepatitis B infection in the neonate lies in the fact that, while in the adult patient the virus is cleared within 6 months in 90% of infected individuals, in neonates 90% become chronic carriers with the risk of post-infective hepatic cirrhosis and hepatocellular carcinoma.

The current recommendations from the government in the UK are for universal screening for HIV at the antenatal booking visit. This has come about because of difficulties in effectively targeting affected women even in areas of high prevalence. There is now clear evidence that the vertical transmission from mother to fetus can be significantly reduced (by two-thirds) by treatment of the mother with antiretrovirals in pregnancy and labour and of the infant for 6 weeks postnatally. Furthermore, the risk of transmission can also be reduced by Caesarean section and avoidance of breastfeeding. It should also be borne in mind that HIV testing performed as part of routine antenatal screening is not used by insurance companies as a marker of high risk. At present, it is not clear what proportion of units in the UK is carrying out HIV screening routinely in all antenatal patients.

Special blood tests

Screening for gestational diabetes mellitus (GDM)

There appears to be no consensus as to who, when, how, or even whether to screen for GDM. Universal biochemical screening has been suggested. Universal screening limited to those over 25 years of age has also been suggested. Screening all pregnant women at 28 weeks gestation would identify those with impaired glucose tolerance or diabetes with a sensitivity of 78% and specificity of 90%. The majority of units decide on who to screen on the basis of clinical risk factors including previous GDM, family history of diabetes (first-degree relative with diabetes), previous macrosomic baby, previous unexplained stillbirth, obesity (BMI > 26), glycosuria on more than one occasion, polyhydramnios and large for gestational age infant in current pregnancy. This policy of selective screening would identify 50% of women with GDM. The timing of testing is also controversial as, the later in pregnancy it is performed, the higher the detection rate since glucose tolerance progressively deteriorates. On the other hand the earlier in pregnancy GDM is diagnosed and hyperglycaemia treated, the greater the likelihood of influencing the outcome.

Screening for haemoglobinopathies

Haemoglobin electrophoresis should be routinely performed in women of ethnic or racial origins with a high incidence of haemoglobinopathies. These include women of Cypriot, Eastern Mediterranean, Middle Eastern, Indian, and Southeast Asian origin where the incidence of thalassaemia is greatest and women of African or Afro-Caribbean origin who are at risk of sickle cell. If a patient herself is affected then consideration should be given to testing her partner as this will have implications on counselling and prenatal testing. Persistent anaemia, where a cause could not be identified, may be an indication for haemoglobin electrophoresis in any woman irrespective of racial origin.

Miscellaneous tests

Other blood tests may be performed on an individual basis. Thus, if there is a history of thyroid disease, thyroid function tests may be required. In patients with hypertension or renal complications of diabetes, baseline urea, creatinine and electrolytes would be advisable. Long-term diabetic control is monitored by means of serum HbA_{1c} estimation. Where epilepsy is poorly controlled despite adequate doses of anticonvulsants, it may be useful to assess serum levels prior to further dose increases or as a means of confirming compliance. Patients with a family or personal history of coagulation disorders may need screening for bleeding disorders or thrombophilia and checking of coagulation factor levels.

Double/triple test

This refers to the estimation of serum-unconjugated oestriol, alphafetoprotein (AFP), and β-hCG in the maternal blood at around 16 weeks gestation (triple test) or the use of AFP and β-hCG (double test) as a screening test for trisomy 21. Down syndrome is the most common chromosomal condition with a birth prevalence of 1 in 700 and has great clinical and societal significance in terms of severity and compatibility with life. Studies have shown that maternal serum (MS) AFP levels in pregnancies affected by Down syndrome are 25% lower than in women with chromosomally normal fetuses and this is independent of age. Similarly, the levels of another hormone produced by the fetoplacental unit unconjugated oestriol (MSuE3), are also 27% lower in pregnancies affected by Down syndrome. The most effective marker to date, however, appears to be the placental-specific product hCG with levels being twice high as normal in pregnancies affected by Down syndrome or other chromosomal abnormalities. While MSAFP and MSuE3 rise between 14 and 21 weeks, hCG levels drop. Because maternal age is independent of the markers, it is used to define risk *a priori*. Given that the three markers are not independent of each other, application of a trivariate Gaussian distribution allows calculation of individual risk with a commercially available software package assisting in the calculations. Different units define different cut-offs as high risk, with cut-off values ranging from 1 in 200 through to 1 in 300. The detection (DR) and false-positive (FPR) rates for the double and triple tests are given in Table 4.1 for the different cut-offs used to define high risk.

The main effect of adding uE3 to the combination testing of β-hCG and AFP is a small reduction in false-positive rate with minimal improvement in detection rate. The management of a screen positive result (i.e. an individual risk greater than the cut-off selected) involves confirmation of a singleton pregnancy, verification of gestational age, and timing of the screening test. If these are correct then the patient and her partner need to be counselled about the options available to them, which include invasive diagnostic testing to obtain a karyotype. On the other hand, if such testing is unacceptable to them due to the risks involved for the pregnancy or because the outcome of diagnostic testing would not alter their attitude towards the pregnancy, the course of action chosen may be to not investigate further. With all types of screening tests there need to be agreed protocols on how abnormal results are managed with adequate time set aside for pre- and post-test counselling and on-going support.

Screening for neural tube defects (NTDs)

It is important at this stage to make the distinction between the double/triple test and the role of MSAFP alone, which is used as a screening tool for open neural tube defect. AFP is produced first by the yolk sac and subsequently by the fetal liver and enters the amniotic fluid by fetal urination. Its level continues to rise till 30–32 weeks after which it declines. During the period of screening (15–20 weeks gestation) the levels of AFP rise at around 15% per week. A level greater than 2.2 multiples of the median (MoM) is considered elevated (MoM is calculated by dividing an individual MSAFP by the median for the gestational week). In addition to open NTD, a raised MSAFP may be a result of abdominal wall defects, congenital nephrosis, upper fetal bowel obstruction, placental or umbilical cord tumours, sacrococcygeal teratoma, multiple pregnancy, gestation more advanced than thought, and bleeding in early pregnancy amongst other causes.

Management of elevated MSAFP includes confirmation of gestation and exclusion of multiple pregnancy along with high-resolution ultrasound to exclude an anatomical cause.

A knowledge of elevated MSAFP in the absence of fetal structural malformation should trigger a modification of prenatal care to provide enhanced fetal and maternal surveillance as it is a marker for adverse perinatal outcomes such as fetal death, intrauterine growth restriction (IUGR), early and late pregnancy bleeding, and preterm delivery while there are conflicting reports as to whether it may be a marker for subsequent development of pre-eclampsia.

Table 4.1 Detection (DR) and false-positive (FPR) rates (%) at birth for the double and triple tests for different cut-off risks

DR for Screening test combination	5% FPR	Cut off risk (at term)					
		1 in 200		1 in 250		1 in 300	
		DR	FPR	DR	FPR	DR	FPR
AFP + uE3 + b-hCG	62.7	60.8	4.4	64.4	5.6	67.3	6.9
AFP + b-hCG	59.3	58.6	4.8	62.6	6.2	65.6	7.5

References

1 Royal College of Obstetricians and Gynaecologists (RCOG) and Royal College of Midwives (1999). *Towards safer childbirth—minimum standards for the organisation of labour wards*, report of a joint working party. RCOG Press, London.

2 Lewis, G. and Drife, J. (ed.) (2001). *Why mothers die 1997–99, the confidential enquiries into maternal deaths in the United Kingdom*. RCOG Press, London.

Chapter 5

Minor symptoms of pregnancy

These can be divided into first, second, and third trimester symptoms.

First trimester symptoms

- Nausea and vomiting are the most common complaints of pregnant women in the first trimester and these are collectively referred to as morning sickness. Morning sickness is believed to be due to high levels of pregnancy hormones secreted by the placenta. In women with multiple pregnancies or molar pregnancy this symptom tends to be exaggerated. It becomes abnormal when vomiting is so severe that it prevents the pregnant woman from adequate fluid and food intake causing severe dehydration, ketonuria, and electrolyte imbalance. This is referred to as hyperemesis gravidarum (see Chapter 7).
    —*Treatment.* Women need to be hospitalized for intravenous feeding and rehydration when vomiting causes ketonuria, dehydration, and electrolyte imbalance. Generally, morning sickness should diminish at about 14 weeks of pregnancy. Conditions such as urinary tract infection, molar and multiple pregnancies, and thyroid disease need to be excluded.
- Tiredness. Women in the early part of pregnancy may feel tired easily. In fact, this may be one of their first symptoms of pregnancy. This feeling will generally ease off towards the second trimester and may return towards the end of pregnancy.
- Frequency of micturition. When the uterus enlarges in the first trimester of pregnancy it presses on the bladder, resulting in decreased capacity and hence giving rise to urinary frequency. Also, urine production by the kidney increases during pregnancy and this in turn increases urinary volume and contributes to frequency. The pressure effect of the uterus eases off by the 14th week when the uterus rises out of the pelvis and the symptom generally improves in the second trimester. Watch out for underlying urinary tract infection, which can also present with increased frequency.
    —*Treatment.* Advise not to drink before bedtime. Avoid caffeine-containing drinks, but have a sensible fluid intake throughout the day.
- Heartburn. Progesterone produced by the placenta in pregnancy causes relaxation of the oesophageal sphincter producing reflux of gastric juices. This produces heartburn.
    —*Treatment.* Advise the wearing of loose clothing and sleeping on two pillows at night and prescribe antacids.
- Constipation. The relaxation effects of progesterone on the smooth muscles of the bowel cause less bowel activity during pregnancy. This may give rise to very troublesome constipation in some women that can continue throughout pregnancy.
    —*Treatment.* Adequate intake of fibre such as fruit and fluids is of help. Avoid powerful laxatives but bulk formula laxatives may be used.
    Note. Iron supplements in pregnancy may cause constipation in some women.

5 Minor symptoms of pregnancy

- Breast changes. From the second month, under the influence of oestrogen and progesterone produced by the placenta, the breasts start to enlarge due to increased fat deposition and glandular proliferation. There is also darkening and increase in size of the nipple and areola with elaboration of Montgomery's follicles scattered around the nipple.
  —*Treatment*. A good support maternity or athletic brassiere will help alleviate breast discomfort.
- Emotional lability. Some women will experience emotional lability and unusual food cravings.
  —*Treatment*. Emotional support from spouse and advice regarding diet.

Second trimester symptoms

- Aches and pains. The majority of these symptoms are benign but a small minority may require medical attention. Aches and pains begin in the second trimester and continue to the end of pregnancy. These are caused by the rapidly enlarging uterus and the increased levels of hormones such as progesterone and relaxin.
  —*Treatment.* Advise sufficient rest periods and the wearing of low-heeled shoes.
- Backache. Progesterone and relaxin produced by the placenta cause softening and relaxation of tendons and ligaments throughout the body. The weight of the womb and fetus in front causes the mother to compensate by arching her back to bring the centre of gravity back between her legs. This imposes considerable strain on the joints on the back resulting in backache. Excessive weight gain and previous back injury can aggravate the situation.
  —*Treatment.* Adopting a proper posture, having sufficient rest, avoiding wearing high-heeled shoes, avoiding lifting heavy objects, bending at the knees instead of the waist, and lifting by using the arms and legs instead of the back should all help to avoid backache. Avoid standing for too long—a foot on a low stool will offset some of the strain on the back. Sleeping on a firm mattress, massage, and using hot pads for the back also help to reduce the backache.
- Lower abdominal and groin pain. Some women may experience aching or sharp pain at the lower abdomen and groin. It may be felt on either side or both sides. This may be pain originating from the round ligaments due to the enlarging uterus pulling on the round ligaments. This pain is felt usually between 16 and 20 weeks and continues till about the 32nd week.
  —*Treatment.* Most abdominal pain during pregnancy is innocuous but any pain that develops suddenly and persists should be paid serious attention. Torsion of an ovarian cyst should be excluded.
- Headaches. Mild headaches are common in pregnancy. Persistent headaches after 20 weeks should raise the possibility of pre-eclampsia. Therefore blood pressure and urine must be checked.
  —*Treatment.* Prescribe simple analgesics like paracetamol after ruling out a pathological cause.
- Calf pain. This is due to muscle spasm and tends to occur at night. Venous stasis due to poor circulation can give rise to dull discomfort. The possibility of deep vein thrombosis should be considered.
  —*Treatment.* Straighten the legs and flex the ankles and toes towards the face to reduce the discomfort. Gentle massage and application of hot pads should ease the pain. If calf pain persists and is associated with swelling of the lower limbs, investigate for deep vein thrombosis.
- Increased vaginal discharge. Leucorrhoea is a white and clear mucoid discharge from the vagina. This is secondary to increased blood flow to the vagina and increased cervical secretions. It becomes pathological when it is associated with an offensive odour or pruritus or when it becomes coloured, blood-stained, or 'watery' in which case it is suggestive of an infection.
  —*Treatment.* Reassurance if physiological. Identify and treat any underlying infection.

5 Minor symptoms of pregnancy

- Braxton–Hicks contractions. These are painless tightenings of the uterus that the pregnant woman experiences after the 20th week and that become more frequent and stronger towards the end of pregnancy. They originate from the top of the uterus and gradually fade off as they radiate downwards. They usually last for between 30 and 60 seconds. This could be confused with pre-term labour, which usually occurs more than 4 times in an hour and is accompanied by abdominal pain or backache. Abdominal pain associated with vaginal bleeding or watery vaginal discharge may suggest an abruption or spontaneous rupture of the membranes.
- The first sensation of fetal movement or quickening can be felt as early as 17–20 weeks. Parous women tend to feel these earlier than primigravidas. It is perfectly normal for no movement to be felt for days in the early part of pregnancy, but after 20 weeks absence of fetal movements should be investigated. Auscultation of the fetal heart sounds using a doptone would allay maternal anxiety and a scan will reveal the growth and liquor volume in relation to the gestational period.

Third trimester symptoms

- Breathlessness. This symptom is felt when the diaphragm is pushed up by the expanding uterus thereby decreasing lung capacity. Progesterone acts on the respiratory centre of the brain causing deep breathing, which allows an increase in tidal volume and thus ensures an adequate oxygen supply to the baby.
    —*Treatment*. Improvement in posture, practising sitting with the back straight and the shoulders relaxed and back and down. Lying on the side when sleeping. This symptom improves with the engagement of the head. *Caution*. Shortness of breath along with rapid pulse and rapid breathing and chest pain or discomfort may raise the possibility of pulmonary embolus.
- Sciatica. Pressure of the pregnant uterus against the two sciatic nerves or sciatica may cause pain, tingling, or numbness running down the buttocks, hip, and thighs.
    —*Treatment*. Adequate rest, warm baths, use of heating pads, change of sleeping positions. An antenatal cradle may be useful. This symptom eases nearer the delivery date. More serious cases should be referred to the orthopaedic surgeon or physiotherapist.
- Sleeplessness or insomnia. This may be due to a very active baby at night or discomfort due to the mother lying flat.
    —*Treatment*. A little exercise prior to going to bed and a drink of warm milk may help mothers to relax. Sleeping on the side with legs and knees bent is the ideal position. Cushions may be used to support the body with additional pillows for the abdomen, upper body, and back. Avoid the use of sedatives.
- Itchy abdomen. This is due to stretching of the skin across the abdomen as pregnancy progresses.
    —*Treatment*. Use of lubricating lotion or moisturisers may help and an anti-itching cream may relieve the discomfort in intolerable cases. If itching continues and is generalized and unrelenting, investigate for possible cholestasis.
- Stretch marks. These are due to both the stretching of the abdomen and changes in tissues beneath the skin as a result of hormonal changes related to pregnancy.
    —*Treatment*. There is no proven treatment. Lubricant creams and ointments have been tried.
- Varicose veins. These may cause slight discomfort and may get worse towards the final stages of pregnancy.
    —*Treatment*. The blood venous circulation in the legs should be improved by regular exercise and the use of compression stockings. Varicose veins become less after delivery.
- Rashes. Rashes are common in pregnancy, but are often not serious. While a few may require treatment, most will disappear after childbirth. PUPP (pruritic urticarial papules and placques of pregnancy) is a skin condition that occurs in about 1 in 150 pregnancies and is characterized by itchy, reddish, raised patches on the abdomen, arms, and legs.
    —*Treatment*. Simple rashes may respond to anti-itching creams. In the case of PUPP a referral to a dermatologist may be useful. Topical steroids are recommended. Most skin conditions will disappear after delivery.

5 Minor symptoms of pregnancy

- Haemorrhoids. These occur in about 1 in every 3 women and may occur for the first time during pregnancy.
  —*Treatment.* Preventive measures such as avoidance of constipation by eating green leafy vegetables and high-fibre foods should be advised from early pregnancy. Increase in regular fluid intake, regular exercises, avoiding long hours of standing or sitting, and sleeping on the side may help. Suppositories or creams may be used for temporary relief. Refer to a surgeon when piles increase in size or become very painful.
- Numbness of the hands. Carpal tunnel syndrome may occur as a result of tissue swelling during pregnancy.
  —*Treatment.* Avoid sleeping with the hands below the face or body. Increase circulation by hanging the affected hand over the side of the bed. Wearing of a wrist splint may be necessary in severe cases. Occasionally, referral to a surgeon may become necessary if there is evidence of neurological deficit.
- Urinary incontinence. This is due to the pregnant uterus pressing on the urinary bladder.
  —*Treatment.* Frequent emptying of the bladder and pelvic floor exercises are of value. Stress incontinence persisting 6 months after delivery should be investigated.
- Weight gain. Women put on about 30% additional weight during pregnancy. Half of this may be during the third trimester. In heavier women watch for diabetes, increased blood pressure, or thromboembolism.
  —*Treatment.* Weight gain is normal. Light exercise and a well balanced diet are good for overall health. Rule out the possibility of diabetes or increased blood pressure if there is a sudden increase in weight.

Chapter 6

Bleeding and/or pain in early pregnancy

This chapter covers uterine bleeding with/without pain before viability (currently 22 weeks). The pregnancy may remain viable (threatened miscarriage) in spite of the bleeding or it may be a feature of non-viability (missed abortion or blighted ovum). The pregnancy may also be partly (inevitable/incomplete miscarriage) or completely expelled (complete miscarriage). Miscarriage is very common, occurring in about 15% of confirmed pregnancies. It may cause significant psychological trauma and therefore counselling and support are very important in management. The term 'miscarriage' is preferable to 'abortion' as the latter may be misunderstood as induced rather than spontaneous.

Miscarriage

Threatened miscarriage

Vaginal bleeding is often minimal and may be associated with mild period-type pelvic pains. The volume of bleeding is usually less than the patient's usual menstrual blood loss. If the bleeding is light and resolves, pregnancy, if viable, usually continues satisfactorily.

Diagnosis

The cervical os is closed, the uterine size corresponds to gestational period on pelvic examination, and ultrasound scan confirms viability of the pregnancy.

Management

- Reassurance that the pregnancy should continue satisfactorily once the bleeding settles. Advise avoidance of strenuous activity but normal daily activities need not be restricted.
- If bleeding continues, repeat ultrasound scan (in about 7 days) to confirm viability. If ultrasound is doubtful, it is necessary to err on the side of caution and repeat after 1–2 weeks depending on circumstances as an inconclusive scan may, for instance, be due to wrong dates.

Inevitable miscarriage

With an inevitable miscarriage, vaginal bleeding is associated with an open internal cervical os (the external os may seem 'open' in multiparous women). The bleeding is usually associated with 'crampy' pelvic pains that may vary from mild to severe.

Diagnosis

Usually clinical, based on bleeding and an open cervical os. Products of conception may be left in the canal. The bleeding usually continues until uterus is emptied.

Management

- Expectant. Await spontaneous completion of miscarriage if the clinical condition permits and the patient wishes.
- Surgical evacuation under general anaesthetic if products of conception are protruding through the os.
- Medical management with prostaglandin analogues, e.g. vaginal misoprostol 200–600 µg.
- Counselling and support should be given as needed.

Incomplete/complete miscarriage

With *incomplete miscarriage* some products of conception may be passed and some may be stuck in the cervical os or the uterus. The os remains open until miscarriage is spontaneously, medically, or surgically completed. It may be necessary to remove tissue stuck in the os or the uterus to prevent further haemorrhage.

- Oxytocin infusion should be given to maintain uterine contraction if the vaginal bleeding is heavy.
- Ultrasound scan, when appropriate, shows retained products of conception.
- Surgical evacuation is usually indicated for incomplete miscarriage.

With *complete miscarriage* pelvic pains and vaginal bleeding reduce spontaneously, the cervical os closes, and ultrasound shows an empty uterus.

Recurrent miscarriage

This is defined as the loss of three or more consecutive pregnancies and affects % of all women.

Associated factors

There are a number of factors implicated or associated with recurrent miscarriage. Chromosomal abnormality (present in 3–5% of partners), congenital uterine abnormalities, cervical incompetence, infection, inadequate secretion of progesterone in the luteal phase, polycystic ovary syndrome and raised lutenizing hormone levels, subfertility and ovulatory defects, autoimmune conditions, and, in particular, antiphospholipid syndrome.

Investigations
- Karyotyping of both partners.
- Karyotyping of any fetal tissue.
- Pelvic ultrasound to assess ovaries and uterine cavity.
- Screening tests for antiphospholipid syndrome.

Further management
- Referral to geneticists if abnormal karyotype.
- Low-dose aspirin + heparin if positive for antiphospholipid antibodies.

There are no other proven treatments but the problem is subject to considerable research.

Missed abortion/blighted ovum

This is failure to expel a dead/non-viable fetus from the uterus. Abdominal pain and vaginal bleeding are usually minimal. Pregnancy symptoms have usually inexplicably resolved. The uterus is smaller than expected for dates. The ultrasound scan shows absence of fetal heart activity. Often, there is a misshapen gestation sac and the fetus may be smaller than expected for dates. With a blighted ovum, a gestation sac is seen on ultrasound but there is no fetal heart activity, yolk sac, or fetal pole.

Management

- Expectant. If very early, the pregnancy may resolve spontaneously. If the patient so wishes, it is reasonable to allow up to 2 weeks for resolution.
- Medical management using misoprostol as for inevitable miscarriage. (Mid-trimester missed abortion is best treated by medical means.)
- Surgical evacuation of uterus is usually necessary for missed abortion or blighted ovum.
- There is a risk of disseminated intravascular coagulation (DIC) with a long-standing missed abortion that has remained in the uterus for 4 weeks or more, especially in mid-trimester. It is therefore necessary to check the coagulation status prior to any intervention.
- Diagnosis is usually unexpected by patient so counselling/support may be required.

Hydatidiform mole

This usually presents as bleeding in early pregnancy. The bleeding may be profuse and accompanied by vaginal expulsion of grape-like tissues. The uterus is large for dates in 50% of cases.

Diagnosis may be incidental, with the finding of typical grape-like material during surgical evacuation of a non-viable pregnancy. More often, an ultrasound scan is requested because of a 'large for dates' uterus, hyperemesis, or slight vaginal bleeding and reveals the typical ultrasound 'snowstorm' appearance with the absence of a fetus (complete mole). Beta human chorionic gonadotrophin (β-hCG) levels are very high and this may result in large, bilateral ovarian (theca lutein) cysts. Pregnancy symptoms may be quite profound due to the high β-hCG levels.

Management

- The uterus is best surgically evacuated and tissue sent for histological confirmation.
- Notify the molar pregnancy register (in the UK, register at Charing Cross, London; Weston Park, Sheffield; Ninewells, Dundee) for follow-up.
- Clinical and biochemical follow-up is essential as there is a risk of malignant trophoblastic disease.
- Advise barrier methods of contraception for a year to allow follow-up.
- Avoid the combined oral contraceptive pill until β-hCG returns to normal.

Hydatidiform mole may recur in future pregnancies.

Other causes of abdominal pain

For discussions of *fibroids* and *ectopic pregnancy* see Chapters 46 and 58, respectively.

Most of the coincidental causes of abdominal pains are related to the hormonal/physiological changes of pregnancy. The approach to management is to exclude a pathological cause and give symptomatic treatment. These conditions include:

- Heartburn.
- Hyperemesis.
- Constipation.

69

More sinister conditions may, however, occur in pregnancy. These are incidental to the pregnancy but diagnosis may be made more difficult because of displacement of abdominal viscera by the gravid uterus, leading to atypical location of pain compared with that of non-pregnant patients. When suspected, surgical opinion should be sought early. These conditions include:

- Appendicitis.
- Cholecystitis.
- Renal colic.
- Inflammatory bowel disease.
- Ovarian cyst accidents (torsion, haemorrhage).
- Sickle cell crisis.
- Pancreatitis.
- Bowel obstruction.

Recommended further reading

1 Royal College of Obstetricians and Gynaecologists (1999). *The management of tubal pregnancies*, 'Green top' guideline no. 21, October 1999. Royal College of Obstetricians and Gynaecologists, London.

2 Royal College of Obstetricians and Gynaecologists and Royal College of Radiologists (1995). *Guidance on ultrasound procedures in early pregnancy*. Royal College of Obstetricians and Gynaecologists and Royal College of Radiologists, London.

3 Fox, R., Richardson, J.A., and Sharma, A. (2000). Early pregnancy assessment. *The Obstetrician and Gynaecologist* 2 (2), 7–12.

4 James, D.K., Steer, P.J., Weiner, C.P., and Gonik, B. (eds.) (1994). *High risk pregnancy: management options*. W.B. Saunders, London.

5 Shervington, J. and Cox, C. (2000). Abdominal pain in pregnancy: diagnosis, surgery and anaesthesia. *The Obstetrician and Gynaecologist* 2 (1), 17–22.

Hyperemesis gravidarum

Nausea and vomiting are both common in pregnancy. Persistent vomiting and severe nausea can progress to hyperemesis. The characteristics of hyperemesis are:

- Prolonged and severe nausea and vomiting, dehydration, ketosis, and loss of body weight.
- Investigations may show hypernatraemia, hypokalaemia, low serum urea, metabolic hypochloraemia, alkalosis and ketonuria, raised haematocrit, and increased specific gravity of the urine.
- There may be associated liver function test abnormalities and abnormal thyroid function tests with biochemical thyrotoxicosis, i.e. raised free thyroxin levels and/or suppressed thyroid-stimulating hormone levels

Pathophysiology

The incidence is 1:1000. The pathophysiology is poorly understood. The risk is increased in youth, non-smokers, primiparas, those working outside the home and in those with multiple and molar pregnancy. A possible direct relationship between severity of hyperemesis, degree of biochemical hyperthyroidism, and the level of human chorionic gonadotrophin (hCG) has been postulated. Transient hyperthyroidism of hyperemesis gravidarum is a self-limiting hyperthyroidism. It resolves by 18 weeks of pregnancy without sequelae and no treatment is required.

Management

Hyperemesis gravidarum may be a result of an underlying disease. Differential diagnosis includes pyelonephritis, hydatidiform mole, red degeneration of fibroids, increased intracranial pressure, an acute abdominal emergency, and hysterical vomiting. In the latter case the patient is likely to complain of vomiting after every meal and of not being able to retain a drop of water. However, she manages to look well physically and her weight is appropriate. Both the patient and her partner are convinced that there is a physical explanation for her symptoms. Psychological explanation may not succeed because of denial of underlying emotional conflict.

Routine investigation should include:
- FBC (packed cell volume (PCV)).
- Urea and electrolytes (U&Es) to help guide the intravenous (IV) fluid regime in addition to an input and output chart.
- Thyroid function tests (TFTs) may help to identify thyroid dysfunction.
- Exclude urinary tract infection by midstream urine (MSU) for culture.
- In protracted or severe cases liver function tests (LFTs) may be deranged.
- Ultrasound will be useful to confirm an intrauterine pregnancy, identify a multiple pregnancy, and exclude a molar pregnancy.

Treatment

- Development of ketonuria in a pregnant woman with severe vomiting should indicate admission to hospital.
- Time should be spent optimizing the woman's psychological well-being.
- IV fluid replacement in the form of normal saline or 5% dextrose saline is required until ketonuria clears and vomiting subsides.
- Potassium and other electrolytes are replaced guided by daily or twice daily U&Es.
- Too rapid reversal of hypernatraemia can cause fetal pontine myelinosis.
- Thiamine (vitamin B_1) supplementation may be required to prevent Wernicke's encephalopathy.

73

Most patients improve with the help of the above measures without long-term sequelae. Conventional anti-emetics are not usually prescribed, especially before 12 weeks gestation, but in these women with hyperemesis it is necessary to wean them to oral feeds. The reluctance to use anti-emetics relates to fears concerning their teratogenic effects. Anti-emetic medication appears to reduce the frequency of nausea and vomiting in early pregnancy. There is some evidence of adverse effects, but there is little information on effects on fetal outcomes.

- Traditional anti-emetics, such as metoclopramide 10 mg every 8 hours IV, may be tried followed by oral anti-emetics.
- Treatment with pyridoxine (vitamin B_1) appears to be effective in reducing the severity of nausea.
- The results from trials of P6 acupressure are equivocal.
- Those resistant to conventional therapy may respond to steroid treatment. There is some evidence that a course of methylprednisolone is more effective than promethazine for treatment of hyperemesis.
- Placing a Dobbhoff nasogastric tube for enteral feeding has proponents. Isomolar feeds are recommended. Parenteral nutrition may be needed in rare instances and the advice of a dietitian would be valuable. This may need to be associated with regular aspiration of the stomach if there is continued vomiting due to delayed gastric emptying.
- When symptoms of hyperemesis gravidarum persist into the second trimester, active peptic ulcer disease from *Helicobacter pylori* should be included in the differential diagnosis.

Chapter 8

Prenatal diagnosis

Congenital abnormalities are common, contributing to 15% of all perinatal deaths and a further 10–15% of deaths in the first year of life in the UK. Of fetal abnormalities, 95% are unexpected, occurring in pregnancies not considered at high risk of those conditions. Screening of whole populations aims to detect abnormalities in low-risk women. For women who have had a previous fetal abnormality, the risk of recurrence may be known and this will guide future testing. When screening test results are of high risk, or the recurrence risk of a previous abnormality is high, a diagnostic test is offered. There is a growing demand for prenatal screening and diagnosis, with families increasingly looking to obstetric and genetic services to assist in their quest for healthy offspring. Prenatal diagnosis is now a major part of antenatal care. It allows for:

- Planning for place and method of delivery.
- Arrangements for repair of structural problems (preferable to deliver in centre with paediatric surgery).
- *In utero* treatment where this is feasible.
- Preparation of parents to cope with a baby with a congenital abnormality.
- Termination of pregnancy (TOP) if requested.

Progress in ultrasound and laboratory techniques has produced an increasing number of conditions for which prenatal diagnosis is available. However, some abnormalities still cannot be diagnosed antenatally and some physical and laboratory-detected abnormalities may be of minor or unknown significance. Even after diagnosis, some women may choose to continue with a pregnancy with a severe or lethal fetal abnormality. Provision of information and support, whatever the choices made by parents, is a major part of any prenatal diagnosis service.

Counselling

Counselling is a major aspect of prenatal diagnosis. Prospective parents may not perceive themselves as being at risk of congenital abnormalities or may not fully comprehend the concept of risk. The finding of a high-risk screening result or ultrasound abnormality is therefore often unexpected by them. Unlike other medical test results, which are given as positive or negative, many screening tests in prenatal diagnosis are reported as a numerical risk. Although health-care staff are advised to categorize these results as high- or low-risk, patients may become aware of the numerical risk and find it difficult to accept the imposition of a cut-off, which they perceive as arbitrary. Carers need to be aware of this and other issues of communication and deal with the circumstances sensitively. Each unit should have a coordinator to serve as a reference point for enquiries on prenatal screening and diagnostic services. The services of a genetics unit, either locally or at a nearby tertiary centre, should be utilized. Support groups of families with similar problems or experiences can be of value to patients.

Screening

Screening tests identify pregnant women at increased risk or likelihood of a fetal abnormality in an apparently normal pregnancy. They have relatively low sensitivity and specificity but, due to their low physical risk, can be offered to whole populations. They are appropriate only when diagnostic tests are available for the specified condition. Screening modalities currently generally available include:

- Biochemical screening.
- Mid-trimester ultrasound scanning.
- First trimester nuchal fold translucency scanning.

Screening is, however, not yet readily or widely available for some common congenital problems, e.g. cystic fibrosis (CF). This is an autosomal recessive condition with a gene frequency of 1 in 20. In spite of its high prevalence, prenatal screening and diagnosis are complicated by the polymorphism of the CF gene. Prenatal diagnosis, when indicated, can now be achieved by using DNA from chorionic villus sampling (CVS), placental biopsy (PB), and amniotic cells. It is currently possible to identify 95% of CF mutations. Advances in laboratory techniques are likely to make screening and diagnosis more readily available in the future.

The most common problems screened for are Down syndrome (DS) and neural tube defects (NTDs). Screening for DS and NTDs is done on a maternal serum sample and the optimal time for taking a serum sample is at 15–16 weeks of gestation.

Biochemical screening
Down syndrome (trisomy 21, 47XX + 21/47 XY +21)

DS is the most common cause of congenital mental retardation, with a birth incidence of 1.5/1000. Associated structural anomalies include ventricular septal defects, anterior abdominal wall defects, typical facies. Life expectancy is reduced (about 60 years) and patients are at increased risk of Alzheimer's and chronic myeloid leukaemia. Biochemical screening for DS is based on a combination of maternal age, human chorionic gonadotrophin (hCG), alpha fetoprotein (AFP), and unconjugated oestriol (uE_3).

Advancing maternal age is the strongest single factor in the incidence of DS. The age-related risk is 1:1376 at 25, 1:424 at 35, 1:126 at 40, and 1:31 at 45 years. DS screening was previously based on maternal age alone and women aged 35 years and over at the estimated date of delivery were offered amniocentesis. However, as a larger proportion of the child-bearing population was under 35 years of age, the maximum detection rate achievable was on the order of 35%. With the risks of amniocentesis, some women at risk by virtue of their age declined the procedure, making the eventual detection rate under 20%. This led to the development of biochemical screening, which can be offered to all pregnant women irrespective of age. Currently available screening utilizes two analytes (hCG, AFP) in addition to maternal age ('double test'), with a detection rate of up to 60% depending on the cut-off used. High hCG, low AFP, and low uE3 are associated with DS but uE3 is no longer commonly used ('triple test' when uE3 is added).

The duration of pregnancy must be confirmed by ultrasound, ideally before the test, to validate the result as wrong dates significantly alter the results. The screening test result is used to recommend invasive/diagnostic procedure, e.g. amniocentesis for women with high-risk results.

Other placental products identified but not in routine clinical usage include pregnancy-associated plasma protein A (PAPP-A), pregnancy-specific beta-1 glycoprotein (SP-1), urea-resistant neutrophil alkaline phosphatase (UR-NAP), and inhibin.

Neural tube defects

The main abnormalities are spina bifida and anencephaly, each with a pregnancy incidence of about 1/1000 in the UK. The widespread use of ultrasound, the option of termination, and the use of folic acid prophylaxis have resulted in very few anencephalic fetuses being born except in instances when women have chosen to continue with the pregnancy in full knowledge of the diagnosis and prognosis.

Anencephaly and open spina bifida leak AFP into maternal serum, leading to elevated levels. This forms the basis of NTD screening. The detection rates of NTDs from serum screening with AFP are 88%, 75%, and 68% for anencephaly, open spina bifida, and all spina bifida lesions, respectively. Raised AFP is also useful in highlighting fetuses with potential growth problems later in pregnancy.

Other causes of raised AFP include:
- Exomphalos/gastroschisis (leakage of AFP).
- Congenital nephroses (defective renal re-absorption).
- Polycystic kidneys (defective renal re-absorption).
- Fetal death (tissue autolysis).
- Fetal teratoma (synthesis of AFP in tumour).
- Duodenal/oesophageal atresia (defective fetal swallowing).

Ultrasonography (U/S)

U/S is now the most common imaging test in prenatal diagnosis with over 90% of UK antenatal patients having a 'routine' scan. It serves as a screening test by checking for soft markers of chromosomal defects and as a diagnostic test by revealing a structural abnormality. However, many women may not appreciate U/S as a screening/diagnostic test, seeing it instead as a 'viewing' of a normal baby. The finding of an abnormality may therefore be unexpected.

The mid-trimester anomaly scan

Currently, most units perform a scan for structural abnormality at 18–20 weeks, this being the optimal time to obtain the best views of all organ systems. It must, however, be borne in mind that some abnormalities may not develop until after 20 weeks and some do not have a sonographic sign.

Although widely practised, the clinical effectiveness and impact on perinatal mortality of routine scanning is still subject to debate. It is well established that the majority of fetal abnormalities occur in pregnancies with few or no risk factors. As prospective parents become more aware of the risk of fetal abnormality, for the majority of patients the main benefit of ultrasound scanning is the reassurance of fetal physical normality. When abnormality is found, *in utero* treatment may be feasible, neonatal treatment can be arranged, or, when appropriate, pregnancy termination undertaken. When treatment is not available, acceptable, or appropriate, parents may value the foreknowledge of the condition and discussion of prognosis.

The sensitivity of ultrasound in detecting abnormalities in various organ systems depends on several factors including the skill and experience of personnel, gestational age at which the scanning is done, and the feasibility of verification of abnormalities. Ultrasound scanning programmes in tertiary centres and centres with obstetricians and radiologists with ultrasound interest achieve higher detection rates than those in other centres. There is better visualization of fetal anatomy after 18 weeks than earlier in the second trimester, with resultant higher detection rates. Regarding verification, this is easily achieved when pregnancy has been terminated for a significant abnormality and post-mortem examination undertaken. For some abnormalities however, particularly mild ones of the heart and urinary tract, the lesion may be asymptomatic, even after birth, and not be diagnosed early, making the collation of sensitivity data very difficult.

Technical difficulties during scanning may also influence detection rates. These include maternal obesity, fetal position, or multiple pregnancies.

Structural abnormalities can be diagnosed in all systems in the mid-trimester. Cardiovascular system (CVS), central nervous system (CNS), and urinary tract abnormalities are among the most common.

Cardiac defects

These have a birth prevalence of 8–10/1000 of which 4/1000 are severe and life-threatening. A four-chamber view may identify 60% of *severe* lesions and a complete fetal cardiac scan identifies 75% of *all* cardiac abnormalities. Detection rates, however, vary widely from 6 to 77%, with a mean of 39%. Much of the variation is due to mild lesions for which postnatal verification may be difficult.

It should be noted, however, that a seemingly normal four-chamber view may be seen at the 18–20 week scan in some cases of serious cardiac abnormalities. This makes it necessary to repeat the scan at a later date, when risk factors, e.g. family, medical, or past history, and other ultrasound abnormalities are identified.

NTDs

Ultrasound in good centres detects up to 95% of *all* spina bifida compared to 75% detection of *open* lesions by AFP screening. The extent of the lesion can also be assessed by ultrasound to allow discussion of prognosis. Of cases of anencephaly 99% will be detected at the 18–20 week scan. The recognized association of frontal bone scalloping ('lemon' sign) and abnormally shaped cerebellum ('banana' sign) aids the detection of neural tube lesions. In a high-risk population, e.g. those with raised AFP, virtually all significant NTDs may be detected by 20 weeks.

Urinary tract abnormalities

These are very common, accounting for 15% of abnormalities diagnosed in the prenatal period. Severe abnormalities include bilateral renal agenesis (Potter's syndrome), infantile polycystic kidneys, bilateral multicystic kidneys, and obstructive uropathies.

- *Potter's syndrome* has an incidence of 0.3/1000, over 90% of which may be detected at the mid-trimester scan, the main features being severe oligohydramnios/anhydramnios and non-visualization of the bladder and kidneys. The condition is incompatible with life, with 40% of fetuses stillborn.
- *Infantile polycystic kidney disease* is an autosomal recessive condition, with an incidence of 1/6000. It has a variable spectrum of severity, such that it may not be apparent on the mid-trimester scan. Prognosis is poor.
- *Multicystic kidneys* have a poor prognosis when bilateral but good prognosis if unilateral with a normal contralateral kidney.
- *Obstructive uropathies*, e.g. urethral stenosis or atresia and posterior urethral valves in male fetuses, may be very severe leading to severe oligohydramnios, gross bladder distension with eventual rupture, and urinary ascites. Prognosis often depends on the degree of obstruction.

The majority of abnormalities are relatively minor, e.g. isolated pelviureteric dilatation. These may carry a risk of neonatal urinary tract infection, but usually require no more antenatal intervention than ultrasound monitoring and paediatric notification. However, as they may remain asymptomatic or resolve spontaneously, diagnostic verification and assessment of the full impact of the lesions is difficult to undertake. Long-term follow-up of these neonates may therefore be necessary.

Gastrointestinal abnormalities

Detection rates for anterior abdominal wall defects (omphalocele and gastroschisis) at the mid-trimester scan, are close to 100%. Isolated oesophageal atresia will result in polyhydramnios and failure to visualize the stomach. However, in 95%, a tracheal fistula coexists, liquor reaches the stomach, and a normal appearance is obtained. Intestinal atresia or obstruction is less detectable

Ultrasonography (U/S) (*continued*)

in mid-trimester as the effects of the pathology become more pronounced at a later stage. Obstruction or atresia is more often diagnosed in late second trimester or the third trimester because of polyhydramnios or an incidental finding of dilated loops of bowel. The association between duodenal atresia/omphalocele and trisomies must be borne in mind.

Thoracic abnormalities

The main non-cardiac abnormality in the thorax is congenital diaphragmatic hernia. This has a birth incidence of 1/2000–5000. It may be diagnosed in the second trimester but is usually more apparent in the third. The defect may be large and the herniation transient, making diagnosis more difficult. The defect is usually left-sided and the heart, although structurally normal, may be displaced to the right by abdominal visceral herniating into the left side of the chest. Normality of the displaced heart and great vessels may then be difficult to determine.

Severe skeletal dysplasias

The incidence is 0.2/1000. Because the femur is measured routinely, shortening of long bones is usually readily noted. Ultrasound detection of severe dysplasias is about 84% and that of musculoskeletal abnormalities in general is about 45%. Examination of the hands and feet is more difficult than that of the long bones. Deformities of the hands, e.g. clinodactyly, and feet, e.g. talipes, are more difficult to diagnose but may be associated with chromosome abnormalities.

Abnormalities of the face and neck

The fetal face is assessed in about 50% of ultrasound examinations, with detection rates for facial abnormalities varying from 25 to 43% in a low-risk population. High-risk populations are more fully assessed and detection rates in this group are likely to be higher. Face and neck abnormalities amenable to ultrasound detection include clefts of lip/palate, Pierre–Robin syndrome, Treacher–Collins syndrome, holoprosencephaly, cyclopia, frontal and occipital encephaloceles, tumours, cystic hygromas, and fetal goitres. Many of these are associated with CNS and chromosome abnormalities and hence a full fetal assessment is necessary. Karyotyping may be indicated.

Markers

The mid-trimester scan may reveal markers of chromosomal abnormality. These markers are on their own not of major significance but may indicate an underlying problem. Significance increases when more than one marker is found or other risk factors coexist, e.g. maternal age or high risk on serum screening. When multiple abnormalities are seen, the overall risk of chromosome abnormality may be as high as 35%.

Markers and the conditions with which they may be associated include:
- Nuchal fold thickening, fetal hydrops, mild ventriculomegaly, duodenal atresia, sandal gap, clinodactyly, and renal pelves dilatation for trisomy 21.
- Echogenic bowel, mild shortening of femur, and cardiac defects for trisomies 18 and 21.
- Cystic hygroma for Turner's syndrome.
- Omphalocele and holoprosencephaly for trisomies 13 and 18.
- Early growth retardation for trisomies 13, 18, and 21

First trimester scanning

Nuchal fold translucency (NFT)

Oedema of the fetal neck, detectable in the first trimester by ultrasound, is associated with cardiac defects, Down syndrome, and other trisomies (Fig. 8.1). NFT screening is best performed between 10 and 14 weeks gestation and, when related with maternal age, the detection rate for DS potentially increases to about 80% compared with 60% for age and biochemical analytes. Introduction of NFT screening into routine practice will have major implications in terms of training of personnel and scanning time. The benefits of large-scale first-trimester screening need to be put in context, as many of the serious abnormalities diagnosed would have spontaneously aborted had they not been detected. Women may potentially be given the extra burden of choosing pregnancy termination for these conditions. Currently, most women are not referred for hospital antenatal care until the second trimester. The place of NFT as a screening test is therefore still being evaluated before its introduction into general use for low-risk populations.

Other abnormalities/limitations in first trimester

First trimester scanning may require a transvaginal probe to achieve optimal views. Abnormalities have been identified in the first trimester in the CNS, heart, gastrointestinal tract, urinary tract, and skeletal system. Care needs to be taken, however, as cranial vault ossification and the return of the intestines into the peritoneal cavity are not complete until about 10 weeks gestation. Anencephaly and omphalocele, for example, may therefore not be confirmed until after 10 weeks. The natural history of some first trimester appearances may not be fully understood until large studies have been undertaken.

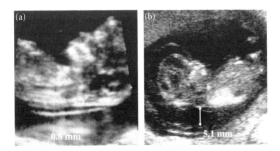

Fig. 8.1 Scans of nuchal fold showing (a) a normal and (b) an abnormal nuchal fold thickness.

Diagnostic tests

These are used to confirm or exclude the existence of a fetal abnormality in pregnancies at increased risk of an abnormality on the basis of past history, family history, or a screening test result.

Ultrasound

Ultrasound confirmation of structural abnormality may follow the identification of specific risk factors, e.g. history or raised maternal serum AFP (MSAFP). A suspicion of abnormality may be raised on the routine mid-trimester scan and confirmed by a more detailed examination. This is particularly relevant to abnormalities that may not be fully apparent at 18–20 weeks that need a repeat examination later to confirm. Some cardiac defects, e.g. hypoplastic left heart, are progressive and may become more apparent in late pregnancy. Microcephaly, bowel atresia, urinary tract obstruction, and problems of liquor volume may not be confirmed until the third trimester.

The sensitivity and specificity of ultrasound increases with the level of skill of personnel. Specialist units with obstetricians/radiologists with ultrasound sub-specialization achieve the highest detection rates, up to 76% overall, compared with up to 36% for smaller units. Management after diagnosis is also more appropriate to the specialist units. Smaller units are encouraged to refer to larger, more specialized units.

Amniocentesis

Amniotic fluid contains fetal cells shed from the gut and skin. Important diagnoses can be made both from the cells and analysis of the amniotic fluid. The procedure is therefore used for:

- Chromosome analysis: most commonly Down syndrome testing for maternal age, high-risk serum tests, and ultrasound markers.
- DNA analysis for genetic disease for which tests have been developed. The list of such conditions is rapidly expanding.
- Enzyme assays for inborn errors of metabolism.
- AFP and acetyl cholinesterase (ultrasound is superior in diagnosing NTDs).
- Diagnosis of fetal infection, e.g. toxoplasmosis, cytomegalovirus (CMV).
- Investigation of fetal lung maturity (lecithin/sphingomyelin ratio or presence of phosphatidyl glycerol).
- Bilirubin (for rhesus iso-immunization).

The main risk of amniocentesis is miscarriage (1% procedure-related risk). This risk is higher when the procedure is performed at 14 weeks or less (early amniocentesis). Risks of respiratory distress and postural abnormalities were reported in some studies but, in the absence of chronic amniotic fluid leakage, these are not significant. Needle injuries are rare, especially when real-time scanning is used.

- Culture failure is rare with a rate of less than 0.5%. Maternal cell contamination occurs in less than 0.2%.
- Results of a full karyotype take about 2 weeks but specific abnormalities such as trisomies, triploidy, and Turner's syndrome can be diagnosed using fluorescent *in situ* hybridization (FISH) with results being available in 48 hours.
- 500 units of anti-D globulin are given to rhesus negative women after the procedure. A larger dose may be necessary, depending on a Kleihauer test result.

Chorionic villus sampling/placental biopsy

The sampling of actively dividing trophoblast cells provides material that yields rapid karyotyping results in about 48 hours. This procedure also instantly provides material for DNA analysis, especially as polymerase chain reaction (PCR) makes small amounts of tissue adequate for testing.

- Chorionic villus sampling (CVS) is performed in the first trimester and placental biopsy (PB) in the second and third trimesters. CVS is performed by transabdominal or transcervical routes and PB by a transabdominal route.
- First trimester diagnosis by CVS allows first trimester TOP, before pregnancy becomes physically apparent, when this option is taken because of fetal abnormality.
- Rh-negative women must be given anti-D globulin.

The most common indications for sampling are:
- Karyotyping when ultrasound findings suggest aneuploidy.
- DNA analysis, particularly for haemoglobinopathies and recessive or X-linked disorders, e.g. cystic fibrosis, Duchenne muscular dystrophy, and haemophilia.

However, with advances in laboratory techniques in the analysis of amniotic fluid, many conditions may now be diagnosed rapidly from simple amniocentesis with its well-established low pregnancy loss rates. This diminishes the need for second trimester CVS/PB in favour of amniocentesis with its lower risks.

Complications of CVS/PB include:
- Pregnancy loss—about 2–3%.
- Maternal cell contamination may lead to false-negative results especially when PCR is used to increase the amount of DNA for analysis.
- Placental mosaicism—1%, usually in direct preparation. Amniocentesis may be needed to clarify.
- Limb reduction deformities appear to be associated with CVS performed before 9 weeks gestation.

Antenatal fetal blood sampling (FBS)

The risks of this procedure are considerably higher than those of amniocentesis, CVS, or PB. It is therefore reserved for conditions in which the information required can only come from testing fetal blood, i.e. fetal Hb, white cells, or specific IgM. Such conditions include fetal hydrops, suspected fetal infection, and rhesus or other blood group antibody problems.

FBS uses a transabdominal approach to obtain fetal blood for prenatal diagnosis. This is done under real-time ultrasound guidance from placental cord insertion, fetal intrahepatic vessels, or fetal heart.
- Anti D globulin must be given to rhesus-negative women.

Complications of FBS include:
- Bleeding from puncture site.
- Haematoma, leading to vascular compression at puncture site.

Diagnostic tests (*continued*)

- Fetal bradycardia from vasospasm.
- Chorioamnionitis.
- Premature rupture of membranes.
- Pregnancy loss (1–2.5%).

Fetal tissue sampling

Most prenatal diagnosis is done with ultrasound, CVS, or amniocentesis but some very rare conditions require histological examination of skin or assay of enzymes restricted to the liver for diagnosis. Fetal tissue biopsies are done under real-time ultrasound guidance.

- Indications for fetal skin biopsy include harlequin ichthyosis, Sjögren–Larsson syndrome, epidermolysis bullosa letalis, epidermolysis bullosa dystrophica, oculocutaneous albinism.
- Indications for fetal liver biopsy include G6PD deficiency (von Gierke's disease), alanine glyoxalate transaminase (AGT; primary hyperoxaluria type 1) deficiency, ornithine carbamyl transferase (OCT) deficiency, carbamyl phosphate synthetase (CPS) deficiency.
- Fetal lung, kidney, and muscle have been biopsied but the quality of currently available ultrasound and advances in DNA analysis make this rarely necessary.

Future trends

- *Pre-implantation diagnosis.* This is feasible in IVF with removal of a single cell from an eight-cell embryo or trophoblast from the blastocyst before implantation.
  - —Advantage. Diagnosis is done pre-pregnancy, reducing the need for pregnancy termination.
- *Fetal nucleated cells in maternal circulation.* Fetal lymphocytes, erythrocytes, and trophoblast cells are present in maternal circulation and harvesting them would provide prenatal diagnosis without a fetal-invasive procedure. Maternal cell contamination is the biggest obstacle.
- *Three-dimensional ultrasound.* This is of value in defining structure, e.g. facial features/abnormalities (facial abnormalities may be associated with chromosome abnormalities), NTDs, and tumours. Availability and use are currently limited as most diagnosis is made with high definition conventional ultrasound.
- *Magnetic resonance imaging (MRI) in pregnancy.* Severely limited by motion artefacts and fetal immobilization is needed. At present this adds little to ultrasound diagnosis.

Recommended further reading

1 Royal College of Obstetricians and Gynaecologists (2000). *Routine ultrasound screening in pregnancy: protocols, standards and training.* Royal College of Obstetricians and Gynaecologists, London.

2 Royal College of Obstetricians and Gynaecologists Working Party (1997). *Ultrasound screening for fetal abnormalities.* Royal College of Obstetricians and Gynaecologists, London.

3 Joint Working Party of the Royal College of Obstetricians and Gynaecologists and the Royal College of Paediatrics and Child Health (1997). *Fetal abnormalities: guidelines for screening, diagnosis and management,* December 1997. Royal College of Obstetricians and Gynaecologists and Royal College of Paediatrics and Child Health, London.

4 Tabor, A. *et al.* (1986). Randomised controlled trial of genetic amniocentesis in 4606 low risk women. *Lancet* i, 1287–9.

5 James, D.K., Steer, P.J., Weiner, C.P., and Gonik, B. (eds.) (1999). *High risk pregnancy: management options.* W.B. Saunders Ltd, London.

6 Brock, D.J.H., Rodeck, C.H., and Ferguson-Smith, M.A. (eds.) (1992). *Prenatal diagnosis and screening.* Churchill Livingstone, Edinburgh.

7 Drife, J.O. and Donnai, D. (eds.) (1991). *Antenatal diagnosis of fetal abnormalities.* Published for the Royal College of Obstetricians and Gynaecologists by Springer-Verlag, London.

8 Wald, N.J., Cuckle, H., Brock, J.H., *et al.* (1977). Maternal serum alphafetoprotein measurement in antenatal screening for anencephaly and spina bifida in early pregnancy. Report of the UK Collaborative Study on Alpha-fetoprotein in Relation to Neural Tube Defects. *Lancet* 1, 1323–32.

9 Souka, A.P. and Nicolaides, K.H. (1997). Diagnosis of fetal abnormalities at the 10–14 week scan. *Ultrasound in Obstetrics and Gynecology* 10, 429–42.

Chapter 9

Infections in pregnancy

There are a number of infections caused by viral, bacterial, and parasitic organisms that are known to cause clinically significant fetal infection resulting in miscarriage, preterm labour, intrauterine death, or long-term sequelae secondary to structural and neurodevelopmental abnormalities. The infections currently screened for routinely are syphilis, rubella, and hepatitis B.

Syphilis

This is a systemic chronic granulomatous infection caused by the spirochaete *Treponema pallidum*. Infection occurs in three stages.

- The first stage of the disease, primary syphilis, is characterized by a painless genital ulcer 10–90 days postinfection that may pass unnoticed if on the cervix and that resolves spontaneously in 2–6 weeks.
- Secondary syphilis involves the widespread dissemination of spirochaetes and is marked by lymphadenopathy, genital condyloma lata, and an extensive maculopapular rash particularly involving the palms and soles, lasting for 2–6 weeks followed by a latent phase of variable duration.
- In the absence of treatment approximately 1 in 3 patients will progress to tertiary syphilis heralded by involvement of the cardiovascular (aortic aneurysms), central nervous (tabes dorsalis, paresis, optic atrophy), and musculoskeletal systems.

Obstetric significance

Treponema pallidum has the ability to cross the placenta and infect the fetus at all stages of the disease, being less common in late disease. Transmission of syphilis is more common with advancing gestation, especially after the 18–20 week stage, and adequate maternal treatment before 16 weeks gestation will virtually eliminate the risk of infecting the fetus. It may well be appropriate to treat the mother in each subsequent pregnancy.

The risk in untreated maternal primary and secondary disease for development of congenital syphilis is of the order of 50% along with risks of prematurity and stillbirth. With early latent syphilis (disease duration < 1 year) the risk is 40%, while with late latent disease (duration of disease > 1 year) the risk is around 10%. The sequelae of congenital syphilis include stillbirth, hydrops, maculopapular rash, hepatosplenomegaly, lymphadenopathy, jaundice, chorioretinitis, and osteochondritis, along with characteristic findings of Hutchinson's teeth, mulberry molars, saddle nose, interstitial keratitis, sabre shins, and eighth-nerve deafness. Thus treatment of syphilis in pregnancy aims to cure maternal disease and prevent congenital infection in the neonate.

Diagnosis

Diagnosis is possible using dark-ground microscopy of a smear from a lesion to detect spirochaetes, but the most common method used for detection of syphilis is serological screening. This consists of an initial screening test involving detection of non-treponemal antibodies using the RPR (rapid plasma reagin) or VDRL (Venereal Disease Research Laboratory) tests, which are both positive in secondary and latent disease and frequently in primary disease. False-positive results may be associated with pregnancy, immunization, systemic lupus erythematosus (SLE), tuberculosis (TB), and leprosy. A positive screening test is then confirmed with a specific anti-treponemal antibody test, the most commonly used being the fluorescent treponemal antibody absorption (FTA-ABS) test, which then remains positive throughout life even after cure.

Management

The treatment of choice is benzathine penicillin G as a single intramuscular IM) dose of 2.4 million units for primary, secondary, and early latent syphilis and the same dose for 3 consecutive weeks for late latent syphilis. Aqueous procaine penicillin may also be used but requires a longer course of daily treatment (600 000–900 000 units for 10–21 days). Penicillin is by far the preferred choice as it offers a cure rate in excess of 98% compared to non-penicillin alternatives, which are associated with failures of prevention of congenital infection in the neonate. Given that about 90% of patients reported to be allergic to penicillin do not have true IgE-mediated hypersensitivity, there is a role for skin testing and temporary desensitization. The patients need to be warned that after the first course of treatment, especially with secondary syphilis, there is a risk of Jarisch–Herxheimer reaction, which may precipitate premature labour, so treatment after 20 weeks is best carried out in hospital. An alternative to penicillin in pregnancy is erythromycin but the lower cure rate means that repeated courses of treatment may be required along with careful assessment of the newborn for signs of active disease that will require treatment. By the third or fourth month posttreatment, quantitative non-treponemal antibody titres must drop at least fourfold—if this is not the case or if titres remain persistently high, the patient needs re-evaluation for neurosyphilis and re-treatment. Contact tracing and treatment must be carried out, together with counselling and testing for other sexually transmitted infections (STIs) including human immunodeficiency virus (HIV) infection.

Rubella

This is also known as German measles. It is caused by RNA togavirus and acquired by respiratory droplet exposure. The affected individual is infectious for the last week of incubation and the first week after the rash appears. After a 2–3 week incubation, a rash with arthralgia, fever, and suboccipital and postauricular lymphadenopathy occurs, but clinical symptoms are present only in 50–75% of those infected. Thus many may have immunity in the absence of a history of symptomatic disease.

Obstetric significance

Rubella infection, though mild or even subclinical, has marked embryopathic consequences when acquired by the fetus *in utero*. Risk of transmission to the fetus with resultant congenital anomalies may be over 80% in the first trimester, dropping to approximately 50% by 13–14 weeks, and around 25% by late second trimester, compared with a less than 10% risk from rubella re-infection. Rubella re-infection may occur in up to 50% of cases of vaccine-induced immunity as opposed to 5% in cases of naturally acquired immunity.

Rubella-associated defects, which are generally attributed to vascular damage or reduced mitotic activity, are present in almost all infants infected before 11 weeks gestation (mainly cardiac defects and sensorineural deafness), in approximately 35% of those infected at 13–16 weeks (mainly deafness), with infection after 16 weeks rarely causing defects. Congenital anomalies may be permanent such as congenital cataracts, glaucoma, heart disease, deafness, microcephaly, and mental retardation along with later development of diabetes, thyroid problems, precocious puberty, and progressive panencephalitis. Other features may be transient findings such as purpura, splenomegaly, jaundice, meningoencephalitis, and thrombocytopenia.

Diagnosis

Rubella is extremely difficult to diagnose because of non-specific rash and commonly subclinical infection, so serological assessment (latex agglutination, fluorescent immunoassay, or enzyme immunoassay) of paired acute and convalescent samples from women with suspect illness or exposure is the main method of diagnosis. During pregnancy, in cases of suspected exposure in a susceptible woman, it is important to confirm serologically the diagnosis in the index case whenever possible. Maternal infection is confirmed by appearance of IgM antibodies or a fourfold rise in IgG antibody titres. Assessment of fetal infection by amniotic fluid culture, IgM in fetal blood, or polymerase chain reaction (PCR) has low accuracy, so counselling is based on the gestation-age risk of congenital infection along with whether this was a primary maternal infection or a re-infection. If maternal seroconversion occurs in the first 12 weeks, then a termination of pregnancy may be offered without invasive prenatal diagnosis. In cases of seroconversion between 12 and 18 weeks or re-infection in the first trimester or where TOP is not an option, fetal blood sampling may be offered to confirm fetal infection, but after 12 weeks the main risk is one of hearing defects. Children with no clinical manifestations but persistent antibodies need to be closely followed up as sensorineural deafness may be of late onset, bilateral, and progressive.

Immunization

All pregnant women should be tested prior to or in early pregnancy to confirm immunity, an expense justified by the significant risk of maternal rubella infection to the developing embryo. Prevention is through childhood vaccination, as well as assessment of the serological status of women pre-pregnancy or while undergoing fertility investigations and treatment. Immunity needs to be confirmed at the time of each subsequent pregnancy. The rubella vaccine is a live attentuated virus preparation and therefore should not be used in pregnancy. There is no evidence that inadvertent use in pregnancy has been associated with congenital infection, and therefore parents can be reassured in such cases or in cases of pregnancy occurring soon after vaccination that the fetal risks are negligible.

Hepatitis B

This is a DNA virus that is hepatotropic, leading to viral liver disease with an incubation period of 2–6 months, though detectable in the circulation from 1 month post-infection. The carriage rate of hepatitis B virus (HBV) varies greatly throughout the world with rates ranging from a low in northern Europe of around 1% to the Far East and tropical Africa where rates of 35% may be encountered. In developed countries the major routes of transmission are through blood and blood products, sexual activity, and IV drug abuse, while vertical transmission at birth is the principal transmission route in developing countries. Approximately two-thirds of acute HBV infections are asymptomatic, subclinical, or associated with minimal, influenza-like symptoms but there may be upper gastrointestinal symptoms such as nausea, vomiting, anorexia, and occasionally right hypochondrium discomfort but with no evidence of jaundice in almost half the cases. HBV infection may be followed by a protracted period of malaise and anorexia, but in a previously healthy individual complete resolution occurs within 6 months in over 90% of cases. By definition 10% become chronic carriers where hepatitis B surface antigen (HBsAg) persists beyond 6 months with presence of symptoms (chronic active hepatitis) or absent symptoms with deranged liver function tests (chronic persistent hepatitis). Rarely, the infection may progress to fulminant infection, hepatic failure, and death.

The severity of hepatitis B in pregnancy in the developed countries is similar to that in the non-pregnant state. However, vertical transmission from mother to neonate has major implications because, under such circumstances, chronic carriage is the norm, with up to 90% of newborn developing chronic active or chronic persistent hepatitis. This has major implications due to the risk of development of cirrhosis and hepatocellular carcinoma over a period of 20–30 years. The majority of infants are infected at birth from maternal blood and body fluids with a small minority infected *in utero* through transplacental bleeds.

Diagnosis

Laboratory diagnosis of HBV infections is based on the detection of a panel of viral-specific antibodies and antigens. HBsAg is a surface antigen from the viral capsule and signifies infectivity while anti-HBs antibody (the antibody to the surface antigen) is a marker of immunological response and cure of infection. HBeAg is an antigen from the core of the virus and implies high infectivity (90% risk of transmission to fetus), while anti-Hbe (antibody to the core antigen) indicates a partial immune response (10% transmission risk).

Management

Treatment of acute HBV infection in pregnancy is symptomatic and supportive to control nausea and vomiting, monitor hydration and uterine activity, and perform liver function tests (LFTs) as well as counselling, testing, and vaccinating family and sexual contacts as appropriate. There is no evidence of associated congenital syndrome or teratogenesis provided the pregnancy survives the acute illness.

Obstetric significance

The impact of vertical transmission of HBV infection along with the low pick-up rate of HBsAg carriers by risk assessment justifies universal antenatal screening for HBsAg carriage at antenatal booking. As the majority of cases of vertical transmission occur perinatally, preventative measures involving active and passive immunization at birth can therefore be put into action in cases of HBsAg carriers identified by antenatal screening. This involves the newborn receiving hepatitis B immune globulin (HBIg) IM within 12 hours of birth along with the first of three doses of recombinant vaccine in the other thigh. The second and third doses of the recombinant vaccines are given at 1 and 6 months and immunity confirmed at approximately 1 year. This policy relies on close cooperation between obstetrician, microbiologist, and neonatologist and is effective in about 90% of cases. Clearly, repeated or additional testing may be required in further exposures/hepatitis-like illness in pregnancy or in high-risk individuals.

Toxoplasmosis

This is caused by the parasite *Toxoplasma gondii* that normally lives within the domestic cat. Infection is often asymptomatic or may produce a lymphadenopathy or present with a glandular fever-like illness in the immunocompetent adult, but in immunocompromised individuals it may develop into severe disseminated illness with chorioretinitis and encephalitis.

Obstetric significance

In the fetus and the neonate, toxoplasmosis leads to a syndrome comprising chorioretinitis, microcephaly/hydrocephaly, intracerebral calcification, and mental retardation as the predominant features. The earlier the infection occurs in pregnancy, the more serious the neonatal consequences with spontaneous miscarriage being common in first trimester infections. With primary maternal infection the risk of transmission rises from 17 to 25% and to 65% from the first through to the second and third trimester, with, overall, 70% of babies born without any damage and a further 10% with chorioretinitis only.

Prevention

Prevention of maternal disease and therefore fetal infection is by avoidance of undercooked meat, unpasteurized milk, and contact with cat litter, as well as thorough washing of garden produce and hands after gardening activities and handling raw meat or vegetables soiled by earth.

Diagnosis

Routine serological testing, although in practice in France where the prevalence of the condition is higher, is of no proven benefit in the UK. Serological testing should be carried out in cases of clinical suspicion and either a fourfold rise in IgG titres between acute and convalescent samples, concurrent high titres of IgG and IgM, or isolated very high IgM titres done by enzyme-linked immunosorbent assay (ELISA) are indicative of acute infection or re-infection.

Management

If maternal infection is confirmed, maternal treatment with spiramycin 3 g/day should be commenced to reduce the risk of transplacental infection (this may reduce transmission by 60%) and consideration should be given to fetal testing and treatment. Fetal infection is confirmed by demonstrating specific IgM at amniocentesis and fetal blood sampling. If fetal infection is indeed demonstrated, ultrasound scanning may be performed at around 22 weeks which may demonstrate ventricular dilatation. Further management depends on parental wishes. TOP is an option in the presence of structural abnormalities but, in cases of fetal infection without ultrasound evidence of fetal damage or where TOP is unacceptable to the parents, treatment with 3-weekly cycles of pyrimethamine sulfadiazine, and folinic acid alternating with spiramycin is recommended for the remainder of the pregnancy along with biophysical monitoring of the pregnancy (for IUGR, ventricular dilatation, and development of microcephaly).

Postnatally, it is important to carry out confirmatory tests (placenta, amniotic fluid, cord blood and maternal blood serology) and a thorough assessment of the neonate including ophthalmic review and cranial radiological assessment (ultrasound and X-ray). It is recommended to continue treatment for a year if toxoplasmosis is suspected. Long-term follow-up is recommended as children asymptomatic at birth may develop problems in later years. Future pregnancies should be delayed until toxoplasma IgM has been cleared, which may take up to 2 years.

Cytomegalovirus (CMV)

A member of the herpesvirus family, the ability of CMV to lie dormant in the host means that its most common manifestation is asymptomatic (95% of cases), its clinical importance in pregnancy being due to intrauterine and neonatal infection. Congenital CMV infection may account for as much as 10% of mental retardation in children up to the age of 6. Primary infection in the adult may present with fever, malaise, atypical lymphocytosis, and lymphadenopathy and rarely may lead to pneumonitis, myocarditis, thrombocytopenia, meningoencephalitis, and hepatitis. The virus can be cultured from urine and excretion of virus may be prolonged from weeks to months and occasionally even longer. Reactivation and re-infection are common sequelae. CMV is transmitted by sexual intercourse, through transfused blood or marrow, and perinatally either transplacentally or by exposure to the virus from the cervix or birth canal. Neonates may acquire the virus through breast milk and, in childhood, transmission may occur through cross-contamination in nurseries, as protracted viral shedding from the urine and respiratory secretions of infected children occurs. Viral shedding occurs more readily in pregnancy and with advancing gestation. Advanced gestation along with primary maternal infection increases the risk of neonatal disease. The incidence of primary infection in pregnancy is around 1–2% and 50–80% of women are seropositive depending on race, parity, and socio-economic status.

Diagnosis

Diagnosis of primary infection is by detecting a significant rise in anti-CMV IgM titres, which may persist for 4–8 months after primary infection, while a recurrent infection may be confirmed by rise in IgG titres.

Management

The management of a patient with confirmed CMV infection in pregnancy will depend on careful counselling of the prospective parents about the risks to the fetus. Appropriate management may involve invasive procedures to determine fetal infection, regular biophysical assessment of fetal growth and health, or consideration of therapeutic termination of pregnancy. Congenital infection is three times more likely to occur after primary infection than after re-infection in the mother, with around 40% of fetuses infected following primary maternal infection in pregnancy. CMV is found in approximately 1% of newborns, of whom 5–10% are clinically affected by one or more features of congenital CMV infection, the most common being hepatosplenomegaly, microcephaly, hyperbilirubinaemia, petechiae, thrombocytopenia, and intrauterine growth retardation (IUGR). A further 5–10% of infected infants, although asymptomatic at birth, will develop long-term sequelae such as sensorineural deafness, microcephaly, low IQ, or seizures, but over 85% of babies born to women with CMV in pregnancy, including 75% of infected infants, will have no CMV-related problems at birth or thereafter. Appropriate clinical and serological assessment and paediatric follow-up should be instituted if infection is confirmed postnatally.

Chicken pox/herpes zoster infection

Varicella zoster (VZ) is a highly contagious DNA virus transmitted through respiratory droplets and close interpersonal contact with a 10–20 day incubation period, the patient being contagious for 48 hours prior to the appearance of the rash and until the vesicles crust over. The incidence of chickenpox (varicella) infection in pregnancy is on the order of 1 in 2000, with 85% of the adult population already seropositive for VZIg. Primary infection leads to chickenpox while reactivation of the dormant virus leads to herpes zoster.

Obstetric significance

In pregnancy VZ infection can have both maternal and fetal consequences. Maternal implications include pneumonia in up to 10% of infected adults, with a 6% mortality risk, with the risks of developing both pneumonia and respiratory complications being higher in pregnancy. Fetal consequences as a result of primary VZ infection in the first 20 weeks of pregnancy include spontaneous miscarriage in the first trimester and a 2% risk of congenital varicella syndrome. The latter is characterized by skin scarring in a dermatomal distribution, eye defects (chorioretinitis, cataracts, micropthalmia), hypoplasia of limbs, and neurological abnormalities (microcephaly, cortical atrophy, mental retardation and dysfunction of bladder and bowel sphincters).

Transplacental passage of the virus increases with gestation age. Thus varicella infection may occur in up to 50% of fetuses whose mothers develop primary VZ infection in the last 1–4 weeks of pregnancy with up to a third of the newborns developing clinical varicella despite high titres of passively acquired maternal antibodies. The main risk to the newborn, however, is with maternal infection occurring up to 5 days prior to delivery or 2 days post-delivery as there has been inadequate time for development and passage of maternal antibodies to the fetus and this leads a significant risk of disseminated VZ infection in the newborn with mortality risks of 20–30%. Finally, babies with no evidence of clinical VZ infection at birth may develop herpes zoster in childhood consistent with an *in utero* primary VZ infection.

Prevention

A live attenuated varicella vaccine has been shown to be effective in preventing chickenpox in adults but is awaiting a product licence in the UK. VZ Ig is known to be effective in preventing or reducing the severity of maternal infection or congenital varicella syndrome if given within 72 hours of contact to a susceptible individual, with some residual benefit if administered within 10 days. It is, however, a blood product with the attendant risks and cost.

Management

The management of a pregnant woman with a suspected varicella contact involves review of the history (certainty of diagnosis in index case, the degree of infectivity, i.e. presence of rash or rash developing within 48 hours, degree of exposure) as well as the susceptibility of the pregnant woman (a history of VZ infection in the past and therefore immune but, even with no clear history, 85% of the adult population have antibodies to VZ). If there is any doubt regarding immunity, then VZ Ig levels can be checked in the routine antenatal booking bloods. If immunity is confirmed no further action is required. If the patient is non-immune and is under 20 weeks pregnant then VZ Ig should be administered as soon as possible, preferably within 72 hours of contact but for up to 10 days post-contact there may be some benefit.

n cases where VZ IgM is detected in the serum, the patient must be counselled regarding the 2% risk of congenital varicella syndrome. A specialist ultrasound assessment at 5 weeks post-infection or at 16–20 weeks (looking for polyhydramnios, microcephaly, hyperechogenic foci in the liver, hydrops fetalis) is recommended along with a neonatal ophthalmic examination at birth. In susceptible women who are beyond 20 weeks at time of exposure, congenital varicella does not occur and the only benefit of VZ Ig administration may be to reduce the severity of maternal infection and risk of VZ pneumonia, though this is not universally accepted.

Pregnant women presenting with VZ infection should be isolated from other pregnant patients or staff and neonates. If delivery occurs within 5 days of maternal infection or the mother develops VZ within 2 days of delivery, the high risk of neonatal VZ infection justifies administration of VZ Ig as soon as possible to the neonate, who should also receive acyclovir if there is any suggestion of neonatal infection. Maternal administration of acyclovir within 24 hours of development of VZ rash may reduce the duration and severity of the illness but this is not recommended in the first trimester due to theoretical concerns of tertogenesis. Pregnant women with primary VZ infection should be advised to look out for respiratory symptoms as this would be an indication for hospitalization and treatment with intravenous acyclovir. If, at around the time of discharge home of the mother and newborn, a sibling has chickenpox then, unless the mother is immune, both she and her newborn should be given VZ Ig.

Parvovirus infection

Parvovirus B19 is a DNA virus and the causative agent of a number of illnesses including aplastic crisis in conditions characterized by accelerated haemolysis such as sickle cell disease, a form of chronic arthropathy in adults, and an exanthematous illness in childhood known as Fifth disease (erythema infectiosum). The latter presents with high fever and a rash giving the appearance of a 'slapped cheek'. Transmission is by respiratory droplets and the incubation period is 4–14 days. Although in children the infection may even be subclinical, the adult form is associated with lymphadenopathy and arthropathy as common sequelae as well as a postviral syndrome of fatigue and depression.

Obstetric significance

The obstetric implications of this condition are due to the transplacental passage of the virus in approximately one-third of cases of maternal infection. Parvovirus infection in early and mid-pregnancy carries a 10% risk of miscarriage, the interval between maternal infection and fetal loss usually being 4–5 weeks but it may be up to 11 weeks. The parvovirus has particular predilection for rapidly dividing bone marrow cells and erythrocytes leading to haemolytic anaemia and haemopoietic arrest, which in turn leads to high output cardiac failure and non-immune hydrops in some cases of maternal infection in the late second and third trimester. If the fetus survives the acute insult (fetal loss being uncommon) or is given supportive treatment, there is no evidence of a congenital syndrome postnatally.

Diagnosis

The diagnosis of the condition in adults is hampered by the variable presentation. Infection is confirmed by demonstrating seroconversion with acute and convalescent sera, IgM antibodies indicative of acute infection being present within a week in the majority of patients and persisting several months, while IgG antibodies appear at 10 days and persist for years. In a previously healthy individual the illness is self-limiting but immunocompromised individuals are at risk of sudden haemolysis and they should therefore be monitored and supportive treatment including blood transfusions given as appropriate.

Management

In pregnant patients with parvovirus B19 infection, treatment is symptomatic for the mother along with ultrasonographic monitoring of the fetus particularly with respect to the development of features of non-immune hydrops, such as ascites, pericardial or pleural effusions, indicative of decompensation. In such cases the options depend on the gestational age and include intrauterine transfusion or delivery and postnatal correction of anaemia in the newborn, although there is now evidence that hydrops may resolve spontaneously *in utero*. Thus specialist fetomaternal assessment is warranted.

Measles

This is an acute febrile illness caused by a paramyxovirus commonly attacking children and conferring lifelong immunity. Characteristic Koplik spots in buccal epithelium along with fever, rash, rhinorrhoea, and conjunctivitis are the most common findings. Rare but serious complications in adults are pneumonia and encephalitis including subacute sclerosing panencephalitis.

Obstetric significance

As with any febrile illness, measles infection may precipitate uterine activity and premature delivery. There is no recognized syndrome of intrauterine measles infection although, if the mother has measles at the time of delivery, there is risk of neonatal measles.

Diagnosis

Diagnosis is clinical based on rash and Koplik spots and serological confirmation through haemagglutination inhibition antibody assay or a complement fixation assay.

Prevention and management

Prevention is by childhood vaccination (which is also effective within 72 hours of exposure). Antenatal management is by treatment of upper respiratory symptoms and fever, with vigilance for uterine activity, whilst appropriate isolation/infection control measures are observed while in hospital.

Listeriosis

This is caused by *Listeria monocytogenes*, a Gram-positive, non-spore-forming facultative anaerobe. The gastrointestinal tract is the major site of entry and preventative measures are centred around avoidance of soft cheese and pates, thorough cooking of raw food from animal sources, thorough washing of raw vegetables and attention to hygiene in storage and preparation of food. Dissemination of the organism throughout the body is usually prevented by the immune system. For this reason listeriosis and some form of depression of cell-mediated immunity (pregnancy being an example) are often found together.

Obstetric significance

The incidence in pregnancy is around 1 in 10 000 and disease in early pregnancy may result in spontaneous miscarriage. Infection is usually in the form of a flu-like pyrexial illness and is self-limiting. Transplacental passage of *L. monocytogenes* (which does not occur in all cases of maternal infection) gives rise to fetal infection with a spectrum of manifestations from spontaneous abortion, amnionitis with brown staining of amniotic fluid, through to premature delivery and early- or late-onset neonatal listeriosis. Fetal infection late in pregnancy may lead to multiorgan morbidity (intraventricular haemorrhage, pneumonitis, hepatitis, neurological handicap) and fetal mortality.

Early neonatal infection due to transplacental spread occurs within 2 days, with an appropriately grown premature infant suffering from congenital pneumonia whereas late-onset disease acquired during passage through the birth canal presents mostly with meningitis. Diagnosis should be suspected in cases of a flu-like illness with pyrexia, uterine irritability, and bloody per vagina (PV) discharge. Vaginal and blood cultures should be taken and the microbiologist warned regarding the clinical suspicions, as *L. monocytogenes* can easily be confused with diptheroids.

Management

Infection is responsive to a wide range of antibiotics including ampicillin, chloramphenicol, co-trimoxazole, and aminoglycosides such as gentamicin. Treatment should continue for 3 to 6 weeks to prevent relapses.

103

Herpes simplex infection

Herpes simplex virus(HSV) is a DNA virus. HSV1 is predominantly responsible for orolabial lesions, while HSV2 is responsible for genital lesions, but there is considerable overlap between the two types. Genital herpes is usually acquired through sexual contact with an infected individual, who may well be asymptomatic, or by orogenital contact. Approximately 20% of the population have been infected by HSV at some time but only one-third have ever had their infection diagnosed. The incubation period is around a week and the severity of the attack is dependent on the presence or not of anti-HSV antibodies in the patient from an earlier exposure. In the presence of antibodies, the attack tends to be of a shorter duration, both in terms of lesions and viral shedding, with fewer constitutional symptoms and complications. Primary genital herpes infection may be quite severe with constitutional symptoms including fever, myalgias, and malaise along with lower motor neuron and autonomic neuropathy leading to bladder atony, urinary retention, and the need for hospitalization.

104 Obstetric significance

Primary HSV causing maternal systemic disease or fever may lead to miscarriage or preterm labour, while the relative immunosuppression in pregnancy may result in generalized viral dissemination. Although no congenital syndrome exists, neonatal concerns are centred around fetal acquisition of HSV in the perinatal period, as the neonatal immunological immaturity may be unable to control the spread of HSV. The majority of neonatal infections occur in women undergoing a primary attack of HSV and occur perinatally, as the fetus emerges through an infected birth canal, with only about 5–10% occurring in the postnatal period. The risk in recurrent disease is low and estimated at less than 5% due to passive transfer of immunity. It should also be borne in mind that the majority of women whose babies are infected are in fact asymptomatic themselves. Neonatal HSV infection presents in the first 2 weeks of life, being limited to eyes and mouth in 25% but with widespread dissemination to multiple organs in 75%. Presenting features include weight loss, poor feeding, fever with multiorgan involvement carrying a high mortality of 70–80% and long term morbidity in survivors including mental retardation and developmental delay.

Diagnosis and management

Laboratory diagnostic methods include tissue culture techniques with a fluorescent antibody test and serological testing.

The management of primary HSV infection in the first and second trimesters of pregnancy is based on symptomatic support with oral or intravenous acyclovir if the mother's condition warrants it. Provided the pregnancy survives the acute episode, no complications are anticipated. A controversial suggestion in some quarters includes the use of continuous acyclovir in the last 4 weeks of pregnancy to suppress viral shedding or recurrence. It has been estimated that, with active primary herpes at the time of delivery, the risk of vertical transmission is around 40–50% and viral shedding may continue for 3–6 weeks. Therefore delivery by Caesarean section would be recommended if the primary attack is within 6 weeks of labour or if visible lesions are present in labour, provided the membranes have not been ruptured for more than 4 hours. In cases of recurrent herpes the risks and duration of viral shedding are less along with a degree of protection conferred to the neonate by passive immunity, so a Caesarean section should be considered only if there are visible lesions and the membranes have been ruptured for less than 4 hours. There is no value of serial cervical cultures towards the end of pregnancy as there is no correlation between the culture result of the latest cervical swab and viral shedding at the onset of labour. In all cases vigilance and observation of the neonate is imperative.

Human papillomavirus infection (HPV)

HPV is a double-stranded DNA virus with over 70 subtypes identified so far. It is the most common sexually transmitted infection. Subtypes 6 and 11 are associated with condylomata acuminata (genital warts) and juvenile laryngeal papillomatosis while subtypes 16, 18, 31, 33, and 35 are associated with cervical intraepithelial neoplasia (CIN), cervical carcinoma, and other lower genital tract precancers and cancers.

Obstetric significance

The significance of HPV infection in pregnancy is related to its association with CIN, the tendency of genital warts to grow rapidly in pregnancy on occasion causing obstruction in labour, and also the risks of perinatal exposure to HPV with the development of juvenile laryngeal papillomatosis. The severity of juvenile laryngeal papillomatosis may range from minor hoarseness in voice to complete obstruction of the upper airways, but a positive maternal history for genital warts is present in only half of the cases. The overall risk of developing juvenile laryngeal papillomatosis following perinatal exposure is minimal and estimated at approximately 0.25%, Caesarean section thus being justifiable only where mechanical obstruction of the birth canal by warts is evident.

Management

In the majority of cases HPV infections are subclinical. The presence of HPV infection may be suspected from characteristic cytological features on cervical screening smears or at colposcopy and is straightforward in cases of genital warts presenting as pale pink or white papillary growths. In general, treatment of genital warts involves excision or destruction of visible lesions by pharmacological, physical, or surgical methods but warts tend to recur due to the presence of latent provirus in epithelial cells. Warts in pregnancy are not treated routinely unless symptomatic. Methods that can be used in pregnancy include application of 80% trichloroacetic acid, which may have to be repeated weekly, and liquid nitrogen cryotherapy as first-line treatments. In refractory cases or for patients with multiple or extensive lesions, treatment under a general anaesthetic with laser or diathermy destruction of warts is an alternative. Use of podophyllin 5-fluouracil, and interferon intradermally are not suitable in pregnancy. Excision of the lesion at time of delivery is not recommended as warts tend to shrink in size following pregnancy and may be very vascular in pregnancy risking significant haemorrhage.

Chlamydia trachomatis

This obligate intracellular organism is responsible for one of the most common sexually transmitted infections in the world and is a significant cause of subfertility. Among the 15 serotypes identified, subtypes D and K are responsible for genital infections while others lead to blindness and lymphogranuloma inguinale. The majority of patients with genital chlamydia infection are asymptomatic, but outwith pregnancy may present with mucopurulent cervicitis, endometritis, acute salpingitis, and acute urethral syndrome. The long-term consequences of chlamydial pelvic inflammatory disease may include subfertility, adhesions, pain, and ectopic pregnancies. Diagnosis is based on culture-independent immunoassay either by PCR detection of DNA or ELISA techniques. Culture of the organism is possible but, due to its intracellular nature, is labour-intensive and very costly and therefore not widely used.

Obstetric significance

The obstetric significance of chlamydia infection is twofold.

There appears to be a modest association (especially of recently acquired infection) with preterm delivery, preterm or pre-labour rupture of membranes, low birthweight, and postpartum endometritis (which all are reduced by maternal therapy to eliminate the infection).

Of neonates born to mothers with maternal chlamydial cervicitis, 50–60% will be colonized, leading to inclusion conjunctivitis in about one-third within the first 2 weeks of life (give prophylactic 0.5% erythromycin or 1% tetracycline ointment) and to approximately 15% developing pneumonia in the first 4 months of life.

Management

Treatment of chlamydial infection in pregnancy is limited to erythromycin 500 mg 6-hourly for 1 week. In the non-pregnant adult, a single 1 g dose of azithromycin or a 1-week course of either doxycycline, tetracycline, or ofloxacin can be used. If erythromycin is not tolerated, alternatives in pregnancy include amoxicillin or clindamycin but these have lower cure rates of 98 and 93%, respectively. Contact tracing for the past 30 days and appropriate counselling and treatment is essential.

Gonorrhoea

This is a common sexually transmitted infection caused by *Neisseria gonorrhoeae*, a Gram-negative intracellular diplococcus. It may cause acute cervicitis, urethritis, bartholinitis, proctitis, pharyngitis, and disseminated systemic infection (more common in pregnancy, with malaise, fever, rash, and septic arthritis). The most common presentation in pregnancy is asymptomatic infection of the cervix.

Obstetric significance

- The obstetric significance of gonococcal cervical infection in pregnancy is the association with prelabour rupture of membranes, premature delivery, chorioamnionitis, and postpartum endometritis.
- Acute salpingitis is rare in the first trimester and even less likely thereafter due to the endometrial cavity being obliterated by the conceptus.
- Although gonococcal infection in pregnancy is not associated with an intrauterine syndrome, 40–50% of babies born to mothers with such infection develop opthalmia neonatarum—hence the importance of diagnosis and treatment of the mother and prophylactic treatment to the newborn.

Diagnosis and management

Diagnosis is based on the presence of Gram-negative diplococci within leucocytes from the infected exudate or discharge and culture of endocervical swab inoculated in Thayer Martin or other selective medium soon after obtaining the specimen.

Treatment depends on the severity of the infection and sensitivities need to be obtained as penicillin-resistant strains, though uncommon, may be responsible. Test of cure, contact tracing, and screening for other sexually transmitted infections are also important. For uncomplicated genital infection a single dose of ciprofloxacin may be adequate but this is not suitable in pregnancy due to adverse effects on the fetus. In pregnancy the recommended regimens include spectinomycin 2 g IM or a combination of probenecid 1 g per os (po) with, either aqueous procaine penicillin G 4.8 million units IM or amoxycillin 3 g orally followed by a 7-day course of erythromycin 500 mg qds (4 times a day). For disseminated infections, hospital admission and intravenous cephalosporins may be required. There is no contraindication to breastfeeding.

Group B streptococcal infection

Group B streptococcal infection (GBS) is one of the most important causes of neonatal bacterial infection and of maternal intrapartum and postpartum infective morbidity. GBS forms part of the normal vaginal flora in about 20% of women of childbearing age. Of infants born to colonized mothers, 60–70% will become colonized with approximately 1% developing invasive disease, the latter group carrying a 20% mortality.

Obstetric significance

A positive culture for GBS at 28 weeks confers a 90–95% chance of carriage at term but eradication is not possible despite multiple courses of antibiotics.

- Women may present with obstetric complications such as preterm labour, prolonged rupture of membranes, or intrapartum fever.
- Neonatal infection may take the form of early-onset disease within the first 4 days presenting with pneumonia or septicaemia and occasionally with concurrent meningitis occurring especially in low-birthweight babies (under 2.5 kg).
- The late-onset form of neonatal disease occurs after the first week of life, 80% presenting with meningitis, and carries a 20% mortality risk and a 50% risk of sequelae including cortical blindness and deafness in survivors.

Diagnosis and management

- Diagnosis is by overnight culture in selective media.
- Given that eradication of GBS despite antibiotics is not possible and universal chemoprophylaxis to all women is not practical, due to cost and risk of anaphylaxis along with development of resistance in the community, management involves selective chemoprophylaxis to women deemed to be at risk. The risk factors identified are based on the observation that the majority of early-onset disease and fatalities occur in low-birthweight and premature infants, those with prolonged rupture of membranes, and especially in the presence of intrapartum fever.
- Presence of GBS on vaginal swabs or GBS bacteriuria at any stage in the pregnancy must always be highlighted, along with a history of a previous infant with GBS as significant risk factors.
- The combination of these risk factors with prematurity, prolonged rupture of membranes, and pyrexia in labour are used to produce protocols for chemoprophylaxis in labour.
- The antibiotics of choice include ampicillin 2 g immediately (stat) followed by 1 g 4-hourly or benzylpenicillin 3 g stat and 1.5 g 4-hourly. In patients allergic to penicillin, clindamycin 900 mg 8-hourly or erythromycin 500 mg 6-hourly are acceptable alternatives.
- If GBS is cultured on vaginal swabs in the presence of preterm rupture of membranes, consideration should be given to the delivery and subsequent treatment of the neonate.
- The neonatal paediatricians need to be informed and the clinical condition of the neonate monitored closely.

Bacterial vaginosis

Present in about 20% of pregnant women, bacterial vaginosis (BV) is one of the most common vaginal infections. It is due to an alteration of vaginal microflora with overgrowth of facultative and anaerobic bacteria that normally form part of the vaginal microflora along with a 1000-fold reduction in *Lactobacillus* species. The organisms that are greatly increased in concentration include *Peptostreptococcus* spp., *Mobiluncus* spp., *Bacteroides* spp., *G. vaginalis*, and *M. hominis* amongst others. A thin greyish, watery, non-pruritic discharge with a fishy odour is the most common presenting feature but half the patients are asymptomatic.

Obstetric significance

It has been reported that there may be an association between BV and preterm labour/delivery, chorioamnionitis, and postpartum endometritis. Recent studies suggest a possible 40–50% reduction in preterm deliveries among women with BV who were otherwise at risk of preterm deliveries and were treated with metronidazole.

Diagnosis

A clinical diagnosis is made on the basis of the presence of three of the following four well established criteria:

- The presence of a thin homogeneous discharge that adheres to the vaginal walls.
- The presence of clue cells on wet prep microscopy.
- A vaginal pH > 4.5.
- The release of a fishy odour on addition of 10% potassium hydroxide to the discharge.

Management

The treatments of choice include metronidazole 200 mg three times daily or 400 mg twice daily for a week or a single 2 g dose of metronidazole, achieving cure rates of > 90%. Clindamycin 300 mg twice daily is an alternative. There are theoretical concerns about the use of metronidazole in the first trimester. Although it crosses the placenta, there is no increase in the risk of congenital anomalies. Metronidazole gel 0.75% may be safely used in the first trimester once daily for 5 days or 2% clindamycin gel once daily for 7 days as an alternative, but systemic treatment with metronidazole may also be required in the second trimester.

Candidiasis

Candidiasis can be caused by a variety of species of *Candida* but almost 90% of cases are caused by *C. albicans*. *Candida* are saprophytic fungi and can be recovered from the vagina of 30–40% of asymptomatic women. *Candida* accounts for 5% of cases of vaginitis in the non-pregnant population, this proportion rising to 45% in pregnancy. The altered vaginal microflora in pregnancy, along with depressed cellular immunity and increased glycogen availability, make for more favourable conditions for candida in pregnancy. Patients present with vulvovaginal pruritus, external dysuria, and a non-malodorous flocculent discharge like cottage cheese.

Diagnosis and management

Diagnosis. Vaginal pH is < 4.5 and microscopy in 10% potassium hydroxide reveals pseudohyphae and mycelial forms.

The mainstay of *treatment* is with the antifungal imidazoles such as clotrimazole, miconazole, etc. These may be administered as creams or pessaries as a single dose or a 3–7 day course. Topical imidazoles do not get absorbed systemically and are safe in pregnancy.

111

Recommended further reading

Adler, M.W. (1997). *ABC of sexually transmitted diseases*, 3rd edn. BMJ Books, London.

Hurley, R. (1999). Infections in pregnancy. In *Turnbull's obstetrics*, 3rd edn (ed. G. Chamberlain), pp. 471–8. Churchill Livingstone, Edinburgh.

Johnson, M.A. and Olaitan, A. (1998). Human immunodeficiency virus in obstetrics. In *Progress in obstetrics and gynaecology*, Vol. 13 (ed. J. Studd), pp. 27–42. Churchill Livingstone, Edinburgh.

Peckham, C.S. and Newell, M.L. (1996). *HIV1 infection in pregnancy*, PACE Review 96/05. Royal College of Obstetricians and Gynaecologists, London.

Royal College of Obstetricians and Gynaecologists (1997). *Chickenpox in pregnancy*, Guideline no. 13, July 1997. Royal College of Obstetricians and Gynaecologists, London.

Sampson, J.E. and Gravett, M.G. (1999). Other infectious conditions in pregnancy. In *High risk pregnancy—management options*, 2nd edn (ed. D.K. James, P.J. Steer, C.P. Weiner, and B. Gonik), pp. 559–98. W.B. Saunders, London.

Stirrat, G.M. (1997). Maternal and fetal infections. In *Aids to obstetrics and gynaecology*, 4th edn. Churchill Livingstone, Edinburgh.

Yankowitz J. and Pastorek, J.G. (1999). Maternal and fetal viral infections. In *High risk pregnancy—management options*, 2nd edn (ed. D.K. James, P.J. Steer, C.P. Weiner, and B. Gonik), pp. 525–58. W.B. Saunders, London.

HIV in obstetrics and gynaecology

Human immunodeficiency virus (HIV) is a retrovirus transmitted via contact with blood or other bodily fluids. HIV infects CD4 lymphocytes, causing their gradual depletion and thus leading to immunosuppression. Carriage of HIV can be asymptomatic but, as CD4 levels fall, symptoms associated with opportunistic infections, tumours, or neurological states can result. Monitoring of HIV is by CD4 levels and viral load. Highly active antiretroviral therapy (HAART) can be given either when symptoms occur or to slow disease progression. Prophylaxis against opportunistic infection is also an important part of treatment. For further details please refer to the *Oxford handbook of clinical medicine*.

Gynaecology

Premalignant change and malignancy

- HIV-positive women are at higher risk of developing lower tract neoplasia. The association is thought to be due not only to immunosuppression but also to sexual behavioural risks and to the interaction of HIV and human papillomavirus (HPV) at a molecular level.
  —As a result of this known increased risk HIV-positive women are advised to have annual cytological surveillance and possibly regular colposcopy.
- Cervical intraepithelial neoplasia (CIN) in HIV-positive women, prevalence 31–63%, is more likely to be extensive, recurrent, rapidly progressive, and non-responsive to standard treatment. Invasive cervical cancer is characteristically high-grade, aggressive, and recurrent. In 1993 cervical cancer was included as an AIDS-defining diagnosis. Cervical disease is more likely to develop with increasing immunosuppression.
- Vulvovaginal lesions are also more common in HIV-positive women. Careful assessment of the whole lower genital tract is necessary in HIV positive women referred for colposcopy. Ideally, vulvoscopy to look for the presence of vulval intraepithelial neoplasia (VIN) should also be performed.

Opportunistic infections

HIV-positive women are at risk of opportunistic infections in the lower genital tract as they are elsewhere. Infection with *Candida* can be a particular problem. Microbiological assessment of *Candida* species and sensitivity to antifungals may be required if the problem is persistent or recurrent. Advice regarding skin care and avoidance of allergens is an essential element of management as well as appropriate antifungals.

Contraception

Contraceptive discussions must include the need to reduce the risk of HIV transmission and also provide effective protection against unwanted pregnancy. Barrier contraception is essential. In addition, another contraceptive may be used to increase contraceptive efficacy. There is no evidence that use of the combined oral contraceptive pill, intrauterine contraceptive device, levonorgestrel intrauterine system, or Depo-Provera alters the risk of transmission.

rtility

Couples with HIV wishing to conceive should be counselled pre-conception regarding the risk of vertical transmission.

In discordant couples either artificial insemination (with a HIV-negative male partner) or sperm washing and artificial insemination (with a HIV-negative female partner) can be considered.

For couples with subfertility problems access to fertility services is still variable and a controversial issue.

Obstetrics

No fetal syndrome is associated with maternal HIV infection, unlike oth[er] viral infections. Vertical transmission is the predominant concern. The rate [of] vertical transmission without intervention ranges from 15 to 35%. Risk [of] transmission is increased with a higher viral load, lower CD4 count, or clinical[ly] advanced disease. In developed countries with appropriate interventions, verti[cal] cal transmission rate can be reduced down to around 2%. The key to reduci[ng] vertical transmission is early detection. Universal screening for HIV has be[en] routinely offered to pregnant women in the UK since the year 2000.

General antenatal care

- Management of pregnant women with HIV should be by a multidisciplina[ry] team including obstetrician, genitourinary medicine or infectious disease physician, and paediatrician.
- Baseline serology for cytomegalovirus and toxoplasmosis should be organized at booking.
- Invasive tests such as amniocentesis should be avoided to reduce the risk o[f] transmission.
- It may be appropriate to consider testing for other blood-borne viruses, such as hepatitis C.

Antiretrovirals

- Zidovudine monotherapy from the 2nd trimester has been shown to decrease transmission by two-thirds. The standard regime involves oral therapy antenatally, intravenous during delivery, then oral to the neonate for 6 weeks. This is recommended for women not warranting treatment outside of pregnancy.
- For women with relatively advanced disease, triple therapy may be more appropriate aiming to reduce viral load and improve CD4 count.
- For women conceiving on treatment, this is often continued with zidovudine added in if not already included.

Delivery

- Elective Caesarean section reduces the risk of vertical transmission compared with that of planned vaginal delivery by 50%, independent of antiretroviral therapy or clinical stage of disease. When combined with antiretroviral therapy, the risk is lowered by 87%. This is thought to result from avoidance of microtranfusions of maternal blood during contraction and avoidance of contact of the fetus with maternal genital secretions or blood. Caesarean section should ideally be performed before the onset of labour and rupture of membranes, although, if presenting in labour, Caesarean section has still been shown to be beneficial.
- It should be remembered that in some countries the risks of surgical delivery to the mother may outweigh the advantage of reducing the risk of vertical transmission.

Breastfeeding

Breastfeeding significantly increases the risk of transmission and as such shoul[d] not be encouraged unless there is no access to safe bottle-feeding.

Surveillance of infant

Previously, serial testing of infants using ELISA (enzyme-linked immunosorbent assay) screening tests was required until 18 months of age as results could be confused due to passive acquisition of maternal IgG antibody. More recently, PCR (polymerase chain reaction) detection of DNA or RNA of HIV antigen has led to much earlier diagnosis.

Infants who have been exposed to antiretrovirals during pregnancies should be reported to the Antiretroviral Pregnancy Register.

Immunization in pregnancy

Immunization may be indicated for short-term (passive) or long-term (active) protection against maternal and or fetal infection.

- Active immunization uses attenuated live organisms, inactivated organisms, or components of the organisms for which immunization is being performed
  —Live attenuated vaccines include poliomyelitis, measles, mumps, rubella and BCG (bacille Calmette–Guérin). These are generally contraindicated in pregnancy.
  —Active immunization produces an antibody response, IgM initially and IgG later.
- Passive immunization utilizes human immunoglobulin to achieve rapid protection but this lasts only a few weeks. Immunoglobulin specific for a condition is obtained from pooled plasma containing the required antibody.
- Except when there is a specific risk of infection, e.g. travel to an endemic area, vaccines containing attenuated or inactivated organisms are avoided pregnancy.
- The main conditions for which immunization may be required in pregnancy include varicella zoster and hepatitis B virus infections.

Rubella

Rubella vaccination is not recommended in pregnancy. Instead, non-immune antenatal patients should be vaccinated after delivery. However, active surveillance in many countries has failed to reveal any case of congenital rubella syndrome in cases of inadvertent vaccination of non-immune women shortly before pregnancy or in early pregnancy. There is no evidence that the vaccine teratogenic and the pregnancy need not be terminated because of such inadvertent vaccination.

Varicella zoster virus (VZV, chickenpox)

VZV is highly infectious and is common in childhood, where it is a mild illness. Over 90% of adults are immune and 80% of persons with no history of varicella infection are found to be seropositive.

- Primary infection in adults, however, can be severe, leading to pneumonia, myocarditis, pericarditis, encephalitis, and adrenal insufficiency.
- Pregnant women are more susceptible to severe illness from primary infection, with pulmonary complications occurring in about 10%.
- Severe illness may precipitate premature labour.
- Fetal infection may occur with a risk of 2–9% if maternal infection occurs before 20 weeks gestation. This may result in the congenital varicella syndrome, comprising of skin scarring, limb hypoplasia, microcephaly, cataracts, neural damage, and growth retardation.
- Primary maternal infection within 4 days of delivery (before or after) carries a 30% risk of disseminated zoster infection in the newborn as transplacental transmission of IgG antibodies would not have been established.

Maternal infection following exposure in pregnancy can be confirmed by the presence of IgM antibodies or a fourfold rise in IgG antibody titres. The pregnant woman should be observed for signs of severe illness.

Varicella zoster immune globulin (VZIG) may be given to exposed non-immune high-risk pregnant women to prevent or reduce the clinical manifestations. VZIG is expensive and therefore used only when strongly indicated.

Antiviral agents, e.g. acyclovir, should also be considered, either alone or along with VZIG.

Neither VZIG nor antiviral drugs remove the risk of congenital malformations in the fetus.

Hepatitis B

Parenteral drug abuse, sexual activity, and transfusion of blood/blood products are the main modes of transmission of hepatitis B, although vertical transmission from an infected mother to the fetus is a major factor in developing countries. Without immunization, up to 90% of fetuses of infected women may become infected. Of these, 5% are infected *in utero* while the rest acquire their infection from maternal blood and body fluids during delivery. Chronic carriage is more common when infection has been acquired perinatally or in childhood.

There are two immunization products for hepatitis B
- Hepatitis B immunoglobulin (HBIG) provides immediate, temporary passive immunity after accidental inoculation or contamination with an infected product.
  —HBIG is given in doses of 500 IU for adults and 200 IU for the newborn.
- Hepatitis B vaccine produces an immune response.
  —Antibody levels of 100 mu/ml are considered protective and less than 10 mu/ml is considered a non-response to the vaccine. A level of 10–100 mu/ml is a poor response and requires a booster dose.
  —HB vaccine is given into the deltoid muscle as vaccine efficacy may be reduced when given into the buttocks.
  —The dosage for HB vaccine is specified by respective manufacturers.
  Pregnant women who are negative for hepatitis B surface antigen (HBsAg) and considered to be at risk of acquiring hepatitis B infection should be offered vaccination with HBIG and HB vaccine during pregnancy.
- HBIG does not suppress the immune response to HB vaccine and neither product is known to cause any fetal abnormality.
- As most fetal infection is postpartum, neonates of carrier mothers or mothers infected during pregnancy should be vaccinated with HBIG within 12 hours of birth, followed by HB vaccine within 7 days and at 1 and 6 months.

Tetanus

Tetanus toxoid and tetanus immunoglobulin are safe in pregnancy and may be used when the risk of acquiring tetanus infection is high for inducing active or passive immunity, respectively. In parts of the world where neonatal tetanus is a major health problem, vaccinating the mother in pregnancy induces transplacental passive immunity in the fetus.

Travel vaccination

Information regarding vaccination when travelling to regions of the world where specific conditions may be endemic and the risk of infection high is found in the leaflet *Health information for overseas travel* published by HMSO London and available from general practitioners, travel agents, and embassies.

- *Hepatitis A* is transmitted by the faeco-oral route and risk of infection comes from travelling to endemic areas. Travellers to areas of moderate to high endemicity are advised to be vaccinated, especially if sanitation and food hygiene is likely to be poor. Hepatitis A vaccine is a formaldehyde-inactivated vaccine and the risks of congenital malformation are low. However, the use in pregnancy has not been fully assessed and it should only be given if there is a definite risk of infection.
  - Human normal immunoglobulin (HNIG) offers short-term immunity against hepatitis A infection and may be a more suitable prophylactic measure for pregnant women travelling for short periods to endemic areas.
- *Typhoid* is also transmitted by the faeco-oral route and therefore is a disease of areas where sanitation and food hygiene is poor. Three typhoid vaccines are available: monovalent whole cell typhoid vaccine, typhoid Vi polysaccharide antigen vaccine, and oral typhoid vaccine.
- *Yellow fever* vaccination is required for travel into highly endemic areas. The immunity conferred lasts at least 10 years and is probably lifelong.
- *Cholera* vaccination is no longer a requisite for travel as it only gives limited personal protection and does not prevent spread of the disease.
- *Rabies* vaccination should only be used in pregnancy if the woman is travelling to a high-risk area and the risk of exposure is high. The appropriate globulin may be used for post-exposure prophylaxis.
- *Meningococcal* vaccine may be used when unavoidable, e.g. during an epidemic or when travelling for long periods to high-risk areas.

Recommended further reading

1 Salisbury, D.M. and Begg, N.T. (eds.) (1996). *Immunization against infectious disease.* HMSO, London.

2 James, D.K., Steer, P.J., Weiner, C.P., and Gonik, B. (eds.) (1999). *High risk pregnancy—management options.* W.B. Saunders, London.

Medical disorders in pregnancy

Anaemia

Plasma volume expansion in pregnancy exceeds the increase in red cell mass, thus leading to a fall in haemoglobin concentration, haematocrit, and red cell count. The haemodilution does not affect the mean corpuscular volume (MCV) or the mean corpuscular haemoglobin concentration (MCHC). During pregnancy there is a two- to threefold increase in iron requirements to meet the demands of haemoglobin synthesis as well as synthesis of enzymes and to meet the demands of the fetus. Pregnancy is also accompanied by a 10–20-fold increase in folate requirements. Platelet count falls in pregnancy, with 5–10% of patients falling in the range $100–150 \times 10^9$/L. Thus, for practical purposes, a count below 100×10^9/L is considered to indicate thrombocytopenia.

In pregnancy a haemoglobin concentration below 10.5 g/dL should be considered abnormal. In the majority of cases anaemia presents in the latter third of pregnancy when demands reach their peak but some women start pregnancy with poor reserves (poor social circumstances and poor nutrition, repeated pregnancies in quick succession) while other situations such as multiple pregnancy are associated with a greater drain on maternal reserves and may result in earlier development of anaemia. Routine screening in pregnancy picks up the majority of cases although occasionally women may present with classical symptoms of lethargy, fatigue, shortness of breath, dizziness, or fainting.

Iron deficiency anaemia

The most common cause of anaemia in pregnancy is iron deficiency resulting from an increased requirement of iron during pregnancy in combination with poor maternal reserves. The increased demands for iron are partly met from increased absorption from the gastrointestinal tract but, if there is no iron supplementation, the shortfall is made up by mobilizing iron stores. The diagnosis of iron deficiency is confirmed by demonstrating a fall in the red cell indices (MCV, MCHC, and mean corpuscular haemoglobin (MCH)). Depletion of iron stores is reflected by a fall in serum ferritin levels.

Management

- Iron deficiency anaemia is treated by oral iron supplementation.
- In certain situations such as multiple pregnancy or where there is a higher risk due to poor maternal reserves, prophylactic supplementation prior to the development of anaemia may be advisable.
- Parenteral iron preparations are only of value in patients who do not tolerate oral supplementation but these preparations do not correct anaemia any more rapidly than do oral supplements.
- The expected improvement in haemoglobin on maximal iron supplementation is around 1 g/dL/week.
- In cases where iron deficiency is diagnosed very near term and correction by iron supplementation is not feasible, blood transfusion may be an alternative option if the anaemia is severe (< 7 g/dL).

Folate deficiency

Folate deficiency is also a common cause of anaemia in pregnancy. Inadequate dietary folate leads to megaloblastic anaemia. Nutritional status, along with conditions such as epilepsy (through the use of anticonvulsants) and haematological problems that predispose to rapid turnover of blood cells (haemolytic anaemia, thalassaemia, hereditary spherocytosis), may all predispose to folate deficiency. A raised MCV along with reduced serum and red cell folate confirms diagnosis of folate deficiency. Folate supplementation at 0.4 mg/day is recommended pre-conception and in early pregnancy as prophylaxis against neural tube disorders (NTDs), the dose being increased to 5 mg/day if the patient is on anticonvulsants or where there is a history of a previous child affected by NTD or where the patient is at higher risk of folate deficiency through haematological disorders such as haemoglobinopathies or haemolytic anaemia.

Vitamin B$_{12}$ deficiency

Vitamin B$_{12}$ deficiency is uncommon in pregnancy and presents in the form of pernicious anaemia that predates pregnancy so treatment should be continued in pregnancy. Vitamin B$_{12}$ deficiency is associated with subfertility and therefore often will have been corrected before pregnancy can be achieved. Rarely, strict vegans and chronic tropical sprue sufferers may present with vitamin B$_{12}$ deficiency. Oral supplementation should be considered with strict vegans and women with diets deficient in animal protein. Anaemia due to haemoglobinopathies is discussed in the section 'Haemoglobinopathies'.

Epilepsy

Epilepsy is the most common neurological disorder encountered in obstetric given that 1% of the general population suffer with it. In the majority of case epilepsy is idiopathic but in rare cases it may be a result of an insult to the brain (trauma, surgery, space-occupying lesion) or a manifestation of a more general ized metabolic disorder. Idiopathic epilepsy can be broadly classified into gener alized seizures (tonic–clonic, absence seizures), partial or focal seizures (complex if associated with loss of consciousness), and special epileptic syndrome such as myoclonic epilepsy. The majority of patients with epilepsy in pregnancy have already been diagnosed. In cases where the first fit occurs in pregnancy the differential diagnosis includes eclampsia, cerebral vein thrombosis, throm botic thrombocytopenic purpura, cerebral infarction, drug and alcohol with drawal, hypoglycaemia, and electrolyte imbalances such as hyponatraemia or hypocalcaemia.

Effect of pregnancy on epilepsy

One-third of women experience an increase in fit frequency, while the remain ing two-thirds experience no change or a fall in fit frequency. Women who are fit-free for many years are unlikely to fit in pregnancy unless they discontinue their medication, while the poorly controlled epileptics are the most likely to deteriorate in pregnancy. The majority of women who have one or more seizures a month are likely to deteriorate. Deterioration of epilepsy in pregnancy may be a result of poor compliance with medication through fear of its terato genic effects, decreased drug levels through nausea and vomiting, as well as reduced gastrointestinal absorbance with increased hepatic and renal clearance There is also increased volume of distribution along with alteration in free drug levels due to fall in albumin levels. Lack of sleep towards term and in labour may also be a contributory factor.

Effect of epilepsy on pregnancy

In general, the fetus is resistant to short episodes of hypoxia and there is no evidence that isolated seizures have a detrimental effect on the fetus. Status epilepticus, however, is dangerous for both mother and fetus and needs to be vigorously treated. The risks from seizures to the fetus are due to maternal abdominal trauma while maternal risks are due to loss of consciousness and injuries sustained during epileptic seizures. Partners or other family members should be aware of how to manage a seizure and, in particular, should be aware of the importance of the recovery position. The women themselves should be advised against taking a bath unattended.

There may well be a genetic predisposition to epilepsy as, even when there is no parental history of anticonvulsant use, children of epileptic parents have a 4% risk of congenital anomalies as opposed to a 3% risk in the general population. If either of the parents have epilepsy, the chances of the child of having epilepsy are of the order of 4%, this figure rising to 15–20% if both parents have epilepsy and 10% with a previously affected sibling.

One of the main concerns regarding the effect of epilepsy on pregnancy stems from the teratogenic potential of anticonvulsant drugs. Phenytoin, primidone, carbamazepine, phenobarbitone, and sodium valproate all cross the placenta and are associated with increased risks of congenital abnormalities. The risk of malformations with any one drug is around three times the background risk and is about 6–7%, increasing to 15% for those taking two or more drugs.

12 Medical disorders in pregnancy

Sodium valproate is associated with NTDs (1–2%) and congenital heart defects.
Phenytoin is associated with orofacial clefts and congenital heart defects while carbamazepine is associated with neural tube defects.
Phenytoin, phenobarbitone, and to a lesser extent carbamazepine and valproate all interfere with folate metabolism and this is thought to be a possible mechanism of teratogenesis.
There is limited data on newer drugs—gabapentin, and lamotrigine appear to be safe while there are some animal studies suggesting a risk for vigabatrin.

Management

Pre-conception management

Pre-conception counselling would be the ideal management and should be part of educating the female patient of reproductive age about her condition. The aim of pre-conception care is to optimize treatment and achieve control of the epilepsy with a single drug, taking into account its teratogenic potential.

- All women on anticonvulsants should be advised to take folic acid at a dose of 5 mg/day for 12 weeks pre-conception and throughout pregnancy.
- If fit-free for several years, a further option maybe to discontinue medication pre-conception and for the first trimester after full counselling concerning the implications of a seizure and, in particular, the implications for driving.

129

Antenatal management

Provided the woman is well controlled on single-agent therapy there is no need to change medication but it is important to stress the significance of complying with it.
General advice should be given regarding adequate sleep and the avoidance of precipitating features.
Prenatal screening should include maternal serum alpha-fetoprotein (MSAFP) and detailed ultrasound, focusing on the detection of congenital anomalies, in particular, NTDs and cardiac malformation. If the latter is suspected, a further scan at 22–24 weeks may be helpful.
The monitoring of serum levels of anticonvulsants is limited to women who continue to have regular seizures on high doses or where compliance is an issue. There is no role for routine monitoring of drug levels in fit-free women.
- Coagulopathies due to deficiency of vitamin K dependent clotting factors have been reported in babies of some women on hepatic enzyme-inducing drugs and, therefore, vitamin K 10 mg/day orally is recommended in such women from 36 weeks gestation.

Postnatal management

- Postnatally, the baby needs to receive vitamin K to reduce the risk of haemorrhagic disease of the newborn.
- There are no contraindications to breastfeeding and in some cases breastfeeding may facilitate drug withdrawal in the babies.
  —Neonates who are being breastfed and whose mothers are on phenobarbitone, primidone, or ethosuximide need to be watched for signs of sedation and poor feeding.

Epilepsy (*continued*)

- If the anticonvulsant dose had been increased in pregnancy, this needs to be gradually reduced to the pre-pregnancy levels over 2–3 months.
- Prior to discharge from hospital, contraception should be addressed. If the woman is on a hepatic enzyme-inducing anticonvulsant (phenytoin, primidone, carbamzepine, or phenobarbitone), a higher dose of oestrogen will be required to achieve reliable contraception. Similarly, higher doses of the progestogen-only pill or a more frequent dosing regimen for Depo-Provera will be required.

131

Heart disease

The pattern of heart disease in pregnancy has changed over the last quarter of century with a reversal in the ratio of rheumatic heart disease to congenit heart disease. This phenomenon is a result, on the one hand, of the dramatic fa in rheumatic heart disease while, on the other hand, a significant improveme in medical and surgical management of congenital heart disease has enable such patients to live to adulthood and reproductive age. Pregnancy leads marked haemodynamic changes such as increased blood volume, increase cardiac output, fall in systemic vascular resistance, and hypercoagulability, name just a few. These physiological changes of pregnancy are well handled the healthy woman but carry the risk of cardiovascular decompensation in thos with heart disease. It is therefore not surprising that heart disease in pregnanc can result in significant morbidity and mortality and in the 1994–6 confidenti enquiry into maternal deaths in the UK, it remains the second most frequen cause of all maternal deaths.

General management

Successful management of the pregnant woman with heart disease requires multidisciplinary approach involving an obstetrician, a cardiologist/obstetr physician, an anaesthetist, and, occasionally, a cardiothoracic surgeon. Ideall pre-conception counselling of women with heart disease would enable discus sion of maternal and fetal risks as well as optimization of maternal cardiovas cular health, including modifying any medical treatment, prior to embarking o pregnancy.

- The risk of the fetus having congenital heart disease is higher if the mother rather than the father has congenital heart disease, with the overall risk being 3–5%, double that of the general population.
- The risk of an affected offspring varies with the type of lesion being highes with aortic stenosis (18–20%) and around 5–10% with an atrial septal defect (ASD).
- Other conditions such as Marfan's syndrome and hypertrophic obstructive cardiomyopathy (HOCM) have a known pattern of inheritance (autosoma dominant).

Unfortunately many pregnancies are unplanned despite patients' knowledge c their underlying problems. Furthermore, there are increasing numbers of immi grant patients who may never have had a medical examination and thus presen in pregnancy with previously undiagnosed cardiac disease. The ability to toler ate pregnancy will broadly depend on the functional reserve of the patien (which can be evaluated using the New York Heart Association (NYHA) hear functional classification), the presence of pulmonary hypertension, and the pres ence of cyanosis. Although the majority of patients (90%) would fall in NYHA classes 1 or 2 (no breathlessness or limitation of physical activity/breathlessnes on severe exertion, slight limitation of physical activity), 85% of maternal death occur in NYHA classes 3 or 4 (breathlessness on mild exertion or marked limi tation of activity/breathlessness at rest, inability to carry out physical activit without discomfort). Chest X-ray can be safely performed with appropriat shielding if deemed appropriate and echocardiography is an invaluable tool t assess not only cardiac anatomy but also ventricular function and to estimat intracardiac pressure gradients.

- Every effort should be made to avoid and correct factors that may contribute to cardiac decompensation such as anaemia, infections, arrhythmias, and hypertension.

During the antenatal period, the patient should be routinely questioned about symptoms and examined for signs of heart failure.

Fetal growth assessment should be regularly performed in patients at risk of intrauterine growth restriction (IUGR).

During labour, it is important to monitor fluid balance and avoid aortocaval compression by use of a wedge or maintaining the patient in the left or right lateral position.

The nature of cardiac monitoring (electrocardiography (ECG), invasive monitoring, oximetry) will depend on the nature of the underlying cardiac condition and its severity, and a plan for intrapartum care should have been made and documented in the patient's records.

Close fetal surveillance throughout labour is recommended.

Caesarean section should be performed for obstetric indications. Operative vaginal delivery to shorten the second stage and avoid blood pressure changes with pushing may be wise in certain patients. Blood loss during delivery should be minimized and promptly replaced.

- Epidural analgesia minimizes changes in heart rate and blood pressure due to pain and, although well tolerated in those with adequate cardiac reserve, should be administered with extreme caution in those with restricted cardiac outputs and right to left shunts.

- During the first 24–72 hours of the postpartum period, significant fluid shifts occur and may lead to congestive heart failure, so close surveillance of fluid balance and oxygen saturations (by pulse oximetry) is advisable to enable early detection of pulmonary oedema.

- Prior to discharge it is essential to discuss and implement plans for effective contraception.

Endocarditis prophylaxis

The American Heart Association classifies cardiac conditions into high- and moderate-risk categories with respect to endocarditis prophylaxis, which is recommended in both these categories.

- Cardiac conditions considered high-risk include prosthetic cardiac valves (including bioprosthetic and homograft), previous history of bacterial endocarditis, complex cyanotic congenital heart disease (tetralogy of Fallot, transposition of great vessels, single ventricle states), surgically constructed systemic pulmonary shunts or conduits.

- Moderate risk of endocarditis is encountered with acquired valvular lesions, hypertrophic cardiomyopathy, mitral valve prolapse with regurgitation, or thickened leaflets.

- Prophylaxis is not warranted for the following groups where the risk does not exceed that of the general population: surgical repair of atrial or ventricular septal defects or patent ductus arteriosus without residual defect beyond 6 months; cardiac pacemakers and implantable defibrillators; physiological or functional heart murmurs; previous rheumatic fever with no valvular dysfunction; mitral valve prolapse without valvular regurgitation.

The current recommendations for treatment are amoxycillin 1 g IV (intravenous) or IM (intramuscular) plus 120 mg gentamicin at the onset of labour or at rupture of membranes. If the patient is allergic to penicillin, vancomycin 1 g IV or teicoplanin 400 mg IV can be substituted for amoxycillin.

Heart disease (*continued*)

Conditions associated with minimal risk of maternal complications

These conditions carry a very small risk of maternal mortality, well below 1%.

- Atrial (ASD) and ventricular septal defects (VSD) are generally well tolerated in pregnancy.
- Most cases of patent ductus arteriosus (PDA) have had surgical correction and pose no problems in pregnancy. Although uncorrected cases of PDA also do well, there is a risk of congestive cardiac failure.
- Similarly, corrected Fallot's tetralogy, porcine valve prosthesis, and pulmonary/tricuspid valve disease also carry low risk of complications.
- In cases of mitral stenosis the outlook depends on cardiac reserve with a good prognosis anticipated with NYHA class 1 or 2 patients.
- Benign arrhythmias are relatively common in pregnancy and include sinus bradycardias, sinus tachycardias, and premature atrial and ventricular contractions. After underlying pathology has been excluded as a cause, the management in healthy asymptomatic patients is observation.
- After investigation, symptomatic and sustained arrhythmias such as supraventricular tachycardia (SVT), ventricular tachycardia (VT), and atrial fibrillation require appropriate anti-arrhythmic treatment using drugs such as digoxin, beta blockers, adenosine quinidine, etc. depending on the underlying arrhythmia.

Conditions associated with moderate risks of maternal complications

These conditions carry a maternal mortality risk of 5–15%.

- Patients with mitral stenosis and NYHA class 3 or 4 may deteriorate rapidly in pregnancy, developing pulmonary oedema. Tachycardia (due to exercise, infection, etc.) in the presence of mitral stenosis leads to reduced diastolic filling of the left ventricle and hence a fall in stroke volume, leading to a rise in left atrial pressures and precipitating pulmonary oedema. Management involves treating the pulmonary oedema with diuretics and reducing heart rate with beta-blockers to improve ventricular filling and atrial emptying, after treating any underlying cause for the tachycardia.
- The severity of aortic stenosis determines the risk it poses in pregnancy—provided the gradient across the valve is less than 100 mm Hg in the non-pregnant state, it is unlikely to cause problems. In cases of moderate to severe disease, symptoms of angina, syncopal attacks, hypertension, cardiac failure, and sudden death may be encountered. Beta-blockers can help to control hypertension and symptoms of angina, dyspnoea, and syncopal attacks. Early signs of emerging left ventricular failure may be a subtle resting tachycardia.
- Patients with mechanical heart valves require lifelong anticoagulation to minimize the risks of valve thrombosis. Anticoagulation of choice with mechanical valves is warfarin and this carries risks of teratogenesis and haemorrhage. Subcutaneous (SC) heparin is inadequate for anticoagulation in the presence of mechanical valve prosthesis but IV heparin is used in the peripartum period.
- Although grafted tissue valves do not routinely require anticoagulation, there is a more rapid deterioration of such valves in pregnancy.
- Patients with corrected Fallot's tetralogy are generally at minimal risk of complications.

Those with uncorrected Fallot's tetralogy but no pulmonary hypertension have a moderate risk of complications. The main maternal consideration is one of paradoxical embolization causing cerebrovascular accidents from right to left shunting—the risks being reduced by SC heparin prophylaxis. The principal fetal problems are secondary to maternal hypoxaemia and can be summarized as IUGR, increased risk of miscarriage, and prematurity (spontaneous or iatrogenic). Maternal oxygen saturations may be improved by reducing physical activity in the latter half of pregnancy—hence the rationale for bed rest.

Coarctation of the aorta is usually diagnosed and corrected prior to pregnancy. The main considerations with an uncorrected coarctation include hypertension, congestive cardiac failure, and angina. Tight control of blood pressure through the use of beta-blockers helps to reduce the associated risks of aortic rupture or aortic dissection.

A risk of aortic root dissection and rupture also exists with Marfan's syndrome, an autosomal dominant condition characterized by clinical features such as high arched palate, arachnodactyly, joint laxity, tall stature, and dislocatable lens of the eye. The risk of complications in Marfan's syndrome is related to family history of aortic rupture and to the degree of pre-existing aortic root dilatation—if the latter is greater than 4–4.5 cm, pregnancy would be contraindicated until after aortic root replacement. Beta-blockers have been shown to reduce progression of aortic root dilatation and also reduce the rate of complications in patients with Marfan's syndrome. In labour an epidural, a shortened second stage, and avoidance of hypertension are recommended along with at least 8-week postnatal vigilance for aortic root dissection.

135

Patients with a previous history of myocardial infarction would ideally need pre-pregnancy assessment of cardiac function (echocardiography and stress test) and counselling on the basis of the results. Consideration of low-dose aspirin, along with avoidance of strenuous activity and vigilance for cardiac failure and arrhythmias is the cornerstone of antenatal management. In the intrapartum period ECG monitoring, supplementary oxygenation, avoidance of fluid overload and exertion, and a shortened second stage would be advisable.

Heart disease (*continued*)

Conditions associated with a high risk of maternal complications and mortality

A significant risk of maternal mortality (25–50%) may be encountered with conditions such as pulmonary hypertension, complicated aortic coarctation and Marfan's syndrome with aortic root involvement.

Pulmonary hypertension associated with pregnancy carries a risk of maternal death of up to 50%; with labour, delivery, and early postpartum periods being the most hazardous times.

- Primary pulmonary hypertension is an idiopathic abnormality of pulmonary vasculature seen primarily in women, whereas secondary pulmonary hypertension is usually a result of longstanding rises in pulmonary pressures due to underlying cardiac causes.
- Eisenmenger's syndrome is an example of the latter where pulmonary hypertension is secondary to an uncorrected left to right shunt of a VSD, ASD, or PDA with subsequent shunt reversal and cyanosis. The increase in blood volume and the fall in systemic vascular resistance can lead to right ventricular failure, with fall in cardiac output and sudden death.
- In both primary pulmonary hypertension and Eisenmenger's complex, the maternal risks justify consideration of termination of pregnancy and this issue should be addressed along with long-term contraceptive plans.
- Where pregnancy is to continue, joint obstetric and cardiological input with early involvement by specialist anaesthetists is likely to offer the best chance for a favourable outcome.
  - The antenatal care needs to address thromboprophylaxis, maternal surveillance, including hospital admission and oxygen saturation monitoring, and fetal surveillance—IUGR being the main fetal concern.
  - Labour and delivery will need to be in a high dependency setting with invasive monitoring planned during the antenatal period. Supplementary oxygen and tight control of blood pressure and fluid balance are imperative.
  - In the postpartum period, high dependency care with monitoring of oxygen saturations, thromboprophylaxis, and vigilance for fluid retention and cardiac decompensation should be among the priorities.

Puerperal cardiomyopathy

This is a rare condition limited to pregnancy. It can occur between the sixth month of gestation and 6 months postnatally, though the most common presentation is in the first month after delivery. Risk factors for this condition include increasing maternal age, hypertension in pregnancy, multiple pregnancies, and a multiparous patient.

- The presentation is usually with shortness of breath, poor exercise tolerance, palpitations, peripheral and pulmonary oedema, and embolic phenomena.
- The diagnosis is based on detection of global dilatation (involving all four chambers of the heart) with marked reduction in ventricular contractility.
- Prognosis is variable with 50% spontaneous recovery with supportive treatment.

- Management is supportive with anticoagulants and angiotensin-converting enzyme (ACE) inhibitors and, where there is evidence that the condition follows myocarditis, immunosuppressive therapy may be of some value.
- In cases of antenatal presentation, elective delivery is recommended.
- In cases that fail to respond, cardiac transplantation may be an option.
- Where the condition resolves, further pregnancy should be discouraged due to risks of recurrence.

Respiratory disease

Physiological changes in pregnancy

During pregnancy there is an increased metabolic rate and therefore increased consumption of oxygen. In order to cope with this increased oxygen consumption and carbon dioxide production, there is a 20–50% increase in ventilation (mainly by increased tidal volume) from the end of the first trimester and this change is maintained throughout pregnancy. The increase in ventilation is thought to be stimulated by the effect of circulating progesterone on the respiratory centre. This leads to a fall in arterial pCO$_2$ and a compensatory fall in serum bicarbonate resulting in a mild compensated acidosis.

Asthma

Asthma is the most common respiratory disease encountered in pregnancy. Asthma is caused by reversible bronchoconstriction caused by smooth muscle spasm in the airway walls with inflammation, swelling, and excess production of mucus. There is often a diurnal variation in severity of symptoms with exacerbations in early morning and at night. Possible provoking triggers include pollen, exercise, emotion, and upper respiratory tract infections. The effect of pregnancy on asthma is variable.

- Patients with mild disease are generally unaffected while those at the severe end of the spectrum are most likely to deteriorate late in pregnancy. Deterioration may also result from cessation of maintenance therapy through anxiety about taking medication in pregnancy.
- Any improvement during pregnancy may be followed by postnatal deterioration.

In general, asthma does not appear to have adverse effects on pregnancy unless the asthma is severe and poorly controlled.

- Although there are theoretical concerns about IUGR with severe poorly controlled asthma, in clinical practice they do not pose a problem.
- Other risks that have been associated with asthma in pregnancy are preterm delivery and hypertension (not pre-eclampsia), but these risks have not been demonstrated consistently.
- The risk of the child developing asthma in later life is around 6–30% and depends on whether the mother is atopic and whether or not the father is atopic and has asthma.

The emphasis on the management of asthma is prevention rather than treatment of attacks. Thus medication needs to be adjusted to control symptomatology. It is essential to educate and reassure patients regarding the safety of asthma medications, including systemic and inhaled steroids, in pregnancy.

- Inhaled steroids such as budesonide (Pulmicort), beclomethasone (Becotide), and fluticasone propionate (Flixotide) all appear safe, though more information is available for the first as compared to the latter two.
- Oral corticosteroids such as prednisolone are safe and, prednisolone being metabolized by the placenta, only 10% of the active drug crosses to the fetus. Oral steroids do increase the risk of gestational diabetes and cause deterioration of blood sugar control if there is already impaired glucose tolerance but this can be managed by dietary modifications and, if required, by insulin administration.

- Other drugs used in the management of asthma include inhaled beta 2 agonists such as salbutamol, terbutaline, and the longer-acting salmeterol, all of which reach the systemic circulation in minute amounts and appear to be safe in pregnancy.
- Similarly, inhaled sodium chromoglycate and inhaled anticholinergic drugs are safe and should not be withheld in pregnancy.
- Methyl xanthines such as theophylline and aminophylline are not used in first-line management of asthma. They readily cross the placenta and, although in large studies there is no significant increase in congenital abnormalities in women receiving theophylline, aminophylline has been shown to be a cardiovascular teratogen in animals. In the relatively small number of women dependent on theophylline, the dose may have to be increased in pregnancy, guided by drug levels.

Management of both chronic and acute severe asthma should be no different from that in the non-pregnant state, including performing chest radiography where indicated.

- During labour there is no contraindication to the use of inhaled beta 2 agonists as there is no evidence that they interfere with uterine activity.
- If patients are on long-term corticosteroids (i.e. > 7.5 mg/day for > 2 weeks) then additional cover with parenteral hydrocortisone should be administered during periods of stress such as labour.
- Prostaglandin E2 used for induction of labour is safe as it is a bronchodilator but caution is required if prostaglandin F2a is needed for intractable postpartum haemorrhage as it can lead to bronchospasm.
- Narcotic analgesia, nitrous oxide, and epidurals are safe and appropriate in asthma.

Cystic fibrosis

Cystic fibrosis (CF) is an autosomal recessive multisystem genetic disease caused by defective function of the CF transmembrane conductance regulation (CFTR) chloride channel. In CF the lungs, gastrointestinal tract, pancreas, hepatobiliary systems, and reproductive organs are affected. It is one of the most common genetic diseases, affecting 1 in 2000 Caucasians. A cycle of recurrent respiratory tract infections leads to bronchial damage, with eventual respiratory failure and death. Advances in the management of cystic fibrosis have led to a marked improvement in life expectancy with patients born now having the potential to reach their 30s and early 40s. They therefore also have the potential of presenting with pregnancy.

- The effect of pregnancy on cystic fibrosis and the risk of developing complications depend on lung function.
  —Where lung function is greater than 50% of the predicted, then pregnancy is likely to be well tolerated.
  —As lung function deteriorates, so does prognosis.
- Low body weights, dyspnoea, and cyanosis are all associated with a poorer outcome, and in one-third of pregnancies pulmonary exacerbations occur that require hospital admission and treatment with IV antibiotics.
- The main maternal morbidity is through poor maternal weight gain (even in those without pancreatic insufficiency), pulmonary infective exacerbations, deterioration of lung function with reduced exercise tolerance, cyanosis and dyspnoea, and congestive cardiac failure.

139

Respiratory disease (*continued*)

- The most common complications due to CF in pregnancy are prematurity (30% less than 37 weeks) and IUGR secondary to chronic maternal hypoxaemia.
- Factors predicting poor obstetric outcome include pulmonary hypertension, cyanosis, arterial hypoxaemia, moderate to severe lung disease, and poor maternal nutrition.

Counselling of women with CF needs to cover a number of aspects.
- There is an obvious risk of the child inheriting CF and this will depend on the genotype of the father. If the genotype of the father is unknown and assuming the carrier rate in the UK is 1 in 25, the risk is approximately 2–2.5%, while if the father is a known carrier the risk of an affected offspring will be 50%.
- Another issue that needs to be addressed as part of pre-conception counselling is the shortened life expectancy of CF patients and the harsh reality that they may not be alive to bring up their child.

The cornerstone of management of pregnancy in CF patients involves a multi-disciplinary approach, with particular attention to maternal nutrition, control of pulmonary infection, avoidance of hypoxia, and fetal surveillance.
- CF patients require a high calorie intake with pancreatic enzyme supplements.
- It is important to bear in mind that 20% of adults with CF have diabetes and a further 15% have impaired glucose tolerance. The latter may deteriorate to gestational diabetes, while insulin requirements are likely to rise in the former.
- Physiotherapy regimes need to be strictly adhered to as in the non-pregnant state.
- Any pulmonary infections must be aggressively treated with antibiotics, which can be modified according to sputum cultures.
- Towards the latter half of the third trimester, breathlessness may become an increasing problem even in the absence of infective exacerbations. If oxygen saturations fall to the low 90s or less at rest, hospital admission for bed rest and supplemental oxygen may be required. This should also prompt fetal growth assessment.
- The aim should be vaginal delivery but instrumental delivery may be indicated to shorten the second stage, as CF patients are particularly prone to pneumothoraces especially with repeated and prolonged Valsalva manoeuvres.
- Breastfeeding should be encouraged.

Sarcoidosis
Sarcoidosis is a chronic multisystem granulomatous disease affecting around 5 per 10 000 pregnancies a year. The patient is often asymptomatic or may present with chest and/or extrapulmonary manifestations.
- The most common extrapulmonary manifestations include anterior uveitis, hypercalcaemia, fever, and central nervous system (CNS) involvement.
- Pulmonary infiltration may gradually progress to pulmonary fibrosis.
- Chest X-ray may be diagnostic with bilateral hilar lymphadenopathy.
- Where the lung parenchyma is involved with no obvious infiltration in the lung fields the diagnosis is made by broncheo-alveolar lavage and transbronchial biopsy.

- Serum ACE inhibitor levels may help in the diagnosis and monitoring of disease activity but not in pregnancy.

Pregnancy does not seem to affect the course of the disease. Any improvement in radiological findings of the disease in pregnancy is often followed by relapse in the puerperium. There appear to be no specific fetal risks. Management of sarcoidosis is as in the non-pregnant state, with extrapulmonary and CNS involvement, along with respiratory impairment being the main indications for steroid treatment. Women need to be reassured about the safety of steroids in pregnancy and, if on long-term steroids, need to receive parenteral cover in labour. Vitamin D supplementation is not advisable as it may precipitate hypercalcaemia.

Tuberculosis (TB)

The rates of TB appear to be on the rise in the UK and USA over the past 2 decades. The main causes of the increased prevalence appears to be the influx of individuals from areas where TB is endemic (Asian and West Indian immigrants) and the increasing numbers of HIV-positive individuals. The onset of the disease is often insidious with cough, haemoptysis, weight loss, and night sweats. The causative organism in the general population is *Mycobacterium tuberculosis*, while, in patients with AIDS, *Mycobacterium avium intracellulare* is an important cause of pulmonary disease. The diagnosis is based on the characteristic chest X-ray appearances as the disease most commonly affects the upper lobes. Culture of the *Mycobacterium tuberculosis* takes 6 weeks but the diagnosis can be confirmed by microscopic examination of sputum (or bronchoscopic washings) for acid-fast bacilli (Ziehl–Nielsen stain).

There is no evidence that TB has a detrimental effect on pregnancy, or that pregnancy adversely affects disease progression. The principles of treatment are similar to those in the non-pregnant patient. Untreated TB poses a greater risk to the mother and her fetus than treatment. A multidisciplinary approach with joint care from a respiratory physician with an interest in management of TB is recommended and chest X-ray should not be withheld where required for diagnosis/management.

Treatment is usually with more than one of the drugs to which the organism is sensitive. The course of treatment needs to be prolonged and supervised to encourage and confirm compliance. The drugs most commonly used in the management of TB in the non-pregnant individual include rifampicin, isoniazid, ethambutol, pyrazinamide, and streptomycin.

- Streptomycin is associated with a high incidence of eighth nerve damage and therefore should be avoided in pregnancy.
- With regard to rifampicin, there have been concerns about teratogenesis but no adverse fetal effects proven so some authorities would recommend avoidance in the first trimester.
- Ethambutol and isoniazid appear to be safe throughout pregnancy, but all patients on isoniazid should take pyridoxine 50 mg/day to reduce the risk of peripheral neuritis.
- There is little information about pyrazinamide and therefore avoidance during organogenesis is recommended unless warranted to treat severe disease.

Respiratory disease (*continued*)

The treatment needs to be carried on for 6 months and usually is modified once sensitivities are available.

During labour and delivery infection precautions need to be taken with active disease but it should be borne in mind that the mother becomes non-infectious within 2 weeks of beginning treatment.

- The neonate should be given BCG (bacille Calmette–Guérin) vaccination.
- Prophylactic treatment with isoniazid is recommended for the baby if the mother's sputum is positive.
- Breastfeeding is permissible when the mother is taking antituberculous drugs as the amounts of drugs excreted in breast milk are negligible.

Pneumonia
Bacterial pneumonia
The incidence of pneumonia in pregnancy ranges from 1.5 to 2.5 episodes per 1000 pregnancies and bacterial pneumonia appears to be no more common than in the non-pregnant population.

- The most common bacterial pathogens are *Streptococcus pneumoniae* (in over 50% of cases), *Haemophilus influenzae* (more common with pre-existing lung disease), spp. *Staphylococcus* (associated with influenza), and spp. *Klebsiella*. Atypical organisms include *Mycoplasma pneumoniae* and *Pneumocystis carinii* pneumonia (PCP) found in association with HIV infection.
- Signs and symptoms of the disease are as in the non-pregnant individual, although reluctance to perform a chest X-ray may delay diagnosis unnecessarily. Other investigations include sputum culture, white cell count, C-reactive protein (CRP), and arterial gases in the breathless patient.
- Maternal and fetal morbidity remain serious complications of pneumonia and therefore it is important that pneumonia is promptly treated.

The principles of management are adequate oxygenation, hydration, and physiotherapy to clear secretion accompanied by appropriate chemotherapy.
- The community-acquired pneumonias (*Streptococcus pneumoniae*, *Haemophilus influenzae*) are best treated with amoxycillin (or erythromycin in the penicillin-allergic patient).
- For hospital-acquired infections, cephalosporins are a better choice while atypical organisms such as *Chlamydia psittaci*, *Mycoplasma pneumoniae*, and *Legionella pneumoniae* are all sensitive to erythromycin.
- Flucloxacillin is the agent of choice for staphylococcal pneumonia (erythromycin if allergic to penicillin).
- Tetracyclines are best avoided especially after 20 weeks gestation as they can cause discoloration to teeth.

PCP is the most common opportunistic infection in patients with AIDS and is associated with adverse obstetric outcome especially if diagnosis is not suspected. If conventional treatment fails or where there is profound hypoxia out of proportion to the radiographic findings, the diagnosis should be considered. Confirmation may require bronchoscopy.

- The treatment of choice for PCP is high-dose Septrin with or without pentamidine.
- There is a theoretical risk of kernicterus or haemolysis from sulfonamides given at term but in practice only long-acting sulfonamides such as sulfadimidine have been implicated in this.
- In women known to be HIV-positive and who have a CD4 count < 200 cells/microlitre, prophylaxis with either Septrin or nebulized pentamidine is recommended.

Viral pneumonia

Viral pneumonia such as influenza pneumonia is more severe in pregnancy. Pregnant women appear to be more susceptible to varicella zoster pneumonia. Varicella zoster (VZ) infection occurs in 0.05–0.07% of pregnancies and of these women 10–20% develop varicella pneumonia. The condition carries a mortality of from 6 to 40%.

- Pregnant women not immune to VZ in whom the infection occurs before 20 weeks gestation should be given VZ IgG as soon as possible after the contact.
- If the infection occurs after 20 weeks gestation there is little risk of congenital varicella but the risk of maternal varicella remains and administration of VZ IgG should be considered.
- Varicella pneumonia at a later gestation appears to be associated with a higher maternal mortality, possibly through increased immunosuppression.
- Women who develop clinical varicella should be treated with acyclovir. Oral acyclovir is safe in pregnancy but caution is needed when using intravenous acyclovir in pregnancy as it readily crosses the placenta.
- If respiratory symptoms develop in a patient with VZ, hospitalization is recommended.
- Maternal and neonatal morbidity and mortality in cases of maternal varicella pneumonia may be improved by the use of intravenous acyclovir and, if required, by mechanical ventilation.

Inflammatory bowel disease (IBD)

The incidence of IBD (ulcerative colitis, Crohn's disease, non-specific colitis, and proctitis) has been on the rise over the last 40 years. The annual prevalence rates for ulcerative colitis are 40–100 per 100 000 population and for Crohn's disease the prevalence rate is 4–6 per 100 000 population. The cause of IBD remains unknown but a multifactorial element involving infection, genetic factors, autoimmunity, and environmental toxins may be implicated.

Clinical features

- Ulcerative colitis is usually confined to the colon and causes liquid diarrhoea, lower abdominal pain, urgency of defecation, and passage of blood or mucus per rectum. Potential complications in ulcerative colitis include colonic dilatation/toxic megacolon, perforation, and malignancy.
- In Crohn's disease, the terminal ileum alone is affected in 30% of cases, the colon alone in 20% of cases, and in 50% of cases both ileum and colon are affected. Colonic involvement presents with symptoms similar to those of UC, while involvement of the terminal ileum is manifest by cramping mid-abdominal pain, diarrhoea, and weight loss. Potential complications in Crohn's disease include perforation, stricture formation, perianal problems, fistulae, and abscess formation.

Effects of pregnancy on disease

In general, pregnancy has little adverse effect on the course of IBD.

- Patients with Crohn's disease limited to the terminal ileum fare better in pregnancy and post partum than those with colonic Crohn's disease or ulcerative colitis.
- Relapses are frequent in pregnancy, especially in the first two trimesters in ulcerative colitis (50% relapse rate—similar to that in the non-pregnant population) and in the first trimester in Crohn's disease, although in about three-quarters of patients Crohn's remains quiescent in pregnancy.

Effects of disease on pregnancy

Female fertility may appear to be reduced as a result of voluntary infertility of the couple, nutritional status, and effects of chronic disease along with psychological problems with sexual dysfunction especially after resective surgery.

- In ulcerative colitis, fertility is affected adversely only in severely active disease with no impairment for quiescent or well-controlled disease.
- In Crohn's disease, amenorrhoea and involuntary infertility correlate with disease activity and normal fertility can be anticipated in well-controlled disease including after resection.

12 Medical disorders in pregnancy

Medical therapy

- Drug treatment in the form of salazopyrine and corticosteroids has no detrimental effect on female fertility (salazopyrine causes reduction in sperm count and increase in abnormal forms, but is a reversible cause of male infertility and therefore a change to 5-aminosalicylic acid alone may be an alternative).
- Earlier reports had suggested a detrimental effect of IBD on rates of spontaneous miscarriage. Recent data show rates of spontaneous miscarriage not significantly different from those in the normal population. With quiescent disease around the time of conception, good fetal outcome is anticipated in 80% of cases.
- In contrast, active disease at conception, first presentation in pregnancy, colonic rather than small bowel disease alone, active disease after resection, and severe disease being treated by surgery are all associated with increased fetal loss and prematurity.
- Women with IBD should be encouraged to aim for pregnancy during clinically quiescent disease and whilst taking minimum medication.

Management

Management of acute attacks and chronic disease is not substantially different from that in the non-pregnant situation. Exacerbation of disease should be investigated by full blood count (FBC), serum albumin (falls in pregnancy), and flexible sigmoidoscopy or rigid proctoscopy to assess activity of colitis. Fresh stool should be sent for culture of pathogenic microorganisms and analysis of their toxins along with screening to exclude parasites.

- Sulfasalazine appears to be safe in pregnancy and breastfeeding and is used for maintenance and induction of remission in women with ulcerative colitis and colonic Crohn's disease but it interferes with folate metabolism and therefore supplemental folic acid is required.
- Supplementation with vitamin B_{12} should be considered especially with involvement of the terminal ileum. Corticosteroids, orally and rectally, are safe in pregnancy, and oral doses of 20–40 mg/day may be required.
- Use of metronidazole in the first trimester is controversial and, although no definitive evidence of adverse effects has been confirmed, its use is generally avoided in the first trimester.
- During pregnancy constipation should be avoided by high fluid intake, a high-fibre diet, and bulking agents.
- Surgical intervention may be required for obstruction, toxic megacolon, haemorrhage, or perforation and should be performed for the same indications as in the non-pregnant patient.
- Vaginal delivery is the preferred option unless there are obstetric indications for a Caesarean section.
  —Severe scarring and inelasticity of the perineum secondary to severe perianal Crohn's or where there is active perianal Crohn's that may delay healing of the episiotomy is an indication for Caesarean section.
  —If abdominal delivery is required, it is wise to anticipate difficulties due to peritoneal adhesions.

Thyroid disease

Thyrotoxicosis

The most common cause of thyrotoxicosis is Graves's disease—an autoimmune disorder associated with the presence of thyroid-stimulating immunoglobulins. Other rarer aetiologies for thyrotoxicosis include autonomous nodules and pregnancy itself, the latter being due to the similarity of the α-subunits of thyroid-stimulating hormone (TSH; thyrotrophin) and beta-human chorionic gonadotrophin (β-hCG). Diagnosis of thyrotoxicosis depends on the demonstration of suppressed pituitary TSH and elevated free thyroxine (fT_4) and free tri-iodothyronine (fT_3). The use of radioactive iodine or technetium is contraindicated in pregnancy.

- Graves's disease accounts for 95% of cases of hyperthyroidism in pregnancy. Thyrotoxicosis may be caused by autonomous thyroid nodules while other rarer causes of hyperthyroidism include subacute thyroiditis and amiodarone or lithium therapy.
- Hyperthyroidism may lead to amenorrhoea and anovulation secondary to associated weight loss but pregnancy may still occur despite thyrotoxicosis. During pregnancy, the disease frequently ameliorates with postpartum flare-up. There have been suggestions that thyrotoxicosis may itself be associated with fetal malformations and that the risk could be reduced by antithyroid treatment.

- Perinatal mortality is higher along with higher incidence of premature delivery and IUGR, all of which can be reduced to the normal range with appropriate treatment.
- Fetal hypothyroidism is a risk with all antithyroid medication so the lowest possible dose to maintain biochemical euthyroidism in the mother should be used with bimonthly checks on free thyroid hormone and TSH concentrations throughout pregnancy.
- Poorly controlled or undiagnosed hyperthyroidism in conjunction with the stress of infection, labour, or operative delivery may precipitate a 'thyroid storm'—a medical emergency characterized by hyperthermia, mental disorientation, and cardiac decompensation. Transplacental passage of thyroid-stimulating immunoglobulin (TSIg) may result in fetal/neonatal thyrotoxicosis in 1–10% of babies of mothers with current or previous history of thyrotoxicosis (including women who have had thyroid ablation) and in these cases serial scans to assess fetal growth, heart rate, and neck are advisable. Management in such cases involves treatment of the mother with antithyroid drugs (and with additional thyroxine if mother is euthyroid), using the fetal heart rate as a guide to adjusting therapy.
- Carbimazole (CBZ) and propylthiouracil (PTU) are the drugs most commonly used in the UK for management of hyperthyroidism.
  - Both drugs cross the placenta but PTU less so than CBZ, and both drugs have the potential, when used in high doses, to cause fetal hypothyroisim and goitre.
  - Neither drug is grossly teratogenic although CBZ occasionally causes aplasia cutis—a scalp defect.
  - The aim of treatment is to achieve clinical euthyroidism, with T_4 at the upper end of the normal range. In newly diagnosed cases initial treatment is with high doses to achieve control, reducing to lowest possible maintenance doses by 4–6 weeks.
  - PTU is preferable in newly diagnosed cases in pregnancy (less transfer across the placenta and excretion into breast milk) but patients stable on CBZ need not be changed to PTU.

—The appearance of a rash or urticaria following the commencement of treatment should prompt changing to an alternative antithyroid agent.
- Women should be seen monthly in cases of newly diagnosed hyperthyroidism, but less frequent thyroid function tests (TFTs) are required if they are on stable doses of antithyroid medication.
- Doses of PTU below 150 mg/day and CBZ below 15 mg/day are unlikely to cause problems with the fetus and do not preclude breastfeeding, but TFTs should be checked at regular intervals in the neonate if the mother is breastfeeding and on higher doses of antithyroid medication.
- Thyrotoxicosis due to toxic thyroid nodules is more difficult to treat in pregnancy as antithyroid drugs will suppress both fetal and maternal thyroid but there are no TSIgs to counteract their effect on the fetal thyroid.
  —Beta blockers are used instead to control symptoms till pregnancy is completed or, alternatively, hemithyroidectomy can be considered in the second trimester.
- Other indications for surgical treatment include dysphagia, stridor, suspected carcinoma, and allergy to antithyroid medication.

Hypothyroidism

This complicates 1% of pregnancies but has often been diagnosed and treated prior to pregnancy. The aetiology may be autoimmune thyroiditis (Hashimoto's disease), viral thyroiditis, congenital absence of thyroid, or iatrogenic following thyroid ablation for hyperthyroidism.

- Autoimmune hypothyroidism ameliorates in pregnancy but recurs after delivery.
- Untreated hypothyroidism leads to anovulatory infertility.
- Hypothyroidism in pregnancy is associated with higher risks of miscarriage, fetal loss, pre-eclampsia, preterm labour, low birthweight, and subnormal neurological development.
- For patients on adequate replacement therapy at the outset of pregnancy who are therefore euthyroid, the maternal and fetal outcomes are good.

Management

The mainstay of management is thyroxine replacement.

- Most patients require 100–150 μg/day and often this requirement is unchanged during pregnancy. In newly diagnosed cases in pregnancy, in the absence of cardiac disease, a dose of 100 μg/day may be an appropriate starting dose.
- Only trace amounts of thyroxine cross the placenta and therefore the fetus is not at risk of hyperthyroidism from maternal replacement therapy.
- TFTs need to be checked each trimester, unless there has been a dose adjustment in which case TFTs should be repeated in 4–6 weeks.

Postpartum thyroiditis

This presents with vague symptoms of fatigue, lethargy, palpitations, or depression, often attributed to the postpartum state. Its incidence is 5–11% and it is more common in women with a family history of hypothyroidism. The condition is due to a destructive autoimmune thyroiditis causing release of preformed thyroxine from the thyroid (accounting for the transient phase of hyperthyroidism) followed by hypothyroidism when the thyroid reserve is depleted. Patients thus may present with transient hyperthyroidism in the first 6–12 weeks postpartum and then develop hypothyroidism 4–8 months postpartum.

Thyroid disease (*continued*)

Treatment should be tailored to symptoms and the majority of patients recover spontaneously.

- In the hyperthyroid phase, treatment is with beta blockers as antithyroid drugs are of no value where the problem is one of release rather than synthesis.
- The hypothyroid phase is more likely to require treatment with thyroxine but this should be withdrawn at 6 months to determine whether the patient has recovered.
- Of the women who develop postpartum thyroiditis, 3–4% will remain permanently hypothyroid while 20–30% of them who are thyroid peroxidase antibody positive will develop permanent hypothyroisim over the next few years so annual screening with TFTs is recommended.

Thyroid nodules

These are present in approximately 1% of women of reproductive age and, of those discovered in pregnancy, almost 1 in 3 may be malignant. Features suggestive of malignancy include a history of growth of the thyroid and radiation to the neck or chest, rapid growth of a painless nodule, a fixed lump associated with lymphadenopathy, voice change, and neurological involvement such as Horner's syndrome. The differential diagnosis may be a toxic solitary nodule, subacute thyroiditis, or a bleed into a cystic lesion.

- Diagnosis involves biochemical assessment of thyroid function and thyroid antibodies and ultrasound to distinguish solid from cystic lesions.
- A raised thyroglobulin level (> 100 µg/L) may elicit suspicion of malignancy.
- Histological diagnosis may be obtained by fine needle aspiration cytology or biopsy of a solid lesion.

Malignancy needs to be treated surgically, postponing any radioiodine treatment till after the end of the pregnancy. Pregnancy has no detrimental effect on previously treated thyroid malignancy.

149

Jaundice

Jaundice complicates about 1 in 2000 pregnancies although there is a much higher frequency in countries where the general incidence of hepatitis is increased.

- Viral hepatitis is the most common cause and may account for up to 40% of cases.
- Other conditions include haemolytic jaundice, recurrent intrahepatic cholestasis of pregnancy (up to 25%), and gall stones (6%).
- Hyperemesis, acute fatty liver, and hypertensive disease of pregnancy are responsible for less than 10% of cases.
- Jaundice may also occur in association with treatment with drugs such as chlorpromazine and, rarely, in severe cases of excessive vomiting.

Diagnosis and management

- A detailed history should be obtained, especially with regard to recent travel abroad, past and current medical or surgical illnesses, drugs, substance abuse, and blood product transfusion.
- Enquiries should be made into family history of jaundice or liver disease, symptoms of pruritus, pain, nausea, vomiting, fever, and colour and consistency of stools.
- Gestation age and estimation of fetal weight and fetal movement and viability should be established.
- Cutaneous manifestations of liver disease, e.g. palmar-erythema and spider naevi, are present in 60% of normal pregnant women. Clinical assessment includes degree of jaundice, hydration status, level of consciousness and cardiovascular stability, and the presence of flapping tremor. Evidence of ecchymoses, ascites, hepatic tenderness, and uterine irritability should be sought and a rectal examination should be performed to observe the colour of the stool.

Hospitalization for investigation and monitoring may be required.

- FBC, urea and electrolytes (U&Es), liver function tests (LFTs), clotting studies, viral hepatitis screen, and urine analysis should be preformed.
- An ultrasound scan of the biliary tract may be useful in the diagnosis.
- Liver biopsy, if indicated at all, should only be performed after correction of any clotting dysfunction.
- Joint management with a physician or surgeon would be useful to identify the aetiology and carry out supportive therapy with maintenance of hydration, nutrition, correction of electrolyte disturbances, correction of coagulopathy, and control of blood glucose levels.
- Intensive care with ventilatory support may be necessary in some cases depending on the aetiology and severity of the disease. It may be necessary to expedite delivery even though the fetus may be premature.

Viral hepatitis

This does not appear to occur more frequently in pregnancy than at other times, nor is it significantly different in its cause or management so far as the mother is concerned. Management of the patient is not influenced by pregnancy and treatment similar to that in the non-pregnant should be given. Prematurity and still births are more common if the disease occurs later in pregnancy. If jaundice occurs earlier, however, it appears to be less harmful. Neither hepatitis B nor hepatitis A virus causes congenital abnormalities so an infection during pregnancy is not an indication for termination of pregnancy. Jaundice due to gallstones is rare in pregnancy but if it does occur removal of the stone(s) would be indicated.

12 Medical disorders in pregnancy

Liver diseases peculiar to pregnancy

- Hyperemesis gravidarum.
- Hypertensive disease of pregnancy.
  - —Vascular changes lead to liver infarction and subcapsular haemorrhage.
  - —Overt jaundice is uncommon, the patient presents with epigastric pain, vomiting, and hepatic tenderness.
  - —Its association with the HELLP (haemolysis, elevated liver enzymes, and low platelet count) syndrome is well recognized and regular platelet counts should be done.
  - —Treatment is by delivery of the fetus.
- Intrahepatic cholestasis of pregnancy.
  - —This presents with pruritus and jaundice.
  - —It usually resolves within 48 hours of delivery and up to 45% of cases recur in subsequent pregnancies and also with the use of the combined oral contraceptive pill.
  - —The most consistent abnormalities on LFTs are slightly raised serum bilirubin and significantly raised alkaline phosphatase and bile acids.
  - —The jaundice is obstructive in origin and is due to intrahepatic cholestasis.
  - —There is a recognized fetal mortality associated with this condition, especially in late pregnancy.
  - —Cholestyramine reduces pruritus.
  - —Fetal assessment in the form of frequent cardiotocographs (CTG) and biophysical profiles is indicated, especially in late pregnancy.
- Acute fatty liver and acute hepatic failure.
  - —Rarely, in late pregnancy a patient will develop vomiting, upper abdominal pain, and jaundice. This may quickly be followed by headaches, mental confusion, and death. The whole duration of the disease may be merely a few days.
  - —The urine is bile-stained and the stools are pale, indicating that the jaundice is obstructive in type. Acute liver failure of this type may arise at other times following drugs or various poisons.
  - —The most prominent histological feature is fatty degeneration in the centre of the liver lobules.
  - —The progress of the condition is so rapid that effective treatment may be almost impossible. Early delivery is indicated at the first appearance of jaundice if the diagnosis is not in doubt.

Autoimmune diseases

Systemic lupus erythematosus (SLE)

SLE is a systemic connective tissue disorder-affecting women nine times more commonly than men. It has an incidence of 1 per 1000 women and is most common during the childbearing years, the average age at diagnosis being 31. SLE is an idiopathic chronic inflammatory disease that affects skin, joints, kidneys lungs, serous membranes nervous system, liver, and other body organs. It is characterized by periods of remission and relapse.

The pathogenesis is unknown but is thought to be multifactorial involving a genetic predisposition and environmental triggers such as viral infection and ultraviolet (UV) radiation. Inappropriate or excess immune activation leads to immune complex formation and deposition of immune complexes causes vasculitis and glomerulonephritis.

The most common clinical complaints are fatigue, fever, weight loss, myalgia and arthralgia, but the symptomatology will vary according to the organ systems that are affected. Joint involvement occurs in 90% of cases, while skin involvement occurs in 80% of patients and 6% have other autoimmune disorders.

The suspicion of a diagnosis of SLE is confirmed by demonstrating the presence of circulating autoantibodies and, in particular, antinuclear antibodies (ANA) present in 96% of SLE patients.

- Antibodies to double-stranded DNA (anti-dsDNA) are the most specific for SLE and the titre of anti-dsDNA is also related to disease activity.
- Patients with SLE may also have antibodies to RNA–protein conjugates referred to as soluble or extractable antigens, since they can be separated from tissue extracts.
- Of the extractable nuclear antigens, anti-Ro and anti-La are of particular importance in obstetrics as they are associated with neonatal lupus syndromes including cardiac lesions such as congenital complete heart block and endocardial fibroelastosis.

Effect of pregnancy on SLE

There is controversy as to whether pregnancy exacerbates SLE and increases the number of flare-ups both antenatally and in the postpartum period. When flare-ups do occur they tend to be in the first two trimesters but diagnosis of a flare-up is hindered as many features of the condition (hair loss, oedema, facial erythema fatigue, anaemia, raised erythrocyte sedimentation rate (ESR), and musculoskeletal pain) also occur in normal pregnancy. Where there is lupus nephritis, pregnancy does not jeopardize renal function in the long term. Even though women with moderate renal impairment usually have uncomplicated pregnancies, the risk of deterioration of renal function is greater the higher the baseline serum creatinine.

Effect of SLE on pregnancy

- SLE is associated with increased risks of spontaneous miscarriage, fetal death, pre-eclampsia, prematurity, and IUGR. Pregnancy outcome is particularly affected by the degree of renal involvement.
- Lupus nephritis in particular is associated with fetal loss, pre-eclamptic toxaemia, and IUGR, especially if hypertension or proteinuria predate the pregnancy.
- Other indicators of increased risk of complications in pregnancy are the presence of anticardiolipin antibodies, lupus anticoagulant, active disease at time of conception, or first presentation in pregnancy.

Management

- Ideally, a woman with SLE should seek *pre-conception* counselling where a full discussion regarding potential obstetric and medical complications can take place, questions can be answered, and a management plan can be formulated.
  —The patient should be in remission and ideally have discontinued cytotoxic medication and nonsteroidal anti-inflammatory drugs (NSAIDs).
  —Assessment to document baseline renal function (urinalysis, serum creatinine, and 24-hour urine for creatinine clearance and total protein), along with FBC (to exclude anaemia and thrombocytopenia) and screening for antiphospholipid antibodies (lupus anticoagulant and anticardiolipin antibodies) should be performed.
- Antenatal care should be undertaken in a combined medical obstetric clinic. Close follow-up is recommended with fortnightly visits in the first and second trimesters and weekly visits in the third.
  —Disease activity needs to be regularly monitored along with fetal welfare by regular fetal biometry combined with umbilical artery Doppler blood flow examination.
  —There is a need to watch for superimposed pregnancy-induced hypertension and fetal growth restriction.
  —In patients with renal involvement, monthly 24-hour urine collections for total protein and creatinine clearance is recommended.
- Disease exacerbation needs to be actively managed and corticosteroids are the drugs of choice.
  —If the patient is on hydroxychloroquine, this needs to be continued since discontinuation may lead to disease flare-up.
  —Azathioprine appears to be safe in pregnancy, though there are theoretical concerns that it may cause chromosomal aberrations in germ cells.
  —NSAIDs are associated with oligohydramnios through their action on the fetal kidneys and may also lead to premature closure of the ductus arteriosus. Both effects may be reversible with early discontinuation of NSAIDs. Under special circumstances it may be warranted to use NSAIDs for pain control but this should be avoided in the third trimester and especially after 32 weeks.
  —The antihypertensive agent of choice is methyldopa with nifedipine and hydrallazine as agents of second choice. Consideration should be given to thromboprophylaxis.
- Delivery at term is recommended in the absence of complications, avoiding postmaturity.
  —In labour continuous electronic fetal monitoring (EFM) should be instituted along with intravenous steroids for patients on chronic steroid therapy.
  —The paediatricians need to be alerted.
- Postnatally, restart maintenance therapy, consider thromboprophylaxis, and watch for exacerbations of SLE.

Autoimmune diseases (*continued*)

Antiphospholipid syndrome

The diagnosis of antiphospholipid syndrome (APS) requires the combination of antiphospholipid antibodies (anticardiolipin antibody (aCL) and/or lupus anti-coagulant (LA)) with one or more of a series of recognized clinical features, the most common ones being a history of thrombosis (arterial or venous), recurrent pregnancy loss (usually late first and second trimester), and thrombocytopenia.

- Other clinical features associated with APS include hypertension, pulmonary hypertension, heart valve disease, and cerebral involvement (epilepsy, cerebral infarction, chorea, and migraine).
- The prevalence of antiphospholipid antibodies in the general population is around 2%. The diagnosis of APS requires positive readings for aCL and/or LA on two occasions at least 3 months apart and there is considerable variation in results between different laboratories.

Management

APS is associated with increased risks of pregnancy loss, thromboembolic disease, and stroke. There is also significant risk of severe early-onset pre-eclampsia, fetal growth impairment, and fetal distress, all of which contribute to increased risk of prematurity. Ideally, these issues should be discussed as part of pre-conception counselling.

- Antenatal management should be in a joint medical–obstetric clinic.
- Aspirin is now generally recommended early in pregnancy (even pre-conception) to prevent failure of placentation in the belief that placental damage occurs in early gestation.
- Controversy surrounds the use of low-molecular-weight heparin (LMWH). In women with a history of previous thromboembolism and a history of APS, the very high risk of further thromboembolism in pregnancy and puerperium justifies thromboprophylaxis with subcutaneous LMWH in the antenatal and postpartum period. Opinion is, however, divided about the use of prophylactic heparin where there is no previous history of thrombosis. The benefits of heparin need to be balanced against the risks of heparin-induced osteoporosis.
- The use of steroids in combination with aspirin is no longer recommended.
- There needs to be close surveillance of fetal well-being and growth by serial biometry and Doppler studies of umbilical artery waveform as well as fetal activity monitoring.
- Maternal surveillance needs to concentrate on screening for pre-eclampsia and detection of signs/symptoms of thromboembolic disease.
- Postnatal thromboprophylaxis should not be forgotten.

Rheumatoid arthritis

Rheumatoid arthritis (RA) is a chronic inflammatory disease affecting synovial joints. It has a 3:1 predilection for females and affects 1 in one to two thousand pregnancies. The characteristic symptoms are joint pains and morning stiffness. RA is a systemic disorder with extra-articular manifestations including fatigue, vasculitis, and pulmonary and subcutaneous nodules as well as affecting the eyes. It is an autoimmune disorder involving immune complexes in the circulation and synovial fluid, leading to progressive damage and destruction of joints. Of RA patients, 80–90% are positive for rheumatoid factor while 30% are positive for antinuclear antibodies.

- *Effect of pregnancy on RA.* Up to 75% of women experience improvement of symptoms in pregnancy, the improvement beginning in the first trimester. Unfortunately, 90% of those who experience remission suffer postpartum exacerbations.

- *Effect of RA on pregnancy.* The main concerns relate to the safety of medication used in the treatment of RA during pregnancy and breastfeeding. In women with anti-Ro antibodies, the infants are at risk of neonatal lupus. Rare complications include atlanto-axial subluxation with general anaesthesia and, in cases of severe limitations of hip abduction, interference with vaginal delivery.

Management

Pre-pregnancy management should concentrate on stabilization of underlying disease at the lowest maintenance doses possible and avoiding teratogenic agents. During pregnancy, increased rest and physiotherapy for symptomatic relief and maintenance of mobility are advisable.

- Paracetamol should be used as the first-line analgesic.
- NSAIDs should, in general, be avoided (see under SLE) but in certain circumstances may be used to control arthritic pain. If they are used, their use should be discontinued after 32 weeks gestation.
- Corticosteroids such as prednisolone should be the first-line medication for worsening disease and are safe in pregnancy but increase the risk of gestational diabetes. Thus blood glucose should be monitored. If patients are on long-term maintenance steroids, parenteral steroids should be administered to cover labour and delivery.
- Sulfasalazine is safe in pregnancy.
- Antimalarials and azathioprine can be used in pregnancy if required for disease control.
- Other disease-modifying agents such as chlorambucil, methotrexate, cyclophosphamide, and Gold salts are contraindicated in pregnancy.

155

Myasthenia gravis

Myasthenia gravis (MG) is an autoimmune disorder characterized by variable weakness and fatiguability of skeletal muscle. It is an uncommon disorder with an incidence of 2–10/100 000, affecting women more than men. The immediate cause of the disease is an autoimmune attack on the acetylcholine receptor complex at the neuromuscular junction with autoantibodies to the human acetylcholine receptor complex present in the serum of three-quarters of patients with MG.

- Ocular muscle weakness resulting in diplopia or eyelid ptosis is the usual presenting symptom, while some patients present with difficulty talking or chewing.
- MG progresses from ocular to generalized skeletal muscle involvement over 1–2 years. Muscle weakness varies throughout the day but tends to be worse towards the end of the day. The long-term course of the disease is variable with periodic fluctuations in severity.
- The diagnosis rests on clinical presentation, physical examination, and confirmatory tests including restoration of muscle vigour after intravenous injection of short-acting anticholinesterase drugs such as endrophonium. Other more sophisticated tests include single-fibre myography and repetitive nerve stimulation studies.
- MG is treatable but not curable. The agent of choice is pyridostigmine, an anticholinesterase that impedes degradation of acetylcholine thus improving muscle function.

Autoimmune diseases (*continued*)

Management

Pre-conception counselling is important to discuss risks of pregnancy and formulate a management plan. There may be a need to adjust medication in pregnancy due to reduced gastrointestinal absorption, increased plasma volume, and increased renal clearance. Patients need to be counselled about the increase in fatigue, especially during the second and third trimester, with the potential of respiratory compromise in late pregnancy.

- Pregnancy should be postponed in women recently diagnosed with MG as this time period represents the greatest risk. There is a high risk of premature delivery, up to 60%.
- Weakness due to MG can be increased by the exertion required in the course of labour and delivery, especially in the second stage of labour.

Treatment of MG in pregnancy does not differ significantly from that in the non-pregnant state.

- The quaternary ammonium compound, pyridostigmine, is the most popular long-acting medication with anticholinesterase activity.
- Prednisolone in high doses is effective in most patients, with slow tapering of dose over many months after improvement.
- Unfortunately, remission appears to be maintained only while the patient is on steroids. Hence pregnant patients with MG on glucocorticoids should be maintained on them throughout pregnancy and the postpartum period.
- It is worthwhile limiting exercise and work and minimizing emotional and physical stress—all factors that may exacerbate MG.
- Any infections should be promptly identified and treated.
- Poor fetal movements and polyhydramnios may raise the possibility of fetal involvement but may be difficult to differentiate from reduced fetal activity due to hypoxaemia—hence the need for regular biometry and biophysical scoring to confirm fetal well-being.
- During labour and delivery anticholinesterase drugs may have to be administered parenterally together with steroid cover if on long-term steroids.
  - Certain drugs such as magnesium sulfate are *absolutely contraindicated* and hypokalaemia (as may occur with beta-sympathomimetics) should be carefully avoided.
- Regional anaesthesia and analgesia is preferable as it limits fatigue and anxiety and is ideal for assisted instrumental deliveries.
- In the postpartum period drug dosages may need to be rapidly adjusted downwards as the effect of volume expansion of pregnancy clears.
- Special care and surveillance of the newborn may be required to detect transient neonatal MG, which is easily treatable with endrophonium and usually resolves by 4 weeks postnatally.

12 Medical disorders in pregnancy

Autoimmune thrombocytopenia (idiopathic thrombocytopenia, IDP)

The incidence is 1 in 1000 pregnancies. If a low maternal platelet count is diagnosed in the first half of pregnancy it is likely to be due to immune thrombocytopenia. The presence of anti-platelet antibodies in the maternal serum is diagnostic.

- The major risks to the mother in this condition usually occur during labour or postpartum and include haemorrhage, particularly from lacerations or from episiotomies, but not usually from the placental site. The incidence is 5–26% and is correlated with the degree of thrombocytopenia. Insertion of an epidural cannula may result in epidural haematoma. These manifestations usually occur when the platelet count is less than 50×10^9/L and clotting characteristics are abnormal. With regards to neonatal thrombocytopenia, which occurs as a result of IgG antibodies crossing the placenta, maternal platelet count is a poor predictor.
- About 10–15% of babies of affected mothers will have platelet counts of less than 50×10^9/L at delivery, although this is not associated with significant morbidity. The perinatal mortality for a baby with ITP is about 5%. Intracranial haemorrhage occurs in less than 1% of all cases and this occurs mostly in the 3% of severely affected babies with platelet counts of less than 50×10^9/L. Caesarean section is not necessarily preventive. The practice of establishing the degree of severity with a fetal blood sampling antenatally or in early labour to decide on the mode of delivery is debated.

Management of ITP

- So long as the booking platelet count is more than 100×10^9/L, regular repeat counts are not necessary until about 26–28 weeks. Thereafter the platelet counts should be monitored at monthly intervals until delivery.
- Platelet counts at booking of less than 100×10^9/L would need weekly measurement. If the platelet count is less than 50×10^9/L, a coagulation screen is necessary to exclude any additional coagulation defect.
- Steroids in the form of prednisolone are indicated for maternal platelet counts of below 20×10^9/L and are preferable in those with counts $< 50 \times 10^9$/L (prednisolone 60–80 mg per day). This usually increases the platelet count to over 50×10^9/L within 3 weeks. Thereafter the dose of prednisolone can be reduced to maintain the platelet count at more than 70×10^9/L.
- An alternative therapy is immunoglobulin at 400 mg per kg per day. Given intravenously, it would give a rapid rise in maternal platelet count that lasts for about 2 weeks.
- During delivery it may be necessary to cover labour and delivery with a platelet transfusion if the platelet count is less than 30×10^9/L. Each unit raises the platelet count by approximately $5–10 \times 10^9$/L.

Coagulation disorders

Pregnancy is associated with changes in all aspects of the haemostatic mechanism (platelets, vessels, coagulation factors, natural anticoagulants, and fibrinolytic system) such that towards the end of pregnancy the overall balance shifts towards hypercoagulability.

- *Haemophilias.* The prevalence of haemophilia is reported to be 13–18/100 000 male population with a ratio of 4:1 between haemophilia A (factor VIII deficiency) and haemophilia B (factor IX deficiency) both of which are X-linked recessive disorders.
  —Female carriers have a second normal gene and therefore do not have significant bleeding problems. Troublesome bleeding may occur in a minority of carriers especially in those with very low clotting factor levels (5–10 IU/dL) that may be a result of extreme lyonization or co-inheritance of another bleeding disorder or where another chromosomal abnormality affects the X chromosome.
  —Male offspring of an affected father will always be affected, while male offspring of a carrier mother may either be affected or normal.
  —Female offspring of an affected male will always be carriers.
  —Haemophilia centres actively seek to educate families and promote the significance of carrier testing which should ideally be performed ahead of puberty when a girl is old enough to understand the implications but before she is sexually active and certainly before her first pregnancy.
- *Von Willebrand's disease* is the most common clinically significant hereditary coagulation abnormality affecting women but it is a milder disorder than haemophilia. Its prevalence in the general population is estimated at 1% and von Willebrand factor synthesis is controlled by a gene on the short arm of chromosome 12.
  —Three major types of von Willebrand's disease are described with both autosomally recessive and dominant forms. Thus both male and female offspring may be carriers or be affected by the condition.
  —Von Willebrand factor is essential for normal platelet activity and acts as a carrier for clotting factor VIII in the circulation.
  —Type III von Willebrand disease is the most severe.
- *Factor XIc deficiency* is an autosomal disorder most prevalent amongst Askenhazi Jews and other families of European extraction. Bleeding is most common amongst individuals with significantly reduced levels of factor XIc. Bleeding problems such as menorrhagia and postpartum bleeds are reported among women with a factor XIc activity around 50% of normal values.

Prenatal diagnosis

Chorionic villus sampling (CVS) in conjunction with fetal genotype analysis by mutation detection or by linked polymorphism is the main method of prenatal diagnosis. Where the mother's DNA analysis is non-informative or there is inadequate information on the family, diagnosis of clotting factor deficiency in the fetal blood obtained by cordocentesis is used. The uptake of prenatal diagnosis for haemophilia is low at 30–35%, the reason often given being that haemophilia is not considered a serious enough disease to justify termination of pregnancy.

Antenatal care

- This should start with pre-conception counselling where the options for prenatal diagnosis and other aspects of the management of the pregnancy should be reviewed.
- Where blood products may be required, it may be appropriate to ensure immunity to hepatitis B. If this is not the case it may be appropriate to

complete a course of hepatitis B (and hepatitis A) vaccination prior to embarking on pregnancy.

The pregnancy should be managed jointly by an obstetrician and a haematologist with interest in haemophilia.

Maternal coagulation factor activity along with Von Willebrand factor antigen and activity should be checked at booking.

Invasive procedures in pregnancy may cause maternal, fetal, or placental bleeding and this includes prenatal diagnostic procedures such as CVS. Thus full discussion of the risks as well as the perceived benefits of each course of action is essential.

In the majority of cases of carriers or potential carriers of haemophilia where prenatal diagnosis has not been performed, fetal gender determination is possible by visualization of the external genitalia from 18–20 weeks.

Maternal coagulation factor activity and (if appropriate) Von Willebrand factor levels should be rechecked at 28 and 34 weeks and at any stage where there is a possibility of surgery or invasive procedures and with miscarriage or accidental bleeding.

Labour and delivery

- In the absence of obstetric contraindications, vaginal delivery at term is the preferred option with early recourse to Caesarean section if labour fails to progress.
- On admission in labour, maternal coagulation factors should be checked aiming for levels greater than 40 IU/L if an uncomplicated delivery is anticipated but levels of at least 50 IU/L if operative delivery becomes necessary. If the maternal levels are below these thresholds, then prophylactic treatment should be given.
- Invasive monitoring, scalp blood sampling, vacuum extraction, and midcavity rotational deliveries should be avoided in cases of Von Willebrand's disease or other autosomally inherited disorders, or where the fetus is known to be an affected male or the sex is unknown in cases of haemophilia carriers.
- Low forceps delivery is considered less traumatic than trying to deliver a deeply engaged head at Caesarean section.
- Epidural anaesthesia is not contraindicated in patients with a normal coagulation screen, provided their clotting factor levels are greater than 50 IU/dL, their platelet count is greater than 100×10^9/L, and their bleeding time is normal.

Postnatal care

- In all patients with hereditary bleeding disorders, it is important to ensure that clotting factor activity and Von Willebrand activity is maintained above 40–50 IU/dL for at least 4–5 days after delivery, to reduce the risk of postpartum haemorrhage.
- A blood sample needs to be collected from the neonate at delivery but sometimes repeat testing at 3–6 months is required for definitive exclusion of some disorders such as mild to moderate haemophilia B or von Willebrand's.
- IM injections must be avoided in neonates with possible inherited bleeding disorders, giving oral prophylactic vitamin K instead along with SC or intradermal administration of routine immunizations.
- Immunization against hepatitis B should be considered in affected neonates, who should also be registered with a haemophilia centre.

Haemoglobinopathies

Sickle cell disease

The sickle cell disorders are a group of inherited abnormalities of haemoglobin synthesis. Although these disorders are more commonly seen in Black people of African origin, they are also seen in Saudi Arabians, Indians, and Mediterraneans. There are in excess of 40 different haemoglobinopathies in this group, all sharing an abnormal form of haemoglobin due to substitution of the glutamic acid residue by the valine residue, at position 6 of the beta-globin chain of the haemoglobin molecule.

- The most commonly found variants are sickle cell anaemia (HbSS, homozygous for sickle cell gene), sickle cell haemoglobin C disease (HbSC, heterozygous for sickle cell and haemoglobin C), and sickle cell β thalassaemia (HbS B thal, heterozygous for sickle cell and β thalassaemia).
- Sickle cell trait (Hb AS) is much more common but does not affect pregnancy in the same way as sickle cell disease. It does, however, have implications for genetic counselling.

The pathophysiological basis of the condition involves distortion of the shape of the red cell into a rigid sickle shape occurring as a result of haemoglobin S forming fibrous precipitates under conditions of deoxygenation. The distorted erythrocytes lead to microvascular blockage and stasis leading to further sickling, stasis, and infarction that may affect any organ in the body (bones, kidneys, lungs, and spleen).

- The sickle crises can be precipitated by cold, infection, dehydration, and pregnancy in addition to hypoxia.
- Their clinical presentation is with haemolytic anaemia and vaso-occlusive symptoms.
- Clinical features include anaemia, infections, acute chest syndrome (fever, chest pain, tachypnoea, leucocytosis and pulmonary infiltrates), retinopathy, leg ulcers, stroke, avascular necrosis of bone, renal papillary necrosis, and splenic sequestration.

Effect of pregnancy on disease

During pregnancy, complications of sickle cell disease are more common especially in the form of acute chest syndrome. Sickle crises may affect up to 35% of pregnancies and there is an increased risk of urinary tract infections (UTIs), pyelonephritis, pneumonia, puerperal sepsis, and anaemia. Pulmonary embolism may be difficult to distinguish from acute chest synrdome. Maternal mortality is estimated at around 2%.

Effect of disease on pregnancy

As there is a risk of the fetus having sickle cell disease the couple needs to be counselled as to whether prenatal diagnosis is appropriate or acceptable to them as it may lead to further ethical and religious dilemmas. These dilemmas are complicated by different variants of the disease and the wide diversity of the clinical course with sickle cell disease both between individuals with the same genotype and any individual during the course of their life. Women with sickle cell disease in pregnancy have a higher risk of miscarriage, IUGR, premature labour, early onset, and accelerated pre-clampsia resulting in higher incidence of fetal distress and delivery by Caesarean section. There is a four- to sixfold increase in perinatal mortality.

Management

Ideally pre-conception counselling with a discussion of risks and a plan for antenatal care along with screening of partner should be undertaken. However, most commonly, the antenatal booking visit is the first opportunity to address issues such as screening the partner, prenatal diagnosis, assessment of maternal health with respect to haematological parameters, and complications associated with sickle cell disease.

- The booking investigations should include quantitative haemoglobin electrophoresis, blood group and antibody screen, liver function tests, antibodies to hepatitis B and C, syphilis and rubella serology, and urine culture.
- A multidisciplinary approach with combined obstetric and haematological input is required setting out a clear management plan.
- Folic acid should be prescribed to aid haemopoiesis and haemoglobin (Hb) level should be checked on a regular basis throughout pregnancy along with estimation of the HbS percentage to consider the need for blood transfusion.
- Urine should be regularly screened for infection.
- Fetal surveillance with ultrasound biometry and umbilical artery Dopplers should be performed from 24 weeks.
- Iron supplementation is indicated only where there is biochemical evidence of iron deficiency, as iron may have accrued from previous transfusions.
- Sickle crises should be managed aggressively with intravenous hydration, antibiotics, adequate analgesia, warmth, and maintaining the patient well oxygenated.
- During labour and delivery and during the first 24 hours postnatally it is essential to ensure adequate hydration and avoid hypoxia.
- Continuous EFM in labour is recommended.
- The use of prophylactic antibiotics in the peripartum period is controversial, but careful consideration should be given to thromboprophylaxis.
- Prior to discharge the issue of contraception should be addressed.

161

Thalassaemias

The thalassaemia syndromes are the most common of the genetic blood disorders, the basic defect being a reduced rate of globin synthesis through deletion of one or more of the α-globin genes or the presence of defective β-globin genes. As a result, the red cells formed have inadequate haemoglobin content. α-Thalassaemia is more common in Southeast Asia, whereas β-thalassaemia is more common in Cypriots, Asians, and a broad band of peoples around the Mediterranean.

- In α-thalassaemia trait, there may be three normal α genes (α+) or two normal α genes (α0). These individuals are asymptomatic, but the latter group may become anaemic during pregnancy.
- In α-thalassaemia major (Hb Barts) there are no functional α-genes and the condition is incompatible with life, the fetus becoming severely hydropic and often born prematurely.
- Patients with β-thalassaemia trait have one defective β-globin gene and are asymptomatic, although they may become anaemic in pregnancy.

Haemoglobinopathies (*continued*)

- Individuals with β-thalassaemia major have two defective β-globin genes and therefore become transfusion-dependent. Survival of these children has improved now reaching the second and third decade. Repeated transfusions gradually lead to iron overload and endocrine, hepatic, and cardiac dysfunction—cardiac failure being a common mode of demise. Puberty is often delayed and incomplete and there have only been anecdotal reports of successful pregnancy in truly transfusion-dependent patients.

α-Thalassaemia major is not compatible with life, while patients with β-thalassaemia major are not encountered in obstetric practice. Patients with α-thalassaemia trait and β-thalassaemia trait need to be counselled preferably prior to pregnancy and their partners screened so that if the partner is also thalassaemia trait/minor then appropriate prenatal diagnosis can be offered to the couple. These patients will need folate supplementation at 5 mg/day and oral iron supplementation if iron-deficient, but no parenteral iron. In cases of severe anaemia, blood transfusion may be required.

163

Renal disease

In pregnancy the glomerular filtration rate (GFR) is increased by 50% because renal plasma flow is increased by 40–50% compared to the non-pregnant state. This is due primarily to volume expansion. Thus creatinine clearance increases to about 150–170 mL/min per 1.73 m². As a result creatinine levels of more than 75 μmol/L and urea levels of more than 4.5 mmol/L merit further investigation. Glycosuria in pregnancy may reflect altered renal physiology and not necessarily imply hyperglycaemia. Abnormal proteinuria is more than 500 mg per 24 hours.

Underlying renal lesions may result in marked increments in protein excretion during pregnancy. This, however, should not be misconstrued as exacerbation of disease. Abnormal blood urate levels are more than 300 μmol/L. There is marked dilatation of the calyces, renal pelvis, and ureters. These changes appear in the first trimester of pregnancy and therefore they result more from hormonal changes brought about by progesterone than from back pressure. Vesicoureteric reflux occurs sporadically. The combination of reflux and ureteric dilatation is associated with a high incidence of urinary stasis and an increased tendency to urinary tract infection and the development of pyelonephritis, especially in women with asymptomatic bacteriuria.

Urinary tract infection (UTI)

True bacteriuria is defined as more than 100 000 bacteria of the same species per mL of urine. The most common infecting organism is *Escherichia coli* and this occurs in 90% of cases. Other organisms frequently responsible include species of *Klebsiella*, *Proteus*, coagulus-negative *Staphylococcus*, and *Pseudomonas*.

Asymptomatic bacteriuria

This is defined as true bacteriuria without subjective evidence of a UTI. It is found in 2% of sexually active women and is more common (up to 7%) during pregnancy. Of patients with asymptomatic bacteriuria, 40% would become symptomatic with UTI and acute pyelonephritis. Acute pyelonephritis can cause fetal growth restriction, fetal death, and preterm labour.

This is an argument for screening all women for bacteriuria at booking. If present on two midstream samples of urine (MSUs), treatment should be given.

- Ampicillin or cephalosporin are the antibiotics of choice. A single dose of amoxycillin 3 g orally is usually effective. One must test for cure after 1 and 2 weeks.
- Coagulase-negative infection (*Staphylococcus albus*) should be treated with flucloxacillin 250 mg tds.
- Sulfonamides *should be avoided* because they competitively inhibit the binding of bilirubin to albumin and can increase the risk of neonatal hyperbilirubinaemia.
- Nitrofurantoin *should be avoided* in late pregnancy because of the risk of haemolysis in the newborn due to possible deficiency of erythrocyte phosphate dehydrogenase in the newborn.
- Tetracyclines *are contraindicated* during pregnancy because they predispose to dental staining and, rarely, may cause acute fatty liver.
- The folic acid antagonist trimethoprim can be an extremely effective antibiotic for UTIs and may be used on a long-term basis in pregnancy with folic acid supplements. A prophylactic dose of 100 mg nightly with 5 mg folic acid is effective in women with a long-term history of UTI.

Pyelonephritis

The presenting picture may consist of malaise with urinary frequency or a more florid picture with a raised temperature, tachycardia, vomiting, and loin pain. Pyelonephritis occurs in 1–2% of all pregnancies. UTIs should be considered in those with hyperemesis and in women admitted with preterm labour. Treatment is with bed rest and plenty of fluids. Antibiotic sensitivity should be identified within 48 hours and an appropriate antibiotic commenced.

- After blood and urine culture, antibiotics such as cefuroxime 1 g every 8 hours can be given IV, or according to sensitivity results, especially if the patient is vomiting and cannot tolerate oral medication. Treatment should continue for at least 2 weeks and an MSU sample should be checked every fortnight for the rest of the pregnancy.
- Recurrent infection commonly occurs in up to 30% of women and 15% continue to have positive urinary cultures. These women require long-term low-dose antibiotics, either cephalosporin, ampicillin, or trimethoprim.
- About 20% of women who have pyelonephritis in pregnancy have underlying renal tract abnormalities and an ultrasound is recommended during pregnancy or an intravenous urogram (IVU) about 12 weeks postpartum.
- Nitrofurantoin, 100 mg every 12–24 hours orally with food, should be given to prevent recurrences. This drug should be avoided if the GFR is less than 50 mL/min. Side-effects include vomiting, peripheral neuropathy, pulmonary infiltration, and liver damage.

Chronic renal disease

- In women with mild renal deficiency with plasma creatinine less than 125 μmol/L and in those without hypertension and proteinuria of 1 g per day there is little evidence that pregnancy accelerates renal disorders.
- Women with moderate renal deficiency with plasma creatinine levels of 125–250 μmol/L may progress to serious renal deterioration with uncontrolled hypertension and increase in proteinuria and may also result in a poor obstetric outcome. Renal function may decline even further in the postpartum period.
- Those with severe renal disease with plasma creatinine levels of more than 250 μmol/L and those with marked anaemia, hypertension, retinopathy, or heavy proteinuria should avoid pregnancy as further deterioration in renal function may be expected and fetal loss is considerable (up to 60%). These women should be managed in close collaboration with renal physicians during the pregnancy.

Care should include visits at least every 2 weeks until 32 weeks and then weekly.

- Blood pressure monitoring may include domiciliary monitoring and ambulatory monitoring to obtain a profile.
- A 24-hour creatinine clearance and protein excretion should be done fortnightly if there is increased excretion on Dipstix testing.
- Uric acid and platelets should be measured at each visit from 26 weeks gestation as an indicator of superimposed pre-eclampsia.

Renal disease (*continued*)

Women on dialysis during pregnancy are prone to complications of fluid overload, hypertension, pre-eclampsia, and polyhydramnios. A 50% increase in dialysis may be needed and life-threatening outcome may be up to 50%. Outcome is better for women with renal transplant as more than 90% of those who go past the first trimester would have successful pregnancies.

Acute renal failure

This condition should be suspected when the urine volume remains inadequate following adequate fluid replacement. Renal failure could be pre-renal or renal due to acute tubular necrosis or acute cortical necrosis. Causes include septicaemia, e.g. from septic abortion or pyelonephritis, haemolysis from sickling crisis or malaria, or hypovolaemia, e.g. in pre-eclampsia, haemorrhage (antepartum, abruptio, or postpartum), disseminated intravascular coagulation (DIC) abortion, or adrenal failure in those on steroids not receiving booster doses to cover labour. Whenever these situations occur the patient should be catheterized and an hourly urine volume should be measured. Management aims to achieve a volume of more than 30 mL/hour output. Monitor renal function with U&Es, and creatinine in addition to urine output. Dialysis may be needed, especially in cases of anuria.

Adrenal disease

The majority of adrenal disorders will have been diagnosed and treated prior to pregnancy. Atypical presentations of hypertension in pregnancy should however prompt consideration of other diagnoses such as phaeochromocytoma or Conn's syndrome.

Phaeochromocytoma

This is a tumour of the adrenal medulla resulting in excess secretion of catecholamines. The incidence of phaeochromocytomas in non-pregnant hypertensive patients is around 1 per 1000, but they are exceedingly rare in pregnancy. Phaeochromocytomas are bilateral in 10% of cases, malignant in 10%, and extra-adrenal in 10%. Hypertension in pregnancy is not uncommon, but atypical features such as excessive sweating, palpitations, anxiety, and headaches may indicate patients that need to be screened for the rare possibility of a phaeochromocytoma. Diagnosis can be confirmed by measuring 24-hour urinary catecholamines or their metabolites such as VMA (vanillymandelic acid) or 5HIAA (5-hydroxyindoleacetic acid). Localization of the tumour is by computerized tomography (CT), magnetic resonance imaging (MRI), or ultrasound. The tumour can also be localized using radiolabelled MIBG (metaiodobenzylguanidine), but MIBG is contraindicated in pregnancy.

The problems associated with phaechromocytomas in pregnancy are the potentially fatal hypertensive crises that may be triggered by the stress of labour or abdominal or vaginal delivery or the pressure exerted by the gravid uterus on the tumour whilst supine. Both maternal and fetal mortality are greatly increased, with maternal mortality of 17% and fetal mortality of 25% in undiagnosed cases. Maternal mortality may be due to arrhythmias, cardiovascular accident (CVA), or pulmonary oedema.

- The management in pregnancy involves medical stabilization with α blockade followed by β blockade to control the tachycardia.
- If the diagnosis is made prior to 24 weeks, surgical management is recommended.
- After 24 weeks, if the patient is medically stabilized, the surgery is probably best delayed to achieve further fetal maturity and surgery may be combined with an elective Caesarean section. Expert anaesthetic involvement is essential with α blockade for at least 3 days preoperatively.
- Postnatally, the patient needs to be monitored for recurrence.

Cushing's syndrome

This condition represents an excess of glucocorticoids and is rare in pregnancy. It is usually associated with anovulation and therefore subfertility. Glucocorticoid excess presenting in pregnancy requires urgent investigation as there is a 10% chance of malignancy of the adrenal cortex. Diagnosis requires demonstration of raised plasma and urinary cortisol comparing it with pregnancy -adjusted ranges along with low levels of adrenocorticotrophin (ACTH). The increased cortisol is not suppressed by dexamethasone, indicating its adrenal origin. Localization of the tumour will require CT or MRI.

Maternal morbidity and mortality are increased with pre-eclampsia being a common finding. There is greater postoperative maternal morbidity due to poor tissue healing. There is an increased incidence of fetal loss, prematurity and perinatal mortality only partly explained by maternal hypertension and diabetes. The neonate is at risk of adrenal insufficiency.

Drugs used in the management of Cushing's syndrome include metyrapone, trilostane, and aminoglutethimide, which block various points in the biosynthetic pathway of cortisol, and cyproheptadine, a serotonin antagonist that is used to inhibit corticotrophin-releasing hormone, but there is very limited experience with the use of these drugs in pregnancy with only anecdotal reports.

- Surgery is the treatment of choice for both pituiutary-dependent and adrenal Cushing's syndrome and has been undertaken successfully in pregnancy.

Conn's syndrome

Primary hyperaldosteronism is caused by adrenal aldosterone-secreting adenoma or carcinoma or bilateral adrenal hyperplasia. It is a very rare cause of hypertension in pregnancy. Diagnosis is based on a low serum potassium < 3 mmol/L) along with raised serum aldosterone and suppressed rennin activity. Full investigation may be postponed till after pregnancy, when radiolabelled selenium cholesterol can be used. Management involves control of hypertension methyldopa, labetalol, or nifedipine) and potassium supplementation for the hypokalaemia. Spironolactone should be avoided in pregnancy as it is an antiandrogen and may affect a male fetus.

169

Addison's disease

This presents as adrenocortical failure with deficiency of glucocorticoids and mineralocorticoids. The most common cause in the UK is autoimmune destruction of the adrenals by adrenal antibodies. Up to 40% of these patients also have other autoimmune conditions such as pernicious anaemia, diabetes, or thyroid disease. Worldwide TB is another significant cause of adrenal failure. Diagnosis is based on a low cortisol (both free and total cortisol levels rise in pregnancy), a raised ACTH, and no response to synthetic ACTH (Synacthen test).

Pregnancy does not affect the course of Addison's disease other than by possibly delaying the diagnosis as some of the features of the condition are commonly encountered in pregnancy. There may be a requirement for increased doses of steroids to cover certain periods of stress such as intercurrent illness, labour and delivery, or surgery. Provided the condition is diagnosed and treated there is no adverse effect on pregnancy.

- Management of Addison's disease in pregnancy should continue as in the non-pregnant individual, with hydrocortisone (20–30 mg/day) and fludrocortisone (0.05–0.20 mg/day), with appropriate additional hydrocortisone at times of increased stress. Clinical well-being and blood pressure provide a good index of adequate steroid replacement.
- Breastfeeding is not contraindicated.

Congenital adrenal hyperplasia (CAH)

CAH is an autosomal recessive disorder with a gene frequency of 1 in 200–400, the most common abnormality being due to 21-hydroxylase deficiency causing reduced cortisol production and increased androgen synthesis. Pregnancies in women with CAH diagnosed in infancy are uncommon as they are often infertile. Many have anovulation associated with polycystic ovaries, while others often have psychosexual difficulties with anatomical problems following corrective surgery (clitoral surgery, vaginal scarring) performed for virilization of the genitalia.

Adrenal disease (*continued*)

In the small numbers of pregnancies in women with CAH, there appears to be a higher than average risk of miscarriage, pre-eclampsia, and IUGR along with higher rates of Caesarean section required because of an android pelvis and in an attempt to avoid the risks of vaginal and perineal lacerations in those with previous history of perineal surgery. During pregnancy, increased surveillance is required for pre-eclampsia and corticosteroid therapy needs to be maintained.

In cases where the fetus is at risk of CAH (i.e. previous child with CAH), a number of options are available.
- Ideally, genetic counselling after the birth of the previous child should have been undertaken along with pre-conception counselling prior to embarking on the current pregnancy. If this is the case, dexamethasone can be started either pre-conception or as soon as pregnancy is confirmed prior to differentiation of the external genitalia.
- Prenatal diagnosis by CVS to determine the sex and, if female, the 21 hydroxylase zygosity should be performed.
- If the fetus is male or an unaffected female, treatment *in utero* will not be required and maternal dexamethasone may be discontinued.
- If the fetus is an affected female the options include continuation with dexamethasone throughout the pregnancy or a termination of pregnancy (TOP).
  —If dexamethasone is continued, maternal oestriol levels should be measured 6–8 weekly to confirm compliance and adrenal suppression and the mother needs to be monitored for impaired glucose tolerance and hypertension.
- Postnatally the child needs to be examined carefully for evidence of virilization and the salt-wasting form of the disease and to receive the appropriate glucocorticoids and mineralocorticoid replacement therapy. Unfortunately, suppression of virilization with this regime is not always successful and parents must be fully counselled regarding the options available to them.

171

Pituitary disorders

Hyperprolactinaemia

This may be a result of pituitary adenomas but a variety of other causes includ normal pregnancy, hypothalamic or pituitary stalk lesions, empty sella syn drome, hypothyroidism, chronic renal failure, and drugs.

Prolactinomas are divided into microprolactinomas (< 1 cm) or macropro lactinomas (> 1 cm in size). Women with primary hyperprolactinaemia ar amenorrhoeic with anovulation and secondary oestrogen deficiency, while oth ers with secondary hyperprolactinaemia have ongoing ovarian activity. Outsid pregnancy the diagnosis is made on the level of serum prolactin in conjunctio with imaging of the pituitary fossa by CT or MRI. In pregnancy prolactin level are greatly raised physiologically and hence this is unhelpful.

Many patients will require treatment with dopamine receptor agonist (bromocriptine or cabergoline) to restore fertility and achieve conception. I patients with a macroprolactinoma, the general advice is to continue with bar rier contraception until imaging confirms shrinkage of the prolactinoma t within the fossa.

- In patients with both micro- and macroprolactinomas, treatment with dopamine receptor agonists should be discontinued upon confirmation of pregnancy.
- Routine visual field testing is not indicated in pregnancy.
- The patient is asked to report symptoms of headache and visual disturbance, which would herald tumour expansion.
  —This can be confirmed by pituitary imaging and treated by bromocriptine
- The risk of tumour expansion and clinical symptoms is 15% for macroprolactinomas and 1.6% for microprolactinomas and is highest in the third trimester.
- Hyperprolactinaemia has no deleterious effect *per se* on pregnancy and breastfeeding is not contraindicated.

Hypopituitarism

Anterior pituitary failure may be the result of pituitary surgery, radiotherapy pituitary or hypothalamic tumours, postpartum pituitary infarction, or autoim mune lymphocytic hypophysitis. The diagnosis is based on a combination o signs and symptoms and confirmed by laboratory investigations. There ar reduced levels of thyroxine, TSH, cortisol, ACTH, follicle-stimulating hormon (FSH), luteinizing hormone (LH), and growth hormone (GH). Furthermore there is a failed response manifest by impaired secretion of ACTH, GH, and pro lactin in response to an insulin stress test. Imaging of the pituitary region i required to exclude a space-occupying lesion.

Pregnancy is possible but gonadotrophin stimulation of ovulation may be required. Once pregnancy is achieved the fetoplacental unit takes over productio of gonadotrophin, oestradiol, and progesterone. Provided the condition has bee diagnosed and adequately treated, maternal and fetal outcome is normal, but a higher incidence of adverse outcome in terms of maternal morbidity and mor tality due to hypotension and hypoglycaemia along with increased miscarriag and stillbirth rate is encountered in inadequately treated cases. Managemen involves replacement therapy with thyroxine and glucocorticoids, but mineralo corticoids may not be required as mineralocorticoid secretion is independent o the pituitary. Lactation may be impaired because of prolactin deficiency.

Diabetes insipidus

Posterior pituitary failure results in diabetes insipidus (DI). Deficient production of antidiuretic hormone (ADH) from the posterior pituitary may be caused by an enlarging pituitary adenoma, a craniopharyngioma, skull trauma, or post-neurosurgery. DI may be nephrogenic in origin due to chronic renal disease or it may be related to pregnancy due to increased vasopressinase production by the placenta or reduced vasopressinase breakdown by the liver as with pre-eclamptic toxaemia or acute fatty liver of pregnancy (AFLP). Pregnancy may unmask previously subclinical DI. Over half the patients with DI show deterioration in pregnancy, possible mechanisms being increased GFR of pregnancy, vasopressinase production by the placenta, and potential antagonism of vasopressin by prostaglandins. DI has no adverse effects on pregnancy, other than possibly a slight increase in uterine contractility owing to the structural similarity of dDAVP to oxytocin.

- Treatment of choice for central DI is intranasal dDAVP (desamino D-arginyl vasopressin) 10–20 μg two to three times a day.
- For nephrogenic DI outwith pregnancy, chlorpropamide increases renal responsiveness to ADH, but is not advisable in pregnancy, carbamazepine being a safer option in pregnancy.

173

Acromegaly

This is rarely encountered in pregnancy. Most patients are infertile due to coexisting hyperprolactinaemia in 40% of cases. Biochemical diagnosis in pregnancy is unreliable. GH-secreting adenomas expand during pregnancy and may cause visual symptoms. GH does not cross the placenta. There is, however, a greater risk of gestational diabetes and resulting macrosomia. Treatment is by surgery or radiotherapy prior to pregnancy. Medical options include the use of bromocriptine, which may work in 50% of cases, and a somatostatin analogue, octreotide, but no data is available on its use in pregnancy.

Rhesus isoimmunization

Rhesus isoimmunization is the condition wherein incompatibility exist between the fetal and maternal blood group antigens such that an immun response occurs. If an exchange occurs between fetal and maternal blood (as a delivery, placental abruption, threatened miscarriage, invasive procedures), the the passage of fetal cells into the maternal system provokes in the mother a antibody response to the fetal red blood cell antigen. This primary respons causes a production of IgM that does not cross the placenta. The fetus is there fore not affected by this process. However, if the mother is subsequently expose to the same red blood cell antigen, her primed memory B cells swiftly produc IgG antibody. Maternal IgG antibodies are actively transported across the pla centa, and bind to the fetal red cell antigen causing red blood cell destruction and ultimately haemolytic anaemia in the fetus.

If severe haemolytic anaemia does develop, then hydrops fetalis may occur (feta ascites, pleural effusions, pericardial effusions, tissue oedema).

There are five rhesus antigens, D, C, c, E, and e, but Rh (D) is the most preva lent. There are also in addition atypical blood group antigens (e.g. Kell, Duffy Kidd) that may occasionally give rise to haemolytic disease of the fetus and new born. In this chapter the discussion will be confined to Rh (D) disease.

Rhesus (anti-D) prophylaxis

Prophylaxis needs to be considered when a Rh (D) negative mother is carrying a potentially Rh (D) positive fetus. When a sensitizing event occurs, exogenou anti-D immunoglobulin should be administered within 72 hours. This binds to the antigenic fetal blood cell and prevents the immunological response devel oping in the mother

Anti-D immunoglobulin, which has been routinely available in the UK sinc 1971, is used when a sensitizing event occurs and the protection is effective fo 6–8 weeks. Despite this, a significant number of cases of Rh (D) immunizatio occur each year. Therefore it has been suggested that routine prophylaxis of al Rh negative women would dramatically affect the incidence of the disease.[1] Thi policy has now been introduced in many units with 500 IU administered at 28 and 34 weeks gestation.

Standard dosages of prophylactic anti-D immunoglobulin are 250 IU before 20 weeks and 500 IU after 20 weeks.

Without a programme of anti-D prophylaxis, 1% of Rh negative women wil have antibodies at the end of the first pregnancy with an Rh positive baby, 7–9% will have antibodies 6 months post-delivery, and a further 7–9% after a secon pregnancy. Therefore, 17% women will have Rh antibodies by the end of thei second pregnancy with an Rh positive baby.

Monitoring the pregnancy

All pregnant women have their blood group determined (ABO and Rh status); and a screen for antibodies is taken.

- If she is Rh positive, the antibody screen is checked at the beginning of the third trimester.
- If she is Rh negative with no previous history of sensitization, antibody screening should be repeated at 28 and 34 weeks.
- If antibodies are present, the paternal blood group is checked. If he is Rh negative, and no doubt about paternity exists, assume an Rh negative fetus, and there is no requirement for further testing.
- If the father is Rh positive, then it will be necessary to determine whether he is homozygous or heterozygous for the D antigen. If he is homozygous, then the fetus will be Rh positive. If he is heterozygous, then there is a 1:2 likelihood that the fetus will be Rh positive.

Antibody levels

If antibodies are present, then serial measurements should be performed every 2–4 weeks.

- An anti-D antibody level of 4 IU or less signifies no or very minimal risk of haemolytic disease in the fetus.
- If the antibody level is above 10 IU at the beginning of the pregnancy or if there is a sudden rise in the antibody level, the risk of fetal haemolytic anaemia increases and further investigation of the pregnancy is mandatory.[2]
- If the father is heterozygous for the D antigen or rhesus isoimmunization occurred in a previous pregnancy, amniocentesis should be considered to determine fetal Rh status.

177

Fetal surveillance

Hydrops fetalis (ascites, pleural or pericardial effusions, soft tissue oedema) is severe consequence of the haemolytic anaemia due to Rh disease. This can b detected by ultrasound examination of the fetus. However, a fetus may b severely anaemic, and not have any ascites.

If Anti-D levels rise above 4 IU, and the fetus is presumed to be Rh positive, feta surveillance should commence weekly. Monitoring consists of:

- Search for indicators of early hydrops: ability to visualize both sides of the fetal bowel; pericardial effusions; enlargement of the right atrium.[3]
- Fetal liver length and spleen perimeter (determined by ultrasound (U/S))
- Doppler assessment of maximum umbilical vein velocity (UV_{max}).

Reduced fetal movement counting and reduced fetal breathing movemer (determined by U/S) may be an ominous sign.

Invasive testing

Where the antibody levels reach 15 IU or more and in the presence of a rhesus positive fetus invasive testing is required.

Amniocentesis

This method was introduced into the management of Rhesus disease by Lile in 1961.[4]

- Bilirubin, the breakdown product of red blood cell haemolysis, is excreted into the amniotic fluid. A sample of amniotic fluid is taken, and the bilirubin is estimated indirectly by measuring the optical density difference at 450 nm (difference in OD_{450}).
- The amniocentesis should be performed under direct ultrasound guidance with particular care to avoid the placenta.
- With the use of the Liley chart, a prediction can be made when further interventions may be necessary, e.g. fetal blood sampling.
- This estimation of bilirubin production is unreliable before 27 weeks, and each invasive procedure may provoke a further rise in maternal antibody level

Fetal blood sampling

This method directly assesses the severity of the disease and is the method o choice. The procedure is performed under direct U/S guidance.

- Usually the umbilical cord is sampled at the placental insertion or at the intrahepatic portion of the umbilical vein. A sample of fetal blood is taken to measure haemoglobin (Hb), haematocrit (HCT), blood group, and direct Coombs' test (DCT).
- If the HCT is more than 2 standard deviations (SD) below the mean for gestational age, an intrauterine fetal blood transfusion is indicated.
- If mild anaemia is present, and HCT > 30%, but the reticulocyte count is high or DCT strongly positive, a repeat fetal blood sample is required in 1–2 weeks (fetus at high risk of fetal anaemia).[2]
- *Timing of fetal blood sample.* If a woman has had a severely affected fetus in a previous pregnancy (and the partner is homozygous for D antigen), fetal blood sampling should be planned for 10 weeks before earliest neonatal or fetal death; fetal transfusion, or birth of severely affected fetus.
  —The procedure should not be performed before 18 weeks gestation unless fetal hydrops is present.
  —If her partner is heterozygous, then amniocentesis at 14 weeks is recommended to determine fetal Rh status.

ntrauterine fetal blood transfusion

trauterine transfusion is indicated when the fetal HCT is > 2 SD below the
ean for gestational age or fetal hydrops is present.[2]

O-negative blood is transfused either directly into the fetal vessel
(intravascular transfusion), or directly into the fetal peritoneal cavity
(intraperitoneal transfusion).

The technique involves the ultrasound-guided insertion of a 20G needle
into the placental insertion of the umbilical vein or intrahepatic vein.

—Intravascular transfusion is more effective in the correction of anaemia
and reversal of hydrops; avoids trauma to intraabdominal organs, and
allows the measurement of the post-transfusion haematocrit.

—Intraperitoneal transfusion is useful at under 20 weeks gestation when
access to fetal vessels is hazardous or when the position of the fetus poses
difficulties in access to fetal vessels.

A combination of both procedures allows increased blood volumes to be
given (lengthening times between transfusions).

ming of delivery

sing the technique of intrauterine transfusion, treatment can proceed well into
e third trimester. Once the fetus has reached 34 weeks, delivery is usually con-
dered as risks of prematurity are likely to be less than the risks of further inva-
ve procedures.

179

eferences

Tovey, L.A., Townley, A., Stevenson, B.J., and Taverner, J. (1983). The Yorkshire antenatal anti-D
immunoglobulin trial in primigravidae. *Lancet* 2, 244–6.

Rodeck, C.H. and Deans, A. (1983). Red cell alloimmunization. In *Fetal medicine: basic science and
clinical practice* (ed. C.H. Rodeck and M.J. Whittle), pp. 785–804. Churchill Livingstone, Edinburgh.

Queenan, J.J. (1982). Current management of the rhesus-sensitised patient. *Clinical Obstetrics and
Gynaecology* 25, 293–301.

Liley, A.W. (1961). Liquor amnii analysis in the management of the pregnancy complicated by rhesus sensitisation. *Annual Journal of Obstetrics and Gynaecology* 82, 1359–70.

Chapter 14

Pre-eclampsia and eclampsia

Pre-eclampsia is defined as pregnancy-induced hypertension ≥ 140/90 mm H developing after 20 weeks gestation in a previously normotensive woman association with proteinuria of ≥ 300 mg/L. In known hypertensive patients, rise in blood pressure (BP) of ≥ +30/+15 mm Hg from baseline may be important. Oedema is present in > 80% of normal pregnant women and should n be included in the diagnostic criterion. The condition resolves by 6 weeks pos partum (usually within 10 days).

Eclampsia (literally *flashing lights*) occurs in 1 in 2000 pregnancies—characterize by the occurrence of convulsions not attributable to other cerebral causes ar occurs in association with the signs and symptoms of pre-eclampsia (exclud epilepsy, subarachnoid haemorrhage, and meningitis).

Aetiology and incidence

Pre-eclampsia/eclampsia is a multisystem disorder originating in the placent The primary defect is the consequence of a failure of the developing trophobla to invade the spiral arteries during the second trimester. These arterial wa then fail to distend to accommodate the required increase in blood flow, a increase in the maternal BP acting as a compensatory mechanism. The mate nal sequelae are a result of the abnormal behaviour of the vascular endotheliur

The incidence of pre-eclampsia is 5–7% of the pregnant population. There is a increased risk in the following cases.

- Patient < 20 or > 35 years of age.
- Family history (first-degree relative).
- First pregnancy with a new partner.
- Hydatidiform mole.
- Multiple pregnancy.
- Maternal obesity (body mass index (BMI) > 32).
- Fetal/placental hydrops (multiple causes).
- Pre-existing diabetes mellitus.
- Pre-existing hypertension and/or renal disease.
- If multiparous: previous severe early-onset pre-eclampsia (< 36 weeks gestation).

There is a lower incidence in smokers (*NB*. Disease severity is often worsened i smokers due to pre-existing vascular endothelial damage).

Prevention

- Calcium supplementation: in those populations with deficiency.
- Sodium restriction and prophylactic diuretics: no place other than in patients with renal disease or salt-sensitive hypertension.
- Magnesium sulfate: pre-eclampsia is not associated with a deficiency of magnesium, and dietary manipulation has no influence on the disease incidence.
- Low-dose aspirin: may be of benefit to those populations at high risk of developing the disease.
- Vitamin C and E supplementation: lowers the incidence of pre-eclampsia i high-risk populations.

Clinical features

The clinical features of pre-eclampsia and eclampsia are extremely variable and unpredictable—a broad spectrum. Pre-eclampsia is often asymptomatic (diagnosed through raised blood pressure (BP) and proteinuria on routine antenatal screening), but clinical features can include: nausea; vomiting; general malaise; headaches (frontal and occipital—may be hard to distinguish from migraine); visual disturbance (photophobia, fortification spectra, flashing lights); epigastric pain (due to liver oedema and pericapsular swelling); irritability and altered conscious state (due to cerebral oedema). Eclampsia is characterised by tonic/clonic seizures. Death may occur from intracerebral haemorrhage or hepatic, renal, or cardiovascular failure.

Examination

A full obstetric examination should be performed, remembering that both mother and fetus are affected.

A brief neurological examination noting the presence or absence of hyperreflexia, clonus (more than three beats), focal neurological defects, and papilloedema plus an abdominal examination noting epigastric and/or hepatic tenderness.

The findings from a vaginal examination yield important information concerning the suitability for induction of labour.

Haematological investigations

These should include full blood count (FBC), urea and electrolytes (U&Es) and uric acid, liver function tests (LFTs), clotting, and group and save serum (G&S).

Hyperuricaemia due to increased production and reduced renal excretion. Rise in plasma levels of > 0.1 mM per week are normal (i.e. 0.3 mM at 30 weeks; 0.36 mM at 36 weeks). Beware of rapidly rising levels, which are a good predictor of poor disease prognosis.

Thrombocytopenia (falling platelet count is a reflection of coagulopathy—and disease prognosis).

Abnormal LFTs. An increase in the enzymes lactic dehydrogenase, aspartate, and alanine transaminase may relate to alterations in liver perfusion or hepatic congestion. Note altered range in pregnancy in comparison with non-pregnant state.

G&S is performed in case delivery by lower segment Caesarean section (LSCS) should prove necessary.

Management

There are two potential patients: the mother and her fetus.
- The main risks to the mother are eclampsia, cerebral vascular damage, renal and liver failure, HELLP, and disseminated intravascular coagulopathy.
  - HELLP (haemolysis, elevated liver enzymes, low platelets) syndrome is a variant of pre-eclampsia with a higher morbidity and mortality (4–12% of patients with severe pre-eclampsia).
  - Disseminated intravascular coagulation (DIC) may be present in severe cases.
- The main risks to the fetus are intrauterine growth restriction (IUGR), intrauterine death (IUD), and iatrogenic preterm delivery.

Mild to moderate pre-eclampsia

Mild to moderate pre-eclampsia is characterized by BP > 140/90 < 160/110 mm Hg and proteinuria > 300 mg/L). It is often asymptomatic, the diagnosis being made on routine antenatal screening. All samples of urine should be tested.
- If proteinuria is confirmed and the patient's condition permits, a 24-hour urine collection should be commenced.
- In such circumstances, BP measurements should be taken at hourly intervals and the trend observed over a period of 4 hours. If the BP is unstable, consider control of BP with antihypertensives and, in rare circumstances, consider delivery.
- Check haematological and biochemical parameters daily if the clinical condition is stable.
- Delay in delivery for 2 or more weeks may reduce the problems of immaturity after birth; however, some patients will achieve little or no gain in that time. If the fetus shows signs of compromise or if the risk of IUD exceeds the risk of prematurity by delivery of the fetus, the pregnancy should be terminated as soon as possible.

Pre-eclampsia has an unpredictable clinical progression—patients may very quickly become very ill. There is no one sign, symptom, or investigation that predicts disease progression. In patient management, consideration of fetal maturity and disease progression is essential. Always ask for senior help in formulating the management plan.

If the condition permits consider:
- If pregnancy needs to be terminated and is < 34 weeks: promote fetal lung maturation by administration of betamethasone 12 mg IM × 2 doses 12 hours apart.
- Transferring care to a unit with adequate neonatal facilities.

Fetal assessment
- Ultrasound to determine fetal growth, size, and presentation is vital for determining mode of delivery and counselling the parents regarding care of the neonate.
- Umbilical artery Doppler. Increased pulsatility index, the reduction or absence of end diastolic flow, suggests fetal compromise.
- Biophysical profile scoring (cardiotocograph (CTG); liquor volume; fetal tone, movements, and breathing movements).

Anti-hypertensive therapy

This may be required in cases of extreme prematurity ≤ 30 weeks. When initiating such treatment, a stepwise and logical approach should be undertaken, as it is difficult to predict how a particular patient will respond to the specific agent chosen. In addition, requirements may increase with the progression of the disease, with changes in treatment being required hourly, daily, or weekly. Start with methyldopa (250 mg to 1 g)/6 hours.

Severe pre-eclampsia

This is characterized by recently developed hypertension ≥ 160/110 mm Hg (mean arterial pressure (MAP) > 125 mm Hg) with proteinuria graded as ++ (> 1 g/L) in the absence of a urinary tract infection (UTI). It is often symptomatic with epigastric pain, headache, malaise, signs of hyperreflexia, clonus, or altered conscious state. Progression of disease is unpredictable and the clinical condition may rapidly worsen. Liaise early with consultant obstetrician, anaesthetist, and paediatricians regarding management. Give H_2 blocker as she may require LSCS.

Principles of management

- Delivery is the only cure. Induction of labour (IOL) or LSCS depending on the clinical picture.
- Close monitoring—one-to-one midwifery care. Summon senior help when needed.
- Strict fluid balance (85 mL total/hour input)—site indwelling urinary catheter. *NB.* Fluid overload leads to pulmonary oedema and at times to adult respiratory distress syndrome (ARDS).
- Stabilize the BP—aim for MAP = diastolic BP + (1/3) systolic BP < 125 mm Hg. Many agents are available. The most commonly employed agent is hydrallazine 5 mg boluses every 10 to 15 minutes until the BP is controlled up to a maximum dose of 20 mg. Other agents include intravenous (IV) labetolol infusion 20 mg (maximum dose 220 mg) or nifedipine 10 mg sublingually (may exaggerate the hypotensive response in patients receiving concomitant magnesium sulfate).
- Magnesium sulfate as eclampsia prophylaxis should be given—MAGPIE (magnesium sulfate for prevention of eclampsia) trial.

Eclampsia

Eclampsia has an incidence of 1:1600–2000 pregnancies. 50% of cases occur postpartum, 25% after 48 hours, but eclampsia may occur up to 10 days after delivery. Call for help and protect the airway.

Treatment

The initial eclamptic fit should be controlled by an IV loading dose of 4 g of magnesium sulfate ($MgSO_4$) to be infused over 20 minutes. $MgSO_4$ comes in a 50% weight/volume (w/v) solution, i.e. 1 g in 2 mL. The initial bolus should therefore be 8 mL of 50% w/v $MgSO_4$ made up to 20 mL with 5% dextrose.

Management (*continued*)

Thereafter, the maintenance dose is 2 g/hour. This volume needs to be deducted from hourly maintenance fluids: 40 mL of 50% w/v MgSO4 made up to 60 mL with 5% dextrose and infused at 6 mL/hour. The infusion may be discontinued after the delivery of the baby and after maternal diuresis has commenced (> 100 mL of urine output for 2 consecutive hours). It is advisable to continue MgSO4 for 24 hours after delivery or the last eclamptic fit.

Magnesium sulfate

- *Contraindications.* Cardiac disease; acute renal failure.
- *Monitoring serum levels.* Therapeutic range 2–3 mmol/L.
- *Monitor deep tendon reflexes* after loading dose plus at hourly intervals whilst on maintenance. *NB.* Check arm reflexes in patients with working epidural.
- *Monitor respiration.* Pulse oximetry whilst on MgSO$_4$. Respiratory rate > 16/min and regular.
- Dose alterations. For oliguria (< 100 mL over 4 hours) or for urea > 10 mmol/L, use a maintenance dose of 1 g/hour and measure MgSO$_4$ levels. For alanine aminotransferase (ALT) > 250 IU/L, measure MgSO$_4$ levels every 2–4 hours.

MgSO$_4$ toxicity

- 4–5 mmol/L. Loss of patellar/biceps reflex, weakness, nausea, feeling of warmth, flushing, somnolence, double vision, slurred speech, hypotension, hypothermia,
- 6–7.5 mmol/L. Muscle paralysis, respiratory arrest.
- > 12 mmol/L. Cardiac arrest.

If toxicity occurs: stop magnesium infusion and give antidote—calcium gluconate 1 g in 10 mL 0.9% saline solution.

Important points to consider

- Delivery is the only cure: antihypertensives only lower the BP, potentially masking the signs, and do not prevent disease progression.
- Do not use ergometrine/syntometrine for management of the third stage. They may cause hypertensive stroke in the mother. Oxytocin 10 IU IV will suffice.
- If eclamptic seizures do not stop with magnesium sulfate a bolus dose of MgSO$_4$ can be given or diazepam 10 mg IV can be given every 10–15 minutes. In status eclampticus, paralyse and ventilate.
- Monitor the patient on the labour ward for at least 24 hours after delivery—observations to be taken half-hourly to start with (BP; temperature, pulse, respiration (TPR); O$_2$ sats; urine output; strict fluid regimens).
- Use intensive therapy unit (ITU) facilities when necessary. Consider invasive monitoring (central venous pressure (CVP)/Swann–Ganz catheter) if there is difficulty with maintaining fluid balance, especially if large-volume blood replacement becomes necessary.

14 Pre-eclampsia and eclampsia

Recommended further reading

1 Witlin, A.G. and Sibai, B.M. (1998). Magnesium sulphate therapy in pre-eclampsia [review]. *Obstetrics and Gynaecology* **95** (5), 883–9.

2 Hayman, R. and Baker, P. (2000). Labour ward management of pre-eclampsia. In *Best practice in labour ward management* (ed. L. Keen, P. Baker, and D. Edelston), pp. 253–94. W.B. Saunders, London.

3 Hallah, M. (1999). Hypertension in pregnancy. In *High risk pregnancy: management options*, 2nd edn (ed. D.K. James, P.J. Steer, C.P. Weiner, and B. Gonik), pp. 639–65. W.B. Saunders, London.

Diabetic pregnancies

Pregnancy is a state of insulin resistance and relative glucose intolerance. The insulin resistance is thought to be a result of placental production of anti-insulin hormones such as human placental lactogen (hPL), cortisol, and glucagon. Fasting glucose levels are reduced, while postprandial glucose levels are elevated in comparison to the non-pregnant state. Insulin production is increased twofold in normal pregnant women, while the insulin requirements of diabetic women also rise. There is also an increase in glycosuria due to lowering of the renal threshold for glucose.

Diagnosis

In the UK the prevalence of insulin-dependent diabetes mellitus (IDDM) is 0.5%, while the prevalence of non-insulin-dependent diabetes mellitus (NIDDM) is 2% (10% in Asian immigrants). Gestational diabetes mellitus (GDM) is diagnosed when the fasting glucose level is greater than 7.0 mmol/L on two occasions in asymptomatic women or a random glucose level is greater than 11.1 mmol/L on two occasions. Borderline cases should undergo an oral glucose tolerance test (75 g) after which diabetes may be diagnosed if either the fasting level is greater than 7.0 mmol/L or the 2-hour value is greater than 11.1 mmol/L. Gestational diabetes mellitus should be used to describe women in whom the criteria for diabetes are met in pregnancy. This latter group will invariably include a proportion (20–30%) of diabetics who were undiagnosed before pregnancy. Impaired glucose tolerance is defined as a 2-hour post-glucose-tolerance-test (GTT) glucose concentration of 8–11 mmol/L with a normal fasting glucose.

Effect of pregnancy on diabetes

Insulin requirements rise in pregnancy, reaching maximal levels by term and being at least two times the pre-pregnancy requirements. In patients with diabetic nephropathy there may be a deterioration of both renal function and proteinuria with a decrease in creatinine clearance in one-third. Any deterioration in renal function during pregnancy is usually reversed after delivery with no long-term detrimental effect on the renal function. Rapid improvement in glycaemic control may lead to worsening retinopathy through increased retinal blood flow. There is a twofold risk of progression of diabetic retinopathy or the first appearance of retinopathy. Tighter diabetic control also leads to an increased incidence of hypoglycaemia, while diabetic ketoacidosis is rare unless associated with hyperemesis, infection, and tocolytic and corticosteroid therapy.

Effects of diabetes on pregnancy

Pre-existing diabetes is associated with an increased risk of congenital abnormalities and this risk appears to be associated with the degree of glycaemic control.

- Specific congenital abnormalities associated with diabetes include sacral agenesis, congenital heart defects, skeletal abnormalities, and neural tube defects.
- If the haemoglobin A_{1c} (HbA$_{1c}$) level is < 8%, the risk of congenital abnormalities is around 5%, whereas when the HbA$_{1c}$ level is > 10%, the risk of congenital abnormalities may be as high as 25% along with an increased risk of miscarriage.
- Perinatal and neonatal mortality figures can be two- to fourfold higher in babies of diabetic mothers. These figures are much lower over the last 2 decades due to improved diabetic control.

15 Diabetic pregnancies

- Babies of diabetic mothers also appear to be at risk of unexplained intrauterine death towards term and this appears to be more common in macrosomic babies.
- The fetus can tolerate hypoglycaemia well but maternal hyperglycaemia may be detrimental to the fetus, while ketoacidosis is associated with a high fetal mortality.
- Babies of diabetic mothers tend to be macrosomic, the incidence of macrosomia being greater with poor diabetic control but not totally eliminated by tight control.
    —Macrosomia carries with it the increased risk of operative delivery, birth trauma, and shoulder dystocia.
- Fetal polyuria and macrosomia are often associated with polyhydramnios, which in turn predisposes to prelabour rupture of membranes as well as preterm delivery.
- Prematurity may pose an added problem as pulmonary surfactant production is slightly delayed in babies of diabetic mothers.
    —Dexamethasone may accelerate pulmonary maturation and should not be withheld despite its deleterious effect on glycaemic control. The issue of glycaemic control can be addressed by regular monitoring of blood sugars and adjusting insulin requirements accordingly.
- Postnatally, babies of diabetic mothers are at risk of hypoglycaemia and neonatal jaundice.
- Diabetic pregnancies and in particular those with pre-existing hypertension are at increased risk of developing pre-eclampsia. This risk reaches almost 30% where there is coexisting nephropathy and hypertension.

Management

Joint obstetric and diabetic management, supported by a multidisciplinary team of specialist dieticians, nurses, and midwives, is required to optimize outcome. Pre-conception counselling is the cornerstone in successful management of diabetic pregnancies. It provides an ideal opportunity to optimize diabetic control prior to pregnancy and thus reduce the risk of congenital abnormalities, as well as to assess the presence and severity of existing diabetic complications and plan antenatal care. Folate supplementation for at least 3 months prior to conception and throughout the first trimester is advisable.

The aim of medical management is to achieve maternal normoglycaemia as far as possible with fasting glucose < 5 mmol/L and postprandial levels of < 7.5 mmol/L. In order to best assess this, regular capillary glucose series ('7 point profile') will be required to make the appropriate adjustments in insulin regime. Dietary advice on a low-sugar, low-fat, and high-fibre diet will improve glycaemic control but tighter control invariably means more frequent hypoglycaemic episodes and patients and partners/relatives should be educated on how to deal with these episodes if not already well versed. In general, short-acting insulin pre-meals and intermediate-acting insulin at bedtime will be required to achieve satisfactory control especially in later pregnancy. The degree of diabetic control needs to be assessed by serial HbA_{1c} measurements, along with ophthalmological examination and appropriate treatment if any retinopathy is detected. Where diabetes is complicated by nephropathy, regular monitoring of renal function is required in the form of serum urea, electrolytes, 24-hour urinary protein excretion, and creatinine clearance.

The increased risk of congenital abnormalities associated with diabetes means that detailed ultrasound screening should be offered in the second trimester.
- It is important to bear in mind that biochemical screening for Down syndrome will be affected by diabetes. Hence this should by interpreted using the appropriate normograms.
- Ultrasound scanning for fetal anomalies at 20 weeks should particularly exclude neural tube defects (NTDs), sacral agenesis, and cardiac malformations. If the latter is suspected, a further scan at 22–24 weeks may be justified as the heart is visualized better at this gestation.
- The frequency of antenatal visits needs to be individualized on the basis of a variety of factors such as glycaemic control, fetal growth and well-being, and the development/worsening of maternal complications such as pre-eclampsia and deteriorating renal function.

Antenatal fetal surveillance

The increased risks of fetal demise *in utero* justify close fetal monitoring especially in the third trimester.
- Serial ultrasound biometry is recommended to detect hydramnios, macrosomia, fetal growth acceleration, or the converse of reduction in growth velocity. Abnormal growth patterns should prompt closer monitoring as they may be associated with uteroplacental insufficiency.
- Umbilical artery Doppler measurements should be used when growth restriction is suspected but are not of value as a screening test.

- The routine use of biophysical profiles is controversial. In women with vascular disease, where there is suggestion of growth restriction or poor glycaemic control, closer monitoring by means of cardiotocography as a screening test for fetal acidaemia may be useful while accepting its limitations.

Labour and delivery

Timing and mode of delivery need to be individualized. Where diabetes is well controlled, there is no vascular disease, and the fetus appears appropriately grown, pregnancy can be allowed to go to term awaiting onset of spontaneous labour.

- Where there are concerns regarding macrosomia or fetal well-being, the risks of intrauterine fetal death need to be weighed against risks of respiratory distress syndrome due to early delivery. Caesarean section rates of up to 50–60% are reported in women with established diabetes and this is hardly surprising when almost half the babies born to diabetic mothers are over the 90th centile.
- Intrapartum care should focus on meticulous diabetic control, continuous electronic fetal monitoring (EFM), and judicious use of oxytocin for poor progression of labour. The target glucose range in labour is 4–7 mmol/L and this is maintained by varying the insulin infusion whilst maintaining a constant rate of 5% dextrose infusion.
- Following delivery of the placenta the infusion rate of insulin needs to be halved as maternal insulin requirements rapidly return to pre-pregnancy levels and, with breastfeeding, even less is required.
- If abnormal glucose tolerance was first diagnosed in pregnancy, a GTT is advisable at approximately 6 weeks post partum.

193

Gestational diabetes

This group includes women with carbohydrate intolerance of variable severity with onset or first presentation in pregnancy. By definition it will include previously undiagnosed diabetics. There is a strong variation in prevalence with the highest incidence of GDM in women from the Indian subcontinent followed by women from Southeast Asia.

Screening for gestational diabetes

There appears to be no consensus as to who, when, how, or even whether to screen for GDM. Universal biochemical screening has been suggested and universal screening limited to those over 25 has also been suggested. The majority of units decide on who to screen on the basis of clinical risk factors including previous GDM, family history of diabetes, previous macrosomic baby, previous unexplained stillbirth, obesity, glycosuria, polyhydramnios, and large for gestational age infant in current pregnancy. The timing of testing is also controversial as, the later in pregnancy it is performed, the higher the detection rate since glucose tolerance progressively deteriorates. On the other hand, the earlier in pregnancy GDM is diagnosed and hyperglycaemia treated, the greater the likelihood of influencing on outcome.

Implications of GDM

GDM is associated with increased perinatal mortality and morbidity but to a lesser extent than pre-existing diabetes. There is no increase in the risk of congenital abnormalities but macrosomia is the main risk factor for adverse outcome. There is an increased risk of operative delivery and maternal risks include a higher incidence of pre-eclampsia. The long-term implications of GDM provide a further justification for screening. Women identified as having GDM have a significantly increased risk of developing NIDDM in later life. This risk has variously been estimated at around 50% over the following 10–15 years. This awareness of the increased risk of developing NIDDM may enable individuals to alter their diet and lifestyle to prevent or delay the development of diabetes. It may also encourage vigilance both by the patient and her physician such that the diagnosis is made early and therefore before the development of microvascular complications.

Management

A combined diabetic–obstetric approach is essential.

- The initial approach is by dietary modification including calorie reduction in the obese patient.
- The need for insulin is heralded by persistent postprandial hyperglycaemia (> 7.5–8.0 mmol/L) or persistent fasting hyperglycaemia (> 5.5–6.0 mmol/L).
- Regular ultrasound scans to assess fetal growth and well-being are recommended though the risks to the fetus are less than in pre-existing diabetes and hence early delivery as a routine should not be advised unless there are other complicating factors.
- Intrapartum management will depend on whether the patient has been on insulin antenatally and, this being the case, how much insulin she has been receiving.
  —Patients who are diet-controlled or on relatively small doses may not require insulin in labour while those on larger doses need to be treated as pre-existing diabetics and therefore may need a sliding scale.
  —Following delivery, any insulin regime can be discontinued.
- Patients with GDM should have a GTT at 6 weeks to assess the degree of glucose intolerance outside pregnancy.

15 Diabetic pregnancies

Chapter 16

Drug use in pregnancy

In the UK about 35% of pregnant women take medication (excluding vitamins and iron) at least once in pregnancy, although only 6% do so in the first trimester. This does not include drugs used in labour. The proportion of women taking medication in pregnancy has dropped from around 80% in the 1960s, the reduction being driven by the continued attention in the news media to drug-induced fetal abnormality. However, the increasing age at which women elect to have children means that more women are already on long-term medication for chronic conditions at the time when they embark on pregnancy. Women suffering from certain medical conditions that were considered in the past to be incompatible with pregnancy (systemic lupus erythematosus (SLE), certain types of heart disease) now have the opportunity of motherhood due to dramatic improvement in medical care and pregnancy outcome.

Timing of exposure and pregnancy outcome

Medication taken in pregnancy can harm the unborn child through teratogenic effects. Teratogenesis is defined as dysgenesis of fetal organs, either in terms of structural integrity or function. Teratogenic effects may take the form of malformations that occur during the period of organogenesis or, subsequently, by causing alterations in the structure or function of organ systems formed during organogenesis. Other manifestations of teratogens include growth restriction or fetal death and carcinogenesis. In addition, some drugs such as retinoids, which are high-grade teratogens, may exert their effect for up to 2 years after the last dose.

The timing of exposure to a particular drug treatment is a critical factor in assessing the nature and extent of any adverse effects. Three important phases are recognized in human development.

1 *Pre-embryonic phase.* This extends from conception to 17 days post-conception (or 3 days after the first missed period). During this period of implantation and blastocyst formation, any adverse effect is an 'all or nothing phenomenon' and the result of an insult will either be death and abortion/resorption or intact survival through multiplication of the totipotential cells.

2 *Embryonic phase.* This period extends from post-conception day 18 to day 55 and is the most crucial period of organogenesis. It is the period of greatest theoretical sensitivity and risk of congenital malformation with rapidly differentiating tissues, so that any damage becomes irreparable. The earlier in this period the insult occurs, the more marked is the likely effect. The following lesions have been identified with time of exposure (approximate days post-conception): anencephaly, day 24; limb reduction defects, days 12–40; transposition of great vessels, day 34; cleft lip, day 36; ventricular septal defects, day 42; syndactyly, day 42; hypospadias, day 84.

3 *Fetal phase.* This phase runs from post-conceptional age 8 weeks through to term. The impact of drugs that can cross the placenta affects fetal growth and development rather than causing gross structural malformations.

Prescribing principles

When prescribing in pregnancy it is important to consider the following principles.
- Drugs should be prescribed only for clear indications and where the benefits (usually for the mother) outweigh the potential risks (usually to the fetus). Question the need for any drug in pregnancy.
- If possible, it is better to try and avoid all drugs (including non-prescription medications) in the first trimester.
- Medication should be used in the smallest effective dose for the shortest period of time required.
- It is preferable to prescribe medication that has been widely used in pregnancy and has a good safety track record, rather than newer agents that may have theoretical though as yet unproved advantages.
- All women of reproductive age are at risk of pregnancy.
- Most drugs with a molecular weight of less than 1500 are capable of crossing the placenta and therefore of potentially affecting the fetus, but very few drugs have been conclusively shown to be teratogenic.
- Encourage pre-conception counselling in all patients with chronic medical disorders and, in particular, those on long-term drug therapy. If this has not been possible, review all drug regimens as early in pregnancy as possible avoiding polypharmacy as far as possible.

Breastfeeding

The vast majority of drugs cross into breast milk. In general terms the doses of drugs reaching the baby are clinically insignificant when one considers dilution of the drug in the mother and the small volumes of milk the neonate feeds on.

Drugs can be considered in three broad categories with respect to breast feeding.
- Drugs that cannot be detected in the baby. Examples include the anticoagulant warfarin and the group of antibiotics known as aminoglycosides, which are not absorbed from the gastrointestinal tract of normal infants.
- Drugs that are detectable in the baby in clinically insignificant amounts, such as non-narcotic analgesics, nonsteroidal anti-inflammatory drugs (NSAIDs), penicillins, cephalosporins, antihypertensive drugs, bronchodilators, and most anticonvulsants except barbiturates.
- Drugs that reach the neonate in sufficient amounts to cause fetal side-effects. Examples in this group include benzodiazepines reported to cause lethargy, barbiturates causing drowsiness, amiodarone with a theoretical risk of hypothyroidism, tetracyclines because of the potential risk of discoloration of teeth, combined oral contraceptive pills (COCP) because of the risk of diminishing milk supply and reduction in nitrogen and protein content, ephedrine associated with irritability, cytotoxic drugs because of immune suppression/neutropenia, and aspirin with its risk of Reye's syndrome.

Management of pregnancy and potential teratogenesis

The risk of teratogenesis is present in two broad groups of patients. The first group comprises patients on long-term medication for a chronic condition. Ideally, they should be counselled prior to pregnancy and made aware of the risks of fetal malformation and how these risks could be reduced. Often, however, this has not been the case. The second group comprises those patients taking a single course of treatment and unaware of early pregnancy.

The management of exposure to potential teratogens in pregnancy relies on accurate determination of the history of exposure including the gestational age at exposure, as well as up-to-date information on the teratogenic potential of the agent in question at the particular gestation of exposure. Accurate dating of pregnancy is essential and this can be performed by a combination of early dating scan and menstrual and conception history. Fetal malformations associated with teratogens affect the central nervous system, cardiovascular system, arms and legs, and orofacial clefting, and there are also multisystem defects. The majority of major malformations are detectable on detailed ultrasound scanning at 18–20 weeks. Where cardiac abnormality is suspected from an earlier scan a repeat scan at around 22 weeks may be helpful. In cases where neural tube defects are one of the manifestations of exposure to a particular teratogen, maternal serum alpha-fetoprotein (MSAFP) estimation may also be of value. Further management will depend on the established risks from exposure to the given teratogen at a particular gestation time along with the wishes of the couple after comprehensive counselling, preferably by experts in the field.

Table 16.1 summarizes the teratogenic and fetal effects of common medications.

Recommended further reading

1 Rubin, P.C., Craig, G.S., Gavin, K., and Sumner, D. (1986). Prospective survey of use of therapeutic drugs, alcohol and cigarettes during pregnancy. *British Medical Journal* **292**, 81–3.

2 Moore, K.L. (1988). *The developing human: clinically oriented embryology*, 4th edn, p. 131. Philadelphia. W B Saunders, Philadelphia.

3 Arulkumaran, S. (1999). *Prescribing for the pregnant patient—is any drug safe? Update on Obstetrics and Gynaecology*. Mount Elizabeth Hospital, 13th Annual seminar, November 1999.

4 Rubin, P.C. (1995). General principles. In *Prescribing in pregnancy*, 2nd edn (ed. P.C. Rubin), pp. 1–8. BMJ Publications, London.

5 Little, B.B. (1999). Medication during pregnancy. In *High risk pregnancy—management options*, 2nd edn (ed. D.K. James, P.J. Steer, C.P. Weiner, and B. Gonik), pp. 617–38. W.B. Saunders, London.

6 De Swiet, M. (2000). Anticoagulants. In *Prescribing in pregnancy*, 3rd edn (ed. P.C. Rubin), pp. 47–64. BMJ Publications, London.

7 Koren, G., Pastuszak, A., and Ito, S. (1998). Drug therapy. Drugs in pregnancy. *New England Journal of Medicine* **338** (16), 1128–37.

Table 16.1 Drugs with proven teratogenic and fetal effects in humans

Category	Drug	Teratogenic effect
Antibiotics	Aminoglycosides	Deafness, vestibular damage
	Tetracycline	Anomalies of teeth and bone
	Quinolones	Animal studies only—irreversible arthropathy
	Sulfonamides	Hyperbilirubinaemia, kernicterus
Anticholinergics		Neonatal meconium ileus
Anticoagulants	Warfarin	Skeletal and CNS defects, Dandy Walker syndrome
Anticonvulsants	Carbamazepine	Neural tube defects
	Phenytoin	Growth retardation, CNS defects
	Valproic acid	Neural tube defects
	Paramethadione, trimethadione	CNS and facial abnormalities
Antidepressants	Lithium carbonate	Ebstein's anomaly, hypotonia, reduced suckling, hyporeflexia
Antihypertensives	ACE inhibitors	Prolonged renal failure in neonates, decreased skull ossification, renal tubular dysgenesis
	Beta blockers	Growth restriction, neonatal bradycardia, and hypoglycaemia
Antithyroid drugs	Propylthiouracil	Fetal and neonatal goitre and hypothyroidism
	Methimazole	Aplasia cutis. Fetal and neonatal goitre and hypothyroidism
Cytotoxic drugs	Aminopterin, methotrexate	CNS and limb malformations
	Cyclophosphamide	CNS malformations, secondary cancer
Diuretics	Frusemide	Decreased uterine blood flow, hyperbilirubinaemia
	Thiazides	Neonatal thrombocytopaenia
Hypoglycaemics		Neonatal hypoglycaemia
NSAIDS	Indomethacin	Premature closure of ductus arteriosus, necrotizing enterocolitis, neonatal pulmonary hypertension
	Salicylates	Haemorrhage
Prostaglandin analogues	Misoprostol	Moebius sequence, abortion, induction of labour
Recreational drugs	Ethanol	Fetal alcohol syndrome (pre- and postnatal growth restriction, CNS anomalies, characteristic facial features)
	Cocaine	Growth retardation, placental abruption, uterine rupture
Systemic retinoids	Isotretinoin, etretinate	CNS, craniofacial, cardiovascular, and other defects
Sex hormones	Danazol and other androgenic drugs	Masculinization of female fetuses
	Diethylstilboestrol	Vaginal carcinoma, genitourinary defects in male and female offspring
Sedatives	Thalidomide	Limb shortening and internal organ defects
Psychoactive drugs	Barbiturates, opioids, benzodiazepines	Neonatal withdrawal syndromes when drugs taken in late pregnancy
	Phenothiazines	Neonatal effects of impaired thermoregulation, extrapyramidal effects

Substance abuse in pregnancy

203

Substances of abuse (psychoactive drugs) are those that lead to relatively rapid effects on the central nervous system (CNS), including changes in the level of consciousness or the state of mind. These include those available for general use, e.g. alcohol, and illegal substances, e.g. cocaine and heroin. Substance abuse in pregnancy has effects on the mother and the developing fetus. Abuse in early pregnancy carries the potential risk of fetal abnormality, while in late pregnancy fetal dependence and neonatal withdrawal are potential complications.

Most users abuse more than one substance. The quality and potency of street drugs vary from time to time and place to place. This is a growing problem as most pregnancies are in young women and young people are the group most likely to be exposed to drugs either on a regular or occasional/experimental basis. Reliable statistics are, however, difficult to obtain as most drug abuse goes undetected and a history of drug abuse may not be given even when specific enquiry is made. UK data on the prevalence of drug abuse come from crime statistics, hospital admissions, special surveys, and Home Office statistics, none of which is comprehensive. One survey estimated that 1–2% of the adult population of several British cities use illicit drugs and the Home Office Addicts' Index has about 20 000 registered addicts.

Definitions

- *Harmful use.* Pattern of use that causes physical (e.g. hepatitis from needle-sharing) or mental (e.g. depression following drug use) damage to health.
- *Tolerance.* Diminishing CNS effects from repeated drug use, such that increasing doses are needed to achieve the same effects.
- *Dependence.* Condition in which the use of a drug takes higher priority for the individual than behaviours that previously had a higher value. Dependence may be physical, psychological, or combined.
- *Withdrawal state.* Physical or psychological symptoms occurring on partial or complete withdrawal of a drug after prolonged use or high dose. It may be complicated by delirium and convulsions.

Maternal problems

Drug abuse has a chronic relapsing course and a mortality risk (usually from accidental overdose) of 10–15% over 10 years. The risk of such overdose is highest after enforced abstinence, leading to loss of tolerance. Other maternal problems include the following.

- *Use of health-care facilities.* Drug abusers are likely to avoid medical and social services facilities. Late booking in pregnancy and poor attendance at antenatal clinic are common problems.
- *Crime.* Drug abuse often results in disinhibition of behaviour and impairment of judgement, leading to violence and criminal activity including theft and prostitution to finance the drug habit. Many of the crimes committed by users are petty in terms of scale but they are vast in terms of numbers.
- *Nutrition.* This is likely to be poor, as funds are diverted to buy drugs. Deficiencies of iron, vitamins, and folic acid may occur.

- *Vascular and skin complications.* Superficial and deep vein thromboses may result from venous injection of drugs. Subcutaneous extravasation or accidental subcutaneous injection may result in tissue necrosis and abscesses.
- *Infections.* Systemic infection may occur from intravenous (IV) injection, including septicaemia, bacterial endocarditis, hepatitis B and C, and HIV. Multiple sexual partners or prostitution predispose to sexually transmitted diseases including heterosexually transmitted HIV.
- *Overdose.* Inconsistent drug quality can produce accidental overdose or withdrawal symptoms, especially with intravenous drug abuse.

Fetal/neonatal problems

The effects of substance abuse on the fetus are not necessarily due to the drugs alone, but are rather a combination of poor nutrition, smoking, poor personal care, and social deprivation associated with drug abuse. Effects observed in childhood may also be partly due to the continuing adverse family and social environment rather than purely a lasting effect of the intrauterine exposure. Problems include:

- Teratogenicity risk with some substances.
- Dating problems result from late booking. Screening tests for fetal abnormality are of limited or no value with late booking and poor attendance.
- Prematurity.
- Intrauterine growth restriction.
- Stillbirth.
- Withdrawal symptoms in neonatal period.
- Vertical transmission of infection.
- Neglect of the baby.

Drugs

Morphine and diamorphine (heroin)

These are natural opiates and are the most widely abused opiates in Western countries. They can be administered by most routes, although abuse is usually by inhalation or IV injection. Clinical effects of opiate use include euphoria, analgesia, respiratory depression, pupillary constriction, constipation, reduced appetite, and reduced libido. Tolerance develops rapidly, leading to the need for increasingly higher doses. However, tolerance also diminishes rapidly such that after a period of abstinence, e.g. hospitalization for detoxification, fatal respiratory depression may result from using a previously tolerated quantity of opiate.

Symptoms of maternal withdrawal include intense craving for the drug, nausea and vomiting, body aches, joint pains, runny nose and eyes, dilated pupils, sweating, pyrexia, insomnia, tachycardia, abdominal pains, and diarrhoea. Withdrawal symptoms usually start about 6 hours after the last dose and reach a peak after 36–48 hours. A person in good health is not likely to suffer fatality from withdrawal symptoms but the great distress caused drives the person to seek further supplies. It should be borne in mind that a drug abuser presenting with non-specific abdominal pain may be exaggerating the symptoms to obtain further opiates, e.g. morphine or pethidine.

Opiates do not carry a teratogenic effect but opiate addiction is associated with intrauterine growth restriction (IUGR) and prematurity. A fetus born to a heroin-dependent mother is likely to develop withdrawal symptoms within 48 hours of birth. Severity is related to the amount and duration of drug used by the mother. Symptoms include irritability, jitteriness, tremors, poor feeding, respiratory distress, sneezing, and a high-pitched cry. The onset of withdrawal symptoms may be delayed when the mother has been on methadone as it is stored in fetal tissues and has a long half-life. The likelihood of neonatal withdrawal symptoms depends on the amount of drugs used in the antenatal period but most babies have minor symptoms if any. Management is mainly supportive and symptoms usually resolve within a few days. There are no substantiated long-term neurological defects in the baby.

Methadone

This is a synthetic opiate similar to heroin. It is available on controlled prescription form in methadone maintenance treatment programmes. Methadone is available in liquid or tablet form but is usually dispensed in liquid form. Patients on methadone may, however, still resort to illicit narcotics to 'top-up', thereby subjecting themselves and their fetuses to the risks that the treatment programmes aim to minimize. Methadone is nearly as potent as morphine and causes similar withdrawal symptoms. Because of its long half-life, methadone withdrawal manifests after 36 hours and peaks after 3–5 days.

Cocaine

Derived mainly from the leaves of the coca plant, cocaine is a potent vasoconstrictor and local anaesthetic. Cocaine can be ingested from chewing coca leaves, smoking coca paste, inhaling or injecting cocaine hydrochloride powder, or smoking crack cocaine, an alkaloid form of cocaine. Because it is a potent vasoconstrictor, nasal inhalation (snorting) leads to delayed absorption. Smoking and IV injection, however, produce a rapid and intense effect. Features of cocaine intoxication include tachycardia, elevated blood pressure, sweating, nausea, and vomiting. Behavioural changes include impairment of judgement, euphoria, agitation, grandiosity, and visual or tactile hallucinations, especially the feeling of insects crawling under the skin (formication, 'cocaine bug').

The euphoria produced by cocaine use is followed by a 'crash', characterized by mood disturbance, anxiety, fatigue, and a craving for more cocaine. Some users will use heroin to alleviate the intensity of the 'crash' following cocaine use. Sudden withdrawal can lead to delirium within 24 hours and withdrawal following chronic use can lead to paranoid and suicidal thoughts.

Although placental vasoconstriction reduces the quantity of cocaine reaching the fetus, the transfer of oxygen and nutrients is similarly impaired. Such placental vasoconstriction may cause spontaneous miscarriage, stillbirth, and placental abruption. Less severe fetal effects include IUGR and subtle neurological signs, persisting for months after birth. The effects appear proportionate to maternal drug use in the second and third trimesters.

Amphetamines

Amphetamines are CNS stimulants, with similar effects to those of cocaine. Fenfluramine and dexfenfluramine are related substances sometimes used as appetite suppressants but can cause psychological dependence. Amphetamine abuse is usually oral, but can also be IV or nasal inhalation, e.g. metamphetamine ('speed'). Amphetamines produce euphoria, excitement, a feeling of well-being, increased confidence, increased drive and energy, and a feeling of alertness and less need for sleep. Physical effects include tachycardia, pupillary dilatation, and raised blood pressure. Effects of chronic use and cessation of chronic use may be similar to those due to opiates. Chronic use of large doses may produce a state similar to schizophrenia.

Amphetamine causes vasoconstriction and hypertension, leading to chronic fetal hypoxia. There may be an association with cleft palate. Like cocaine, it increases the risks of placental abruption, IUGR, preterm delivery, and perinatal mortality. Neonatal effects include hyperactivity, tremors, poor feeding, and disordered sleep.

Hallucinogens

These include lysergic acid diethylamine (LSD), dimethyltryptamine (DMT), mescaline, phencyclidine (PCP), and 3,4-methylenedioxymethamphetamine (MDMA, 'Ecstasy'). These are usually taken orally in tablet or capsule form. Physical effects include sweating, pupillary dilatation, blurring of vision, tachycardia, palpitations, tremors, and loss of co-ordination. Psychological effects may depend on the personality of the user and include anxiety, depression, impairment of judgement, paranoid thoughts, and life-threatening delusions. Hallucinogens have been responsible for people jumping off tall buildings under the delusion that they could fly. MDMA produces feelings of euphoria, sociability, and intimacy. MDMA deaths have been attributed to hyperthermia, cardiac arrhythmias, intracerebral haemorrhage, and toxic hepatitis. Tolerance to MDMA develops quickly but no clear withdrawal syndrome has yet been described.

Drugs (*continued*)

Solvent abuse (glue sniffing)

Solvents, petrol, adhesives, butane gas, and paint thinners give off psychoactive vapours that can be inhaled either directly or from plastic bags. The latter route carries the additional risk of loss of consciousness or suffocation. Toxicity from these substances can cause death. Physical effects include dizziness, blurring of vision, poor coordination, poor concentration, slurring of speech, ataxia, muscle weakness, and tremors. Psychological effects include apathy, psychomotor retardation, and impairment of judgement and social functioning. Some solvents may cross the placenta, leading to growth restriction, microcephaly, prematurity, perinatal mortality, and developmental delay.

Cannabinoids

The major active substance in this group is tetrahydrocannabinol. The main source is the cannabis plant, the leaves of which may be smoked or chewed. Cannabinoids can lead to marked psychological dependence but not physical dependence. Cannabinoids can cause euphoria, anxiety, suspiciousness (sometimes leading to delusions of persecution), impairment of judgement, and social withdrawal. There are no substantiated fetal effects. Cannabis use may, however, be a gateway to the abuse of harder drugs with more established negative maternal and fetal effects.

Benzodiazepines

Benzodiazepines are commonly prescribed to patients of all ages and initial exposure may occur in the form of medically indicated prescription. Subsequent abuse of benzodiazepines is usually from illicit procurement. The quality and purity are variable and high doses are common. Neonatal withdrawal effects include hypotonia, feeding difficulties, and respiratory depression.

Alcohol

Total abstinence or minimal consumption of alcohol is recommended in pregnancy. Excessive consumption can lead to permanent fetal damage. Alcohol intake of over 140 g (14 units) per week may lead to fetal alcohol syndrome (FAS). Features of FAS include IUGR, microcephaly, typical facies, mild to moderate mental restriction, and increased perinatal mortality.

Tobacco

Tobacco is the substance most commonly abused in pregnancy. Complications include increased risk of placental abruption, low birth weight, neonatal death, and sudden infant death syndrome. The risk is related to the number of cigarettes smoked per day.

17 Substance abuse in pregnancy

Management

Management of opiate addiction is more formalized than for other substances of abuse but the principles are similar. Management in pregnancy is based on a multidisciplinary approach involving obstetricians, midwives, neonatologists, addiction counsellors, social workers, and health visitors. Genitourinary medicine input will be necessary for HIV-positive women. All efforts should be made to keep the pregnant woman within the service, reducing the risk to herself and the fetus and improving her long-term prospects of being weaned off her addiction.

- It is important to avoid a judgemental approach as this may drive the woman away from the needed care.
- The risks to the mother and fetus should be carefully outlined.
- The woman should be reassured of confidentiality. It is useful to have a record of friends and family who know of her addiction, as their support may be valuable.
- Recommending cessation of drug abuse is often counterproductive but this is the only way forward for some substances, e.g. cocaine, hallucinogens, amphetamines, and solvents, as there are no substitutes to use as replacement.
- Screen for hepatitis B and C, sexually transmitted diseases, and HIV after appropriate counselling.
- Screen for fetal abnormality and IUGR by ultrasound in the second and third trimesters, respectively.
- The labour ward should be informed and the neonatal unit alerted to the delivery of a baby who may have withdrawal symptoms.

Many mothers will use their opiate before coming into hospital for labour and delivery. This complicates fetal monitoring and analgesia in labour and potentiates neonatal withdrawal. Epidural analgesia is preferable to using more opiates in large doses.

When necessary, drug use can be confirmed from analysis of urine sample, although hair analysis is more informative in investigating long-term abuse.

Planned withdrawal

Eventual drug withdrawal is the ultimate aim of a treatment programme but will not succeed on its own without psychological treatment and social support. Treatment is usually done in psychiatric units or special treatment clinics. Return to drug abuse after such hospitalization carries a high risk of accidental overdose due to loss of tolerance.

Drug maintenance

This approach is adopted for patients unwilling or unable to give up drug abuse. A less addictive drug with a slower action/longer half-life is prescribed. This form of management is of particular use in opiate addiction, with methadone used as the alternative. There are no suitable substitutes for many abused substances, e.g. cocaine, amphetamines.

Maintenance therapy removes the need to obtain illicit supplies and the associated criminal tendencies. It needs to be combined with social and psychological support to enable eventual withdrawal. It should, however, be borne in mind that some subjects on maintenance programmes continue to use illicit drugs and supplement these with the supplies from the maintenance programme.

They may also obtain large amounts by registering in more than one centre. Regular urine or hair testing can be used to monitor compliance. Many pregnant women return to illicit opiates, especially after delivery. Relapse is usually related to the circumstances that made the woman an addict in the first place.

Harm reduction

This is a more controversial approach that aims to reduce the risk of serious infections, e.g. HIV, for drug abusers not willing or able to change, by offering education/counselling and practical help. The practical help includes the supply of sterile syringes and needles or advice to adopt non-injection modes of drug use.

Recommended further reading

Puri, B.K., Laking, P.J., and Treasaden, I.H. (1996). Psychoactive substance use disorders. In *Textbook of psychiatry*, pp. 119–137. Churchill Livingstone, Edinburgh.

Frischer, M. (1992). Estimated prevalence of injecting drug use in Glasgow. *British Journal of Addiction* 87, 235–44.

Gelder, M., Gath, D., Mayou, R., and Cowen, P. (1996). The abuse of alcohol and drugs. In *Oxford textbook of psychiatry*, pp. 438–81. Oxford University Press, Oxford.

Walker, J.J. (1999). Drug addiction. In *High risk pregnancy—management options*, 2nd edn (ed. D.K. James, P.J. Steer, C.P. Weiner, and B. Gonik), pp. 599–616. W.B. Saunders, London.

Llewelyn, R.W. (2000). Substance abuse in pregnancy: the team approach to antenatal care. *The Obstetrician and Gynaecologist* 2 (1), 11–16.

British Medical Association (1998). *The misuse of drugs*. Harwood Academic Publishers, Amsterdam.

Chapter 18

Multiple pregnancies

The incidence of twins in the UK is 11/1000 pregnancies and that of triplet 1/4000. There is an increasing incidence as a consequence of assisted reproductive techniques.
- Incidence following clomiphene treatment, 5–10%.
- Incidence at 20 weeks following 3-embryo transfer:
  —*In vitro* fertilization (IVF)—zygote transfer, 32%.
  —Zygote intrafallopian transfer (ZIFT), 27%.
  —Gamete intrafallopian transfer (GIFT), 16%.

The incidence of triplets as a consequence of assisted reproductive techniques is
- IVF—embryo transfer (ET), 4.1%.
- GIFT, 4.3%.

The incidence of monozygous twins is 3.5/1000.

Predisposing factors and mechanisms

Predisposing factors include the following.
- Previous history.
- Family history of twins.
- Increased maternal age (< 20 yrs, 6.4/1000; > 25 yrs, 16.8/1000; > 35 yrs, 19.1/1000).
- Induced ovulation and IVF.
- Race (Japanese, 6.7/1000 pregnancies; Nigerian, 40/1000).

Dizygotic (DZ) twinning is due to the duplication of the normal process of conception, implantation, and further development arising from the fertilization o two ova from the same or opposite ovaries. Each fetus has its own membrane both chorion and amnion, and its own placenta (dichorionic, diamniotic).

Monozygotic twinning (MZ) is a departure from the normal process of development, the varieties depending on the time after fertilization when splitting occurs in the embryo.
- Less than 3 days (8-cell stage): implantation at separate sites; same structural arrangements as in DZ pregnancies but identical fetuses (MZ—dichorionic, diamniotic).
- 4–7 days (formation of inner cell mass): single placenta; if the amnion has not developed, each embryo will develop its own amniotic membrane (monochorionic, diamniotic).
- > 8 days (*rare*).
  —Prior to primitive streak formation: single amniotic cavity and chorion (monochorionic, monoamniotic).
  —After primitive streak formation: conjoined twins.

Whenever there is a single chorion, vascular anastamoses inevitably connect the two circulations with frequent pathological sequelae.

Determination of zygosity at birth
- Twins of opposite sex are DZ.
- A single chorion on examination of the placenta and membranes = MZ.
- Dichorionic twins of like sex may be DZ or MZ and genetic markers are required.

Diagnosis

Suspect with hyperemesis gravidarum, large for dates, 3 or more fetal poles, 2 or more fetal heart sounds on auscultation. Definitive diagnosis is by ultrasound scanning. In current obstetric practice, multiple pregnancy is identified in the first trimester at the time of dating scan or when scan is done for nuchal translucency.

Complications

Pregnancy
Maternal complications
As with singleton pregnancies, but increased risks of minor and major compli
cations at all stages. The following are increased: symptoms of early pregnancy;
risk of miscarriage; anaemia (greater iron and folate requirements); polyhy
dramnios (12% of multiple pregnancies); pre-eclampsia (5% singletons, 25%
twins); musculoskeltal problems; antepartum haemorrhage; placenta praevia;
preterm labour; postpartum haemorrhage.

Fetal complications
- There is increased incidence of neural tube defects, bowel atresia, and
  cardiac anomalies. Congenital abnormalities are twice as common as in
  singletons especially in MZ twins (conjoined 1:200; acardia 1:100).
- Vanishing twin syndrome (1st trimester: prognosis good for remaining
  twin).
- Perinatal mortality 36.7/1000 (singletons 8/1000; triplets 73/1000).
- Intrauterine growth restriction (IUGR; less than 10th centile, incidence of
  25–33%).
- Antepartum fetal demise: psychological sequelae + risk of disseminated
  intravascular coagulation (DIC; 25% incidence).
- Acute polyhydramnios is more common in MZ pregnancies (10–15% of all
  twin pregnancies but 4–35% of monochorionic diamniotic pregnancies)
  and twin-to-twin transfusion syndrome with placental arteriovascular
  anastamoses with unequal vascular distribution of blood.
  —The donor twin becomes anaemic, hypovolaemic, oligohydramniotic,
    and growth-restricted and may develop hydrops.
  —The recipient becomes polycythaemic, hypervolaemic, and polyuric
    with polyhydramnios. Ascites and pleural and pericardial effusions
    may result.
  —Mortality of ≥ 79% (preterm labour and preterm prelabour rupture of
    membranes (PPROM) contributing); cord accident and death of the
    co-twin are other causes.

Complications of labour
Intrapartum
- Pre-term labour is more common (43.6% before 37 weeks as compared
  with 5.6% for singletons). Mean duration of pregnancy decreases as
  number of fetuses *in utero* increases.
- Increased risk of pulmonary oedema with tocolysis (β sympathomimetics).
- Cord accident following pre-labour rupture of the membranes—mainly
  prolapse.
- Cord entanglement and knotting in monzygotics (perinatal mortality of up
  to 50%); mortality from asphyxia for a twin is 4–5 times that for a
  singleton.
- Malpresentation (cephalic/cephalic, 40%; cephalic/breech, 40%;
  breech/breech, 10%; cephalic/transverse (TV), 5%; breech/TV, 4%; TV/TV,
  1%).
- Increased risk of operative delivery—either as an elective procedure or as an
  emergency before or after delivery of the first twin.
- Risk of bleeding from undiagnosed vasa praevia.
- Twin entrapment (1:817 twin pregnancies—typically with MZ twins).
- Risk of postpartum haemorrhage (10% twin versus 5% singletons).

Postpartum
- There is a higher incidence of postnatal depression in mothers of twins.
- Breastfeeding twins is physically and psychologically demanding.
- There may be financial difficulties.

NB. The Twins and Multiple Births Association (TAMBA) and other support groups may be helpful.

Management

Antenatal care

A wide range of practices are seen and are acceptable. Shared care is usually appropriate with increased frequency of visits to detect complications such as pre-eclampsia. Iron and folate supplements are useful from the 2nd trimester onwards. Aim to determine chorionicity in the first trimester by scan in view of increased risks to monochorionic twins.

- Detailed anomaly scan at 19 weeks and cardiac anomaly scan at 22–24 weeks. No benefit from routine bed rest.
- No place for prophylactic cervical cerclage. Routine screening for gestational diabetes at 32 weeks gestation.
- Fetal assessment includes serial ultrasound scanning for growth and well-being at 24, 28, 32, 34, and 36 weeks.
- Increase in surveillance as required for acute hydramnios—consider serial therapeutic amniocentesis, indomethacin, or nonsteroidal anti-inflammatory drugs (NSAIDs).
- Laser ablation of aberrant placental vessels is useful in twin-to-twin transfusion syndrome. Although the rate of fetal loss is reduced by such treatment to 40–50%, neurological, cardiac, and renal sequelae are common in survivors.
- Nuchal fold measurements for Down screening may be performed (serum screening is of little help), with amniocentesis for confirmatory diagnosis.
- It is uncommon for twin pregnancies to be allowed to progress beyond 40 completed weeks.
- Labour is often induced prior to this for fetal or maternal reasons.

Labour/delivery

- Consider induction of labour for pregnancy complications.
- Intravenous (IV) access.
- Full blood count (FBC) and group and save serum (increased risk of operative delivery and postpartum haemorrhage (PPH)).
- Continuous monitoring. When feasible, site a fetal scalp electrode on the first twin.
- Epidural minimizes the risks of pushing prior to full cervical dilatation and enables operative procedures without recourse to general anaesthetic, e.g. internal podalic version or lower segment Caesarean section (LSCS).
- Staff present at delivery to include two midwives, a senior obstetrician, anaesthetist, a pediatrician, and a neonatal nurse.
- Vertex/vertex presentation: aim for vaginal delivery.
- Vertex/non-vertex presentation: optimum mode of delivery uncertain, but vaginal delivery preferred. Spontaneous vaginal delivery (SVD) of first twin with either external cephalic version or internal podalic version of the second twin. No randomized trials to confirm whether elective LSCS or vaginal delivery is the safest.

Higher-order multiple deliveries

- The recommendation is to deliver by elective LSCS as there is increased morbidity and mortality due to problems with fetal monitoring in labour.
- An oxytocin infusion is mandatory if there is uterine inertia, especially after delivery of the first twin (10 IU in 1litre of 0.9% saline solution to run at 1 mIU/min, increasing in doubling doses every 5 minutes to restore adequate uterine activity (i.e. 3–4 contractions lasting 40 seconds per 10 minutes)).
- Consider intervention to aid delivery of second twin if time between the deliveries exceeds 30 minutes.
- Active management of the third stage with intramuscular (IM) syntometrine (0.5 mg ergometrine and 5 IU syntocinon) is recommended as a prophylactic measure against uterine atony followed by 40 IU of oxytocin in 500 mL 0.9% saline solution to run over 3–4 hours.

Postnatal

Persistence with and help in establishing breastfeeding. Ensure extra help is available in the community if required.

Recommended further reading

1 Walters, W. (1995). Multiple pregnancy. In *Turnbull's obstetrics*, 2nd edn (ed. G.V.P. Chamberlain), pp. 329–52. Churchill Livingstone, Edinburgh.

2 Crowther, C.A. (1999). Multiple pregnancy. In *High risk pregnancy—management options*, 2nd edn (ed. D.K. James, P.J. Steer, C.P. Weiner, B. Gonik), pp. 129–53. W.B. Saunders, London.

3 Neilson, J.P. (1995). Multiple pregnancy. In *Dewhurst's textbook of obstetrics and gynaecology for postgraduates*, 5th edn (ed. C. Whitfield), pp. 439–54. Blackwell Science, Oxford.

Breech presentation

Breech presentation is the most common malpresentation. The incidence of breech presentation is higher in early pregnancy: 40% at 20 weeks; 25% at 32 weeks; and only 3% by term. It is normal in pregnancy for the buttocks and feet to come to lie in the fundus, perhaps because the fundus has more space and the heavier head gravitates to the lower pole.

Conditions predisposing towards breech presentation include contracted pelvis; bicornuate uterus; fibroid uterus; placenta praevia; multiple pregnancies; poly-hydramnios; oligohydramnios; spina bifida (baby cannot kick well); or a hydro-cephalic baby (the 'lower segment' is too small). Ultrasound may show the cause and influence the management, although, in the vast majority, no cause can be identified.

Types of breech presentation

The breech may present in one of three ways.
- Extended breech presentation is the most common, i.e. flexed at the hips but extended at the knees, the buttocks presenting to the pelvic inlet.
- Flexed breeches sit with hips and knees both flexed so that the presenting part is a mixture of buttocks, external genitalia, and feet.
- Footling breeches are the least common. One thigh is flexed and one is extended so that the foot or knee would descend first through the cervical os into the vagina. This type has the greatest risk (5–10%) of cord prolapse.

The position of the fetus is described by using the sacrum as the denominator (occiput is the denominator for a vertex presentation).

Diagnosis

Diagnosis should be made antenatally. The mother may complain of pain under the ribs. On palpation the lie is longitudinal, a broad pole is felt in the pelvis, and in the fundus there is a smooth, round mass (the head) that can be ballot-ted. The fetal heart is best heard at the level of the umbilicus or above. If the diagnosis is uncertain in late pregnancy, vaginal examination may resolve it but if doubt still remains, an ultrasound examination should be made.

Management

Breech presentation is associated with an increased risk of perinatal mortalit
and morbidity due principally to prematurity, congenital malformations, an
birth asphyxia from cord compression or trauma. Caesarean section for breec
presentation has been suggested as a way of reducing the associated fetal prob
lems. Recent evidence recommends the policy of planned Caesarean section fo
breech presentation. Despite the large Canadian trial recommending Caesarea
section as safest for the baby, some mothers may elect to have an assisted breec
delivery. Breech presentation, whatever the mode of delivery, is a signal fo
potential fetal handicap and this should influence antenatal, intrapartum, an
neonatal management.

Reducing the incidence of breech presentations

External cephalic version (ECV) should be offered after 36 weeks. The benefi
and risks of ECV at term should be explained to women with an uncomplicate
breech presentation at term. ECV is best carried out with the mother awake an
facilities for emergency delivery should be available nearby. Cardiotocograph
should be done prior to ECV. Tocolysis has been shown to be effective bot
when used routinely and when used selectively. The breech is manoeuvre
through a forward, less commonly a backward, somersault to become a cephali
presentation if vaginal delivery is planned. There is compelling evidence tha
ECV at term increases the chances of a cephalic birth. With ECV there is an 80%
reduction in the odds of a non-cephalic presentation at birth and a reduction c
over 50% in the rate of Caesarean sections. Anti-D should be administered t
women who are rhesus-negative and a Kleihauer test should be done to detec
the 1% who may need additional anti-D.

- Factors that increase the likelihood of ECV include multiparity, flexed
  breech presentation, adequate liquor volume, and a station of the breech
  above the brim.
- Contraindications to ECV include placenta praevia, multiple pregnancy,
  antepartum haemorrhage (APH), small for dates babies, and mothers with
  uterine scars, pre-eclampsia, or hypertension (risk of abruption is increased).
- Theoretical risks of ECV include placental separation, cord entanglement,
  pre-labour rupture of the membranes, precipitation of labour,
  transplacental haemorrhage with rhesus sensitization if the mother is
  rhesus-negative with a rhesus-positive baby.

Planning the mode of delivery

Policies for term breech pregnancy management, where ECV was contraindi
cated, declined, or failed, should be based on available evidence and the choic
of the woman. If assisted vaginal delivery is preferred, there should be a carefu
selection of patients.

- A trial of vaginal breech delivery is more likely to be successful if both
  mother and baby are of normal proportions. The size of the fetus should be
  between 2000 and 3500 g.
- The presentation should be either frank (hips flexed, knees extended) or
  complete (hips flexed, knees flexed, but feet not below the fetal buttocks).
  Ultrasound examination after 36 weeks is useful in confirming the above.
- There should be no evidence of feto-pelvic disproportion with a 'clinically
  adequate' pelvis. Clinical judgement is adequate (there is little evidence tha
  objective measurement of pelvic size correlates with the chance of vaginal
  delivery). If pelvimetry is required computerized tomography (CT)
  scanning may be preferable to X-ray because the radiation dose is less.

19 Breech presentation

- Vaginal delivery should probably only be allowed when labour is spontaneous, Caesarean section being preferable to induction of labour.
- Whatever the indication the most important factor in determining whether or not a vaginal delivery is achievable is the efficiency of uterine activity producing cervical dilatation and descent of the breech.

Intrapartum breech management

When vaginal breech delivery is planned the mother should be advised to present as soon as labour starts or the membranes rupture. Vaginal examination is performed at the time of admission to exclude cord presentation. The length of labour is the same as in a vertex presentation. Epidural anaesthesia is recommended.

Delivery technique

- At full cervical dilatation the mother is encouraged to bear down when the buttocks and anus of the baby come into view over the mother's perineum without retraction.
- After an episiotomy is performed (under local infiltration in cases without epidural), the mother is encouraged to push the child to the level of the umbilicus.
- Abducting the baby's hip joint and flexing the knee helps to deliver the legs. It is important to keep the back sacro-anterior.
- Bearing down efforts with contractions are encouraged to help descent occur until the scapulae are visible.
- The arms may be delivered by adduction at the shoulder and flexion at the elbow. If this is unsuccessful the Lovset manoeuvre can be carried out by holding the baby with the thumbs on the sacrum and index fingers on the anterior superior iliac spines. The baby is turned in a clockwise (to deliver the posterior shoulder by rotating it below the symphysis pubis) and then anticlockwise direction to enable descent of the opposite shoulder.
- The trunk is allowed to hang until the nape of the neck becomes visible. The trunk is then swung upwards through 180° until the mouth comes into view or the delivery achieved by either the Mauriceau–Smellie–Viet manoeuvre (a finger is placed in the mouth and two fingers over the maxilla to flex the head and deliver) or by the application of Neville Barnes forceps for the aftercoming head.
- The mouth, nose, and pharynx are cleared of secretions as they come into view.

225

Management of the preterm breech

Management of preterm (less than 37 weeks) breech delivery is an area of clinical controversy. The poor outcome for very low birth weight infants is mainly related to complications of prematurity and probably not the mode of delivery. The decision about the mode of delivery should be made after close consultation with the woman and her partner.

Conclusion

Elective Caesarean section is recommended for breech presentation. However, mothers may choose to deliver vaginally or the woman may come in advanced labour with breech presentation necessitating that the accoucheur be trained in assisted breech delivery. This is done by practice with mannequins, assisting senior personnel in assisted breech delivery, and performing the sequence needed in vaginal delivery at the time of delivering a breech by CS.

Antepartum haemorrhage

Antepartum haemorrhage (APH) is defined as bleeding from the genital tract after the 22nd week of pregnancy. It complicates 2–5% of all pregnancies and is an important cause of fetal and maternal morbidity and mortality. Dangerous causes are placental abruption, placenta praevia, and vasa praevia. Other causes include additional bleeding associated with a 'show' (blood loss associated with the release of the mucous plug from the cervix that occurs prior to the onset of labour), cervicitis, trauma, vulvovaginal varicosities, genital tumours, and infections.

Management

Women with APH should always be admitted to a hospital with adequate facilities for transfusion, delivery by Caesarean section, and neonatal resuscitation. Initial management depends upon the severity, the cause of bleeding, and gestational age. Rhesus-negative women will require anti-D.

- Resuscitation with intravenous fluids and blood transfusion is the first priority in women who are haemodynamically unstable and intravenous (IV) access should be secured in all patients with two large-bore (size 14) IV cannulae.
- History and examination are important to determine the likely cause of the bleeding and evaluate the patient's general condition.
  —Digital vaginal examination should be avoided until placenta praevia has been excluded by ultrasound or an examination in theatre with facilities for delivery by Caesarean section.
  —In those with minimal bleeding, speculum examination after an ultrasound examination to exclude placenta praevia may help to identify local causes of bleeding.

Investigations
- Take blood for full blood count (FBC), group and save of serum (G&S), or cross-matching.
- If placental abruption is suspected, a coagulation profile and urea and electrolytes (U&Es) should be performed.
- If the woman is rhesus-negative ask for a Kleihauer test.
- Arrange an ultrasound scan to exclude placenta praevia. A major placental abruption with placental separation may be seen on ultrasound, but will be clinically obvious based on symptoms and signs. Ultrasound should only be done only when maternal and fetal conditions are stable.

Placenta praevia (PP)

The placenta is partly or completely inserted in the lower uterine segment. This complicates 0.5% of pregnancies. The cause of PP is unknown but it is more common in older women, multiparas, after a previous Caesarean section, in smokers, and in women with a previous history of PP (recurrence risk of 4–8% after one PP). Only 3% of women with a low-lying placenta seen on the midtrimester ultrasound scan will have PP at term (the lower uterine segment develops in the second half of pregnancy). PP is classified as major (type III and IV) and minor (type I and II) (Fig. 20.1).

- In type I, the placenta is low but does not reach the cervical os.
- In type II the placenta reaches the cervical os.
- In type III the placenta covers the os asymmetrically.
- In type IV the placenta covers the os completely.

Maternal and fetal risks

- Placenta praevia carries risks to the mother from massive obstetric haemorrhage (most commonly as a result of postpartum haemorrhage), complications of surgery and anaesthesia, air embolism, and postpartum sepsis.
- The major risk to the fetus is from iatrogenic preterm birth but there is also an increased incidence of intrauterine growth restriction (IUGR), congenital malformation, malpresentation, fetal anaemia, and cord complications. The perinatal mortality rate was reported as 100% at less than 27 weeks, 19.7% between 33 and 36 weeks, and 2.6% after 36 weeks but is likely to be less with current management.

Presentation and diagnosis

Presentation is as unprovoked painless vaginal bleeding or bleeding after sexual intercourse. Without routine scanning one in six cases present for the first time in labour. Malpresentation is common. The uterus is soft and non-tender (although abruption can occur in women with PP). The first bleed is usually (but not always) smaller.

Diagnosis is as follows.

- Avoid vaginal examination as this may cause catastrophic bleeding.
- Ultrasound scanning is safe and generally reliable although false-negative scans occur in 7% of cases. The latter are more common when the placenta is posterior, the bladder is too full, the fetal head obscures the low edge of placenta, or the sonographer is inexperienced.
- Magnetic resonance imaging (MRI) may be useful in cases of posterior placenta praevia.
- Where there is still doubt the diagnosis should be confirmed or excluded by examination in theatre at term if there is no bleeding.

Management

Management depends on the clinical condition, type of PP, and gestational age.

- Steroids should be given to women who are under 36 weeks gestation to help fetal lung maturity.
- Immediate resuscitation and delivery is required if the bleeding doesn't settle or is causing maternal or fetal compromise or when the gestation is more than 36 weeks.

20 Antepartum haemorrhage

Hospitalization and expectant management is usually advised for patients with types III and IV PP—if the bleeding is not life-threatening and the fetus is not mature. A wide-bore cannula should be inserted and 4 units of blood must be ready for transfusion with any bleeding. This conservative management is continued until 37 weeks.

Delivery is by Caesarean section, which should be performed by an experienced obstetrician. The woman should be counselled about the possibility of hysterectomy if uncontrolled bleeding occurs. This is more likely when there has been a previous Caesarean section and the placenta is anterior.

In minor degrees of anterior PP, examination in theatre after 37 weeks with amniotomy followed by syntocinon can be considered.

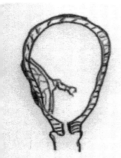
Type 1 placenta praevia

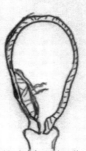
Marginal placenta (type 2)

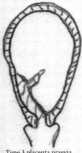
Type 3 placenta praevia

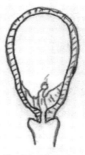
Type 4 placenta praevia

Fig. 20.1 Different types of placenta praevia.

Placental abruption ('accidental haemorrhage')

Placental abruption is bleeding following premature separation of normally si uated placenta. The incidence varies from 0.43 to 1.8%. It may be revealed (wit vaginal bleeding) or concealed (with no bleeding). The cause is unknown in th majority of cases. It can be caused by direct trauma or sudden decompressio of the uterus after membrane rupture in patients with polyhydramnios or mu tiple pregnancy. Abruption is more frequent where there is maternal hyperte sion or a history of abruptions in the present or past pregnancies. It is mo common in older women, those of high parity, cigarette smokers, substanc abusers, and anaemic patients.

Maternal and fetal risks

- Cases severe enough to produce coagulopathy are associated with a maternal mortality rate of 1%. Complications for the mother include hypovolaemic shock, acute renal failure, disseminated intravascular coagulation (DIC), postpartum haemorrhage, and feto-maternal haemorrhage.
- For the fetus, perinatal mortality varies from 4.4 to 67.3% depending on neonatal facilities and the size of abruption. IUGR and preterm delivery ar common. Anaemia and coagulopathy may occur as complications.

Presentation and diagnosis

Presentation is as abdominal pain with or without vaginal bleeding and uterin contractions, uterine tenderness, and fetal distress. The pain is sharp, severe, an sudden in onset. In severe cases there may be signs of shock, increasing abdom inal girth, or a rising fundal height and the uterus is described as irritable an tender, which may later become woody and hard. Signs of shock may be out proportion to the observed blood loss. Posterior abruptions may present backache. The fetus may be difficult to palpate or monitor. Fetal distress death may happen. Up to 50% of cases are in labour at the time of presentatio If the membranes are ruptured, blood-stained liquor is seen.

Diagnosis is usually made on clinical grounds. Ultrasonography is not an accu rate diagnostic tool, but it is useful in cases of minor abruption for monitorin the cases managed conservatively.

Management

Management depends on the severity, associated complications, maternal an fetal condition, and gestational age.

- Immediate delivery is required in severe cases, whether the fetus is alive or dead. Vaginal delivery (by induction or allowing labour to continue) is usually preferred if the fetus is already dead or where there is no evidence of maternal or fetal compromise. Caesarean section is carried out in 15–25% of cases.
- Blood coagulation failure occurs in 5% of cases and this must be diagnose and treated before any operative procedures are undertaken.
- The prognosis for the fetus following a significant abruption is inversely proportional to the length of time from bleed to delivery and the fetal condition may deteriorate with little warning.

Conservative management should only be undertaken after 34 weeks for minor degrees of bleeding and the pregnancy is treated as high risk with serial ultrasound scans to monitor growth and delivery by 40 weeks.

There is an increased risk of postpartum haemorrhage after delivery.

Postpartum management after a large abruption is supportive with regular monitoring of urine output, blood pressure and pulse, and coagulation profile.

Acute abdominal pain in pregnancy

Abdominal pain is a common complaint during pregnancy. The most common cause is the physiological onset of labour. Labour pain is intermittent and associated with uterine contractions. When these occur with cervical dilatation and descent of the presenting part, the diagnosis is usually straightforward but this may be preceded by a latent phase of some length. Remember that pathological causes of abdominal pain such as abruption may precipitate labour. Other physiological causes of abdominal pain during pregnancy include musculoskeletal pain from round ligament stretching and symphysis pubis pain.

Pathological condition related to pregnancy

- *Early pregnancy complications* such as ectopic pregnancy and miscarriage were discussed in Chapter 6.
- *Placental abruption* occurs in 0.5–1% of all pregnancies. There is separation of the placenta and retroplacental bleeding. The patient usually presents with sudden onset of abdominal pain with or without vaginal bleeding and uterine irritability. If the placenta is posterior, symptoms of backache may predominate. On palpation the uterus is tender and palpation of fetal parts may be difficult because of uterine irritability and increased tonus. Retroplacental bleeding may be seen on ultrasound, but is a late finding and the diagnosis in these cases has usually already been made clinically. Abruption may lead to coagulopathy (33–50% of severe cases) and fetal death (up to 60%). Postpartum haemorrhage (PPH) is also common.
- *Uterine leiomyoma.* Uterine fibroids may cause severe abdominal pain in pregnancy as a result of red degeneration or when a pedunculated fibroid torts. The mainstays of management are pain relief (parenteral if needed) and bed rest, as most cases are due to red degeneration and may resolve with time. Rarely, the pain may be severe enough to require laparotomy for diagnosis and treatment.
- *Chorioamnionitis.* Although pre-labour rupture of the membranes usually precedes chorioamnionitis, infection may be present without ruptured membranes and cause abdominal pain.
- *Uterine rupture.* Rupture of the gravid uterus is rare (1:1500 deliveries in the UK). It usually occurs during labour but may precede it. It is associated with a high fetal mortality (30%) and significant maternal mortality (5%). Most cases are due to rupture of Caesarean section scars but it can also occur in cases of pregnancy developing in a rudimentary horn, with excessive oxytocin use, in obstructed labour, high parity, and following other surgical trauma (such as previous uterine perforation). Rupture of the uterus should be suspected in women at risk who present with constant abdominal pain, tenderness, fresh vaginal bleeding, and fetal distress with or without maternal shock. The management should be resuscitation, prompt laparotomy, delivery by Caesarean section, and repair of the uterus or hysterectomy.

21 Acute abdominal pain in pregnancy

- *Severe uterine torsion.* The uterus rotates axially by 30–40° to the right in 80% of normal pregnancies. Torsion may occur when this rotation extends beyond 90° causing severe abdominal pain, shock, a tense uterus, and urinary retention in the later half of pregnancy. In 80–90% of cases there is a predisposing factor such as a fibroid, congenital uterine anomaly, adnexal mass, or a history of pelvic adhesions. Maternal vasovagal shock and possible fetal distress are the main risks of severe uterine torsion. The diagnosis is suggested by a displaced urethra on catheterization. Conservative management is by analgesia and altering maternal position but laparotomy and delivery by Caesarean section will be required in those cases that do not resolve with conservative management.

- *Ovarian tumours.* Ovarian cysts have the potential risk of torsion, rupture, or haemorrhage, which may cause severe abdominal pain, especially when torsion leads to infarction. Once ovarian torsion is diagnosed, a laparotomy should be carried out. If the adnexum is necrotic it should be removed taking care not to 'untwist' it. Ovarian cystectomy can be carried out if the adnexum appears viable.

Pathological conditions unrelated to pregnancy

- *Acute appendicitis* complicates about 1/1000 of pregnancies. There is no increase in incidence during pregnancy but mortality is higher. During pregnancy the caecum and appendix are displaced upwards and to the right with advancing gestation. The pain is less well localized and tenderness, rebound tenderness, and guarding are less obvious. This leads to delay in diagnosis and treatment and an increased incidence of perforation (15–20% of cases), peritonitis, and sepsis. When perforation occurs, maternal and fetal mortality reach 17 and 43%, respectively (compared to 5–10% for simple appendicitis). Ultrasound scan may be of value in excluding degenerating fibroids, twisted ovarian cysts, ureteric obstruction, and placental abruption. Early surgical referral and laparotomy by an experienced surgeon is essential.
  —In the first trimester this can be through McBurney's incision.
  —In the second and third trimester a right paramedian incision at the site of maximum tenderness should be used.
- *Cholecystitis.* Gallstones grow rapidly during pregnancy due to biliary stasis. Acute cholecystitis complicates about 1 in 1000 pregnancies. Presentation is with sudden onset of right upper quadrant or epigastric colicky pain with associated nausea, vomiting, and fever. Jaundice is uncommon. It is important to differentiate cholecystitis from severe pre-eclampsia and acute fatty liver and appendicitis. The diagnosis can be made on the basis of the clinical features, biochemical tests, and the presence of stones in the biliary tree on ultrasound scan. The treatment is by using the appropriate antibiotics, adequate analgesia, and fluids. Where possible, cholecystectomy is deferred until after the puerperium.
- *Intestinal obstruction* occurs in 1/2500–1/3500 of pregnancies. Of cases 60% are due to adhesions. Other causes include volvulus intussception, hernia, and complications of Crohn's disease. The presentation is usually in the second or third trimester with colicky abdominal pain, nausea, vomiting, constipation, and abdominal distension. The diagnosis can be made by observation of distended loops of bowel with fluid levels on erect and supine abdominal X-rays. Like appendicitis, delay in diagnosis is common and carries maternal and fetal mortality rates of 10–20% and 30–50%, respectively. Conservative management is by nasogastric suction, intravenous fluids, and analgesia but a midline laparotomy may be required to correct the cause of the obstruction. Caesarean section can be carried out at the same time if pregnancy is sufficiently advanced. Careful attention to fluid and electrolyte balance is essential.
- *Crohn's disease.* Patients complain of abdominal pain, diarrhoea, anaemia, and weight loss. Rectal bleeding and the passage of mucus may occur. Rectal bleeding by itself is more likely to be due to haemorrhoids in pregnancy. The diagnosis is confirmed by sigmoidoscopy and rectal biopsy. Treatment is as in non-pregnant patients and sulfasalazine and steroids should be continued during pregnancy.
- *Peptic ulceration.* Pregnancy reduces the risk of peptic ulceration. However, acute upper abdominal/epigastric pain may rarely be caused by a perforated peptic ulcer. Management is by laparotomy and repair.

21 Acute abdominal pain in pregnancy

- *Acute pancreatitis.* Acute pancreatitis is rare in pregnancy (1 in 4000 pregnancies). The presentation is with upper abdominal pain radiating into the back and associated with vomiting. A raised serum amylase concentration will confirm the diagnosis. Management is by intravenous fluid and electrolyte replacement, suppression of pancreatic activity, analgesia, antibiotics, nasogastric suction, and laparotomy if conservative treatment fails.
- *Acute pyelonephritis* occurs in 1–2% of pregnant women. Obstructive uropathy and stasis are predisposing factors. The diagnosis is made by clinical features (fever, loin tenderness, urinary frequency) and positive culture from midstream urine. Ultrasound findings may show hydronephrosis. Treatment should be as an in-patient with intravenous antibiotics, fluids, and adequate analgesia.
- *Urolithiasis* occurs in 0.03–0.5% of pregnancies. Urinary calculi in pregnancy normally present with sudden-onset abdominal pain that is severe enough to warrant hospital admission, associated with urinary tract infection and haematuria. Ultrasound scan findings of hydronephrosis or a calcified area are suggestive of renal calculi. Intravenous urography for the purpose of diagnosis is not contraindicated at any stage of pregnancy. The management should be conservative with intravenous fluids, antibiotics, and effective analgesia. If a calculus is large enough to cause obstruction, surgery may be required.
- *Acute fatty liver of pregnancy.* This occurs in 1–10 000 to 1–15 000 pregnancies. The symptoms are sudden abdominal pain, nausea, vomiting, and jaundice. The serum bilirubin is raised with abnormal liver enzymes and associated leucocytosis, thrombocytopenia, hypoglycaemia, and coagulation defects. The management is correction of fluid, electrolyte, and coagulation abnormalities and prompt delivery.
- *Severe pre-eclampsia* and HELLP (haemolysis, elevated liver enzymes, and low platelet count) syndrome may present with epigastric pain due to distension or haemorrhage stretching the liver capsule. This is discussed in Chapter 14.
- *Miscellaneous.*
  —Sickle cell crises in women who have homozygous SS or SC disease can present with acute abdominal pain during crises.
  —Porphyria and malaria may also present with abdominal pain.
  —Bleeding into the rectus muscle and subsequent rectus sheath haematoma formation following rupture of a branch of inferior epigastric vessels may be caused by coughing or trauma. This may cause sudden and severe abdominal pain.
  —Rare conditions resulting in intraabdominal haemorrhage can cause acute abdominal pain in pregnancy. These include rupture of utero-ovarian veins, rupture of aneurysms (splenic, hepatic, renal, aortic), and rupture of uterine veins requiring urgent laparotomy. These cases will present with clinical symptoms and signs suggestive of intraabdominal bleeding.

Preterm labour

241

Pre-term labour is defined as the onset of labour prior to 37 completed weeks of gestation. The incidence of preterm delivery is around 7%, although a proportion of these deliveries will be iatrogenic.

Causes and prevention

Certain groups of women are at particular risk of preterm labour. Multiple pregnancies account for a growing proportion of such deliveries since the advent of modern methods of assisted conception. These pregnancies have their own particular determinants of risk, and are dealt with in Chapter 18.

- Those with a *previous history of preterm labour* should be considered at risk of recurrence and the events surrounding their previous delivery should be carefully examined for any indicators of causation. At particular risk are those whose history suggests cervical incompetence, indicators of which may include previous cervical surgery or surgical termination of pregnancy, *in utero* exposure to diethyl stilboestrol, recurrent late second trimester miscarriage, or a rapid, painless progression to full dilatation. The use of cervical cerclage to reduce the risk of preterm delivery may be considered.
  —The Macdonald (without reflecting the bladder upwards) or Shirodkar (after dissecting the bladder upwards) are the most commonly utilized cervical sutures.
  —Abdominal cerclage is increasing in popularity in difficult cases, where the vaginal approach has failed or is difficult.
  —All carry risks, such as iatrogenic pre-labour rupture of membranes or of inducing preterm labour or spontaneous abortion.
  —Those inserted vaginally may act as a focus for infection.
  —Randomized controlled trials to assess the benefits of cervical cerclage are always confounded by the difficulties of differentiating cervical incompetence from other precipitants of preterm delivery. However, the evidence suggests that, with careful case selection, prophylactic cervical cerclage can result in improved perinatal outcome in those with cervical incompetence, but there is no evidence supporting the use of cervical cerclage in the presence of preterm labour.
- *Infection* is likely to play a significant part in the onset or promotion of preterm labour in many cases, and bacterial vaginosis is recognized as a contributory factor in a proportion of cases of preterm labour.
  —There is no evidence that the treatment of bacterial vaginosis in women without a history of preterm labour provides any reduction in preterm delivery rate.
  —However, in those with a previous history of preterm delivery, the treatment of bacterial vaginosis results in some reduction in the preterm delivery rate, although there is no resultant alteration in measures of neonatal outcome.
- Pregnancies complicated by *polyhydramnios* are at risk of preterm labour. Women with this complication should be counselled accordingly and management tailored to take account of this risk.
- *Placental abruption* may precipitate preterm labour. Significant placental abruption may result in acute fetal and/or maternal compromise necessitating precipitant delivery regardless of gestation. Lesser clinically evident abruption may permit at least temporary conservative management to permit the promotion of fetal maturity. The only evidence of a silent abruption may be threatened preterm labour. This possibility should

therefore always be considered in women with spurious preterm labour, as the presence of placental abruption may result in isoimmunization of the rhesus-negative mother or in adverse pregnancy outcome (such as late intrauterine death or intrauterine growth restriction). Appropriate investigation and follow-up is therefore important in these women, even after the acute threat of preterm labour is over.

The presence of *extrauterine irritants* may precipitate preterm labour, and signs of its onset should be anticipated and tocolysis considered if required. Relatively common precipitants may include intraabdominal surgery, appendicitis, or severe urinary tract infection.

Diagnosis

Preterm labour is diagnosed when progressive cervical shortening and dilation occur prior to 37 completed weeks of gestation.

Contractions that may be regular and/or painful may occur, but may be absent or minimal in the presence of cervical incompetence. Contractions in the absence of cervical change constitute threatened preterm labour. The prediction of preterm labour would clearly provide benefits in the provision of appropriate care. No specific test, however, has yet been developed that provides a prediction influencing perinatal outcome.

The fetal fibronectin test, which determines levels of fetal fibronectin in cervical mucus, may give some assistance in determining those most at risk of delivery within the next 10 days, but such information is frequently confounded and rarely permits alteration in management in those with threatened preterm labour.

The assessment of cervical competence in those whose history suggests incompetence may become feasible in time. However, clinical assessment is notoriously poor, and the predictive value of ultrasound evaluation has so far varied between trials. Ultrasound findings such as funnelling of the internal os during a maternal Valsalva manoeuvre are being assessed. Transvaginal ultrasound assessment of the cervix may prove to be useful in the management of those considered at risk of cervical incompetence.

243

Management

The mainstays of management of preterm labour involve the promotion of fetal maturity with consideration of causative factors endangering the mother or fetus. Prompt assessment of mother and fetus is required in the presence of preterm labour.

- Signs of acute fetal or maternal compromise may require immediate delivery, regardless of the gestation. Such situations would include maternal haemodynamic instability in the presence of placental abruption, signs of established chorioamnionitis, or evidence of acute fetal compromise at a gestation compatible with neonatal viability (e.g. after 24–26 weeks, depending on neonatal facilities).
- In the absence of the above problems, attempts to arrest the progress of labour to improve fetal maturity may be appropriate, but tocolysis is unlikely to be successful in advanced labour with regular or painful contractions.
- Steroid injection, however, should be considered unless delivery is imminent, as the time to delivery can be difficult to predict in preterm labour, and there may be sufficient time for significant improvement in respiratory compliance to occur, courtesy of transplacental uptake of betamethasone.

Tocolysis

Tocolysis should be considered if there are no contraindications to its use and labour is not advanced (i.e. < 4 cm dilatation without significant effacement). The aim of tocolysis is to allow time for the steroids administered to take effect. There is no evidence that outcome is further improved by prolonging tocolysis beyond 48 hours after steroid administration. Indeed, as most tocolytic drugs have significant side-effects of varying severity (e.g. pulmonary oedema with beta-sympathomimetics), their prolonged use should be strongly discouraged.

The choice of optimal tocolytic drug remains the subject of much research. The most commonly used drugs and their complications are detailed below.

- *Beta-sympathomimetics.* Intravenous (IV) ritodrine remains the most commonly used tocolytic. Its use results in prolongation of pregnancy by up to 48 hours in a significant proportion of the preterm labour in which it is used, but it results in no significant improvement in perinatal mortality or morbidity. Its complications include maternal tachycardia, arrhythmias, cardiac ischaemia, hyperglycaemia, hypokalaemia, hyponatraemia, tremor, and pulmonary oedema. It is hence poorly tolerated by many women. Relative contraindications to its use include multiple pregnancy, diabetes mellitus, antepartum haemorrhage, and pre-eclampsia. Its administration is by IV infusion of 1 mg/hour, increased until contractions cease and thence titrated against contractions and side-effects until sufficient time after steroid administration has lapsed or the threat of preterm labour has ceased.
  —Oral salbutamol was traditionally used to maintain tocolysis following the cessation of ritodrine. There is no substantive evidence to support its use above placebo.
- *Glyceryl trinitrate patches.* These nitric oxide donors result in a reduction in uterine muscle contractility. Their efficacy is less well tested than that of ritodrine, but a number of studies have demonstrated reasonable tocolysis with improved tolerance in comparison. Their main side-effects are severe headache, tachycardia, and flushing. A 5 mg patch may be replaced by a 10 mg patch if contractions are not controlled after 2 hours. Once effective control is achieved, the patch requires changing after 24 hours.

- *Nifedipine.* This calcium channel blocker also reduces myometrial contractility. There is good evidence for its effectiveness as a tocolytic, both in the acute phase of preterm labour and in the further prolongation of pregnancy, but again its use in either capacity results in no improvement in perinatal mortality. Its side-effects are generally minimal and include headaches, flushing, and hypotension. It is administered orally, with a starting dose of 10 mg/hour, falling to 20 mg 8-hourly once control of contractions is achieved (various studies have used differing regimens, but the dosages have been broadly similar to this).

- *Magnesium sulfate.* This membrane stabilizer has been used as a tocolytic. No advantages in efficacy have been demonstrated above those of ritodrine or nifedipine, and fetal and maternal nervous system suppression may occur. The therapeutic band of serum concentration is relatively narrow, and toxicity may occur at varying levels in different women.

- *Indomethacin.* This cyclo-oxygenase inhibitor acts as an antiprostaglandin to reduce the stimulation and promotion of preterm labour. It may also help to reduce the threat of preterm labour in women with significant polyhydramnios by additionally reducing fetal renal output. The majority of evidence for its beneficial use is in this scenario with polyhydramnios. Its complications include premature closure of the fetal ductus arteriosus and oligohydramnios. It is administered orally or as rectal suppositories (1–3 mg/kg body weight of the mother).

- *Oxytocin antagonist.* Atosiban is a new agent available for delay of labour. Clinical trials have suggested efficacy similar to that of beta-sympathomimetics, but fewer treatment discontinuations due to very much reduced side-effects and no adverse events.

Recommended further reading

1 Steer, P. and Flint, C. (1999). ABC of labour care: preterm labour and premature rupture of membranes. *British Medical Journal* 318, 1059–62.

2 Lockwood, C.J. and Kuczynski, E. (1999). Markers of risk for preterm delivery. *Journal of Perinatal Medicine* 27, 5–20.

3 Medical Research Council/Royal College of Obstetricians and Gynaecologists (1988). Multicentre randomized trial of cervical cerclage. Interim report. *British Journal of Obstetrics and Gynaecology* 95, 437–45.

4 Gibbs, R.S. and Eschenbach, D.A. (1997). Use of antibiotics to prevent preterm birth. *American Journal of Obstetrics and Gynecology* 177, 375–80.

5 Lamont, R.F. (1999). The prevention of preterm birth with the use of antibiotics. *European Journal of Pediatrics* 158 (suppl. 1), S1–4.

6 Moore, M.L. (1999). Biochemical markers for preterm labor and birth: what is their role in the care of pregnant women? *MCN, American Journal of Maternal/Child Nursing* 24, 80–6.

7 Leitich, H., Brunbauer, M., Kaider, A., Egarter, C., and Husslein, P. (1999). Cervical length and dilatation of the internal cervical os detected by vaginal ultrasonography as markers for preterm delivery. *American Journal of Obstetrics and Gynecology* 181, 11465–72.

8 Gyetvai, K., Hannah, M.E., Hodnett, E.D., and Ohlsson, A. (1999). Tocolytics for preterm labour: a systematic review. *Obstetrics and Gynecology* 94, 869–77.

9 Keirse, M.J.N.C., Grant, A., and King, J.F. (1989). Preterm labour. In *Preterm labour: effective care in pregnancy and childbirth*, Vol. 1 (ed. I. Chalmers, M. Erkin, and M.J.N.C. Keirse), pp. 694–745. Oxford University Press, Oxford.

10 Smith, P., Anthony, J., and Johanson, R. (2000). Nifedipine in pregnancy. *British Journal of Obstetrics and Gynaecology* 107, 299–307.

Chapter 23

Preterm pre-labour rupture of membranes

Preterm pre-labour rupture of membranes (PPROM) is defined as the spontaneous rupture of the fetal membranes prior to 37 weeks gestation in the absence of regular painful contractions.

Causes/risk groups

PPROM may be precipitated by a number of factors. An inflammatory process, particularly infective in origin, may alter the composition of the amnion or chorion or the intraamniotic pressure may be raised, e.g. in the presence of polyhydramnios or in the presence of uterine irritability. The conditions that therefore predispose to PPROM are:

- Polyhydramnios.
- A previous history of PPROM.
- Bicornuate uterus.
- Known infection with *Chlamydia* or bacterial vaginosis (particularly with a history of previous preterm ruptured membranes or labour).

Women with these conditions should be considered at risk of PPROM and advised to self-present if they suspect this has occurred. There is evidence that women with bacterial vaginosis and a previous history of preterm labour or ruptured membranes will have their recurrence risk reduced by treatment of the bacterial vaginosis (metronidazole is the drug of choice, with better results than clindamycin cream). Chlamydial infection should always be treated, with contact tracing, if it is detected.

Diagnosis

It is important that an accurate diagnosis is made, as women with PPROM require careful surveillance until delivery to detect and treat infection or fetal compromise promptly. Conversely, it would be unfortunate to subject a woman to such close surveillance and potential prolonged hospitalization on the basis of a false-positive diagnosis.

- If the history is suggestive of PPROM (gush or trickling of fluid vaginally, remote from micturition), a clean speculum examination should be performed, looking for the pooling of liquor in the upper vagina or trickling from the cervical os. (A digital examination should be avoided for fear of introducing infection.) This may be assisted by performing the examination when the woman has been semi-supine for a period of time to allow pooling of liquor, and by use of a maternal Valsalva manoeuvre to increase intraabdominal pressure.
- Cord prolapse should be excluded and high vaginal and endocervical swabs taken, including an endocervical swab for detection of *Chlamydia* by ELISA (enzyme-linked immunosorbent assay) or culture.

23 Preterm pre-labour rupture of membranes

Management

- *Tocolysis*. Once PPROM is confirmed, labour may intervene spontaneously. This is most likely in the first 48 hours. Tocolysis in the presence of ruptured membranes should only be undertaken with extreme caution and in the absence of any evidence of infection and in cases of extreme prematurity or at the lower bounds of viability. Short-term tocolysis may provide an opportunity for the positive effects of steroids to work.

- *Oligohydramnios*. In those in whom PPROM occurs very remotely from term (e.g. in the latter part of the second trimester), the presence of significant and sustained oligohydramnios carries a poor prognosis, particularly being associated with pulmonary hypoplasia. Serial ultrasound scanning has a role to play in determining the persistence of severe oligohydramnios. In these patients, the offer of a termination of pregnancy may be considered, as even those fetuses that survive *in utero* may not be viable once delivered, due to the difficulties with effective ventilation. Transabdominal and transcervical amnio-infusion has been tried with variable success rates.

- *Chorioamnionitis*. If labour does not occur in the more mature fetus, then a balance needs to be found between avoiding the complications due to iatrogenic prematurity and those due to chorioamnionitis. At initial assessment, any signs of chorioamnionitis should be excluded (fetal or maternal tachycardia, maternal pyrexia, tender or irritable uterus, offensive liquor, or maternal leucocytosis), as should any signs of fetal compromise (cardiotocograph). Obstetric ultrasound scanning will again be useful to assess residual liquor volume and any obvious fetal or uterine abnormalities that may have contributed to rupture of membranes or that may influence the subsequent management.

- In those who demonstrate no signs of infection or fetal compromise, conservative management to achieve improved fetal maturity is likely to be the optimal course. Close liaison with the neonatologists is essential, both in terms of informing and preparing the parents, and to ensure that appropriate neonatal care is available from the moment of delivery. This may require *in utero* transfer to another unit if such facilities are not available.

- Careful ongoing surveillance for the onset of chorioamnionitis or fetal compromise is essential.
  —At least twice-daily fetal heart rate monitoring is important, as fetal tachycardia is commonly the first sign of developing chorioamnionitis.
  —In the third trimester, CTG (cardiotocograph) may be the optimal way to effect this, as signs of fetal compromise may be detected.
  —Four-hourly observations of maternal pulse and temperature should be performed, and full blood count (FBC) should be checked twice weekly to detect leucocytosis, or on any occasion where symptoms or signs suggest the onset of infection.
  —Non-specific inflammatory markers, such as erythrocyte sedimentation rate (ESR) or C-reactive protein (CRP), have been used in surveillance, but add little to improve infection detection rates.
  —Equally, the value of repeated high vaginal swabs is dubious in the absence of any signs of infection, and the repeated examinations may, in fact, promote ascending infection.

23 Preterm pre-labour rupture of membranes

Prophylactic antibiotics are used in women with preterm ruptured membranes with a view to prolong the pregnancy. Subclinical infection may be a precipitant of the condition and the argument for antibiotics would seem logical, but improved outcome has not been demonstrated in recent trials. The risks of allergic reaction with the antibiotics and increase in resistant strains should be kept in mind. In the presence of clinical infection, the prompt use of appropriate intravenous antibiotics is essential.

Steroids. The use of maternally administered intramuscular betamethasone to promote fetal maturity has been widely credited with reduced mortality and morbidity in the premature neonate. However, their use in the presence of PPROM has been debated. There are arguments that steroids may facilitate the more rapid onset of infection by immune downregulation and that signs of infection may be masked by the steroids (antipyrogenic effects and leucocytosis). However, if these effects are considered during surveillance of the patient and the above level of surveillance is closely adhered to, the benefits of steroids prior to 34 weeks gestation far outweigh their disadvantages. Furthermore, the use of prophylactic antibiotics when steroids are used helps to counter the effects of any immune compromise.

Care of the fetus. During conservative management, placental function should be monitored with fortnightly growth scans, liquor volume, and surveillance by umbilical artery Doppler and CTG.

Labour and delivery. Delivery should be effected at the onset of any signs of chorioamnionitis or fetal compromise, or when adequate maturity is attained (ideally 37 weeks). Delivery may be vaginal if there are no other contraindications and there is sufficient time to achieve this safely.

Maternal complications. The maternal effects of prolonged hospitalization should not be forgotten, both in terms of psychological and social effects (particularly if there are already children at home) and in terms of the risk of thromboembolic disease. Risk factors for deep vein thrombosis (DVT) and thromboprophylaxis should be carefully considered.

Recommended further reading

Grieg, P.C. (1998). The diagnosis of intrauterine infection in women with preterm premature rupture of the membranes (PPROM). *Clinical Obstetrics and Gynecology* 41, 849–863.

Allen, S.R. (1998). Tocolytic therapy in preterm PROM. *Clinical Obstetrics and Gynecology* 41, 842–8.

Richards, D.S. (1998). Complications of prolonged PROM and oligohydramnios. *Clinical Obstetrics and Gynecology* 41, 817–26.

Ernest, J.M. (1998). Neonatal consequences of preterm PROM. *Clinical Obstetrics and Gynecology* 41, 827–31.

Mercer, B.M. (1998). Management of preterm premature rupture of the membranes. *Clinical Obstetrics and Gynecology* 41, 870–82.

Chapter 24

Term pre-labour rupture of membranes

The spontaneous rupture of membranes prior to the onset of labour constitutes an abnormal situation. The majority of women who demonstrate this phenomenon will establish in active labour spontaneously within the following 48 hours. Pre-labour rupture of membranes presents a number of potential complications and management dilemmas.

Diagnosis

Most patients with pre-labour rupture of membranes will present with a history of fluid loss vaginally. This may constitute a sudden gush of fluid or a steady trickle remote from micturition. Although liquor may be seen on the patient's underwear or sanitary towel, urinary incontinence may confound the diagnosis. Hence a speculum examination should be performed to confirm the diagnosis of ruptured membranes, at which liquor should be seen pooling in the upper vagina or trickling from the cervical os. Transiently raising intraabdominal pressure by asking the woman to cough or perform a Valsalva manoeuvre may help to demonstrate this if liquor is not immediately obvious.

The presence of other vaginal discharge may confuse the detection of liquor, and detection aids, such as Amnicator sticks (colour change from orange to dark blue due to alkaline liquor as opposed to acidic vaginal secretions), have been advocated to clarify diagnosis, but may lead to overdiagnosis (e.g. contamination with blood, semen, etc.).

Management

Evaluation

Following speculum examination to confirm the diagnosis and exclude cord prolapse, any evidence of fetal or maternal compromise must be ruled out. A fetal cardiotocograph (CTG) should be commenced. Evidence of possible fetal hypoxia, such as meconium-staining of the liquor or a suspicious or pathological CTG, should lead to expedition of delivery, by induction of labour or Caesarean section as deemed appropriate. Any signs of chorioamnionitis indicated by fetal tachycardia, maternal tachycardia, maternal pyrexia or rising leucocyte count, and uterine tenderness or irritability must be sought. Unstable lie of the fetus should be identified as it is associated with the risk of cord prolapse whilst the onset of contractions is awaited.

Conservative management

If none of the above problems are identified, then conservative management is a reasonable approach, to allow the possibility of spontaneous onset of labour.
- A high vaginal swab should be taken at speculum examination. Prolonged rupture of membranes may be followed by pyrexia in labour or by neonatal infection, and early identification of pathogens facilitates optimization of antibiotic therapy.
- The timing of induction of labour, if it does not commence spontaneously, remains a matter for debate and a source of variation in protocols between different units. The majority of units intervene 24–36 hours after pre-labour rupture of membranes to allow time for the spontaneous onset of contractions and to reduce the risk of chorioamnionitis.

24 Term pre-labour rapture of membranes

Labour and delivery

The mode of induction of labour also varies, with either prostaglandins (vaginally, or in some units, orally) or synthetic oxytocin (syntocinon). In the presence of ruptured membranes, there is no difference in the mean induction to delivery interval whether prostaglandin or syntocinon is used. However, the protocols of most units differentiate between an unfavourable cervix, where the use of prostaglandins is favoured, compared with a favourable cervix, when use of intravenous syntocinon infusion is preferred.

Fetuses who have marked oligohydramnios secondary to pre-labour rupture of membranes may demonstrate cord compression, with corresponding CTG changes (variable decelerations with shouldering) with uterine contractions. Amnio-infusion has been used in some centres to alleviate the effects of cord compression, but it is rarely practised in the UK.

Recommended further reading

1 Parry, S. and Strauss, J.F. (1998). Premature rupture of the fetal membranes. *New England Journal of Medicine* **338**, 663–70.

2 Duff, P. (1998). Premature rupture of the membranes in term patients: induction of labour versus expectant management. *Clinical Obstetrics and Gynecology* **41**, 883–91.

3 Mozurkewich, E. (1999). Management of premature rupture of membranes at term: an evidence-based approach. *Clinical Obstetrics and Gynecology* **42**, 749–56.

Chapter 25

Intrauterine growth restriction

Intrauterine growth restriction (IUGR) is a failure of the fetus to achieve t
expected weight for a given gestational age. The term 'small for gestational ag
(SGA) refers to any baby whose birthweight is below the tenth centile for t
given population. Many SGA babies will have reached their full growth pote
tial and hence not be growth-restricted. Conversely, some babies with IUC
may have a birthweight well above the tenth centile for the population but ha
failed to achieve their optimum birthweight as a result of a pathological proce
The terms are hence not synonymous,[1] and this chapter examines how to ide
tify the growth-restricted fetus in order to permit appropriate surveillance a
intervention.

Causes of IUGR/SGA can be classified as: constitutional (i.e. SGA b
not IUGR); chromosomal; uteroplacental; environmental (infection, drugs);
syndromic.

Available diagnostic tools[2]

- The *history* should include: previous obstetric history (particularly looking
  for previous growth restriction, adverse outcomes, or maternal medical
  problems); medical history (connective tissue disease, thrombotic events,
  endocrine disorders); drug history (therapeutic and recreational); family
  history (congenital abnormalities, thrombophilias); antepartum
  haemorrhage/history suggesting abruptio placentae; personal or close
  family history of recent viral illness; fetal movements.
- *Palpation* is an important part of routine antenatal care, and each visit afte
  24 weeks should include a measurement of symphysis–fundal height. This
  measurement in centimetres should equate to the gestation in weeks. A
  measurement more than 2 cm different from that expected requires furthe
  assessment of the fetus. Gross oligo- or polyhydramnios may be evident o
  abdominal palpation.
- *Ultrasound scanning*
  —Biometry. Measurements of biparietal diameter, head circumference,
    abdominal circumference, femur length, and cerebellum may be valuabl
    in the diagnosis, differential diagnosis, and surveillance of growth-
    restricted fetuses. Interpretation of an isolated set of measurements may
    be misleading.
  —Anatomy. Structural abnormalities may raise the suspicion of
    chromosomal abnormalities causing growth restriction.
  —Liquor volume. The amniotic fluid index is the sum of the deepest pool
    each quadrant and provides the most reproducible measure of amniotic
    fluid volume for the differential diagnosis or surveillance of IUGR.
- *Doppler waveform analysis*. The umbilical artery resistance index may be
  raised in the presence of raised placental resistance due to growth
  restriction of uteroplacental origin. Measurement of this parameter can ai
  in differential diagnosis (although abnormal umbilical artery Doppler
  waveforms can also occur in the presence of aneuploidy) and in the
  surveillance of a growth-restricted fetus during conservative management.
  In IUGR of uteroplacental origin, a compensatory fall in resistance index o
  the middle cerebral artery Doppler may occur. The absence of uterine
  artery Doppler waveform notching at 20 weeks gestation provides
  reassurance in a pregnancy with previous severe IUGR of uteroplacental
  origin (recurrence rate then only 2%).

25 Intrauterine growth restriction

Invasive fetal testing. Amniocentesis or placental biopsy facilitate karyotyping if aneuploidy is suspected, and samples can be rapidly analysed for the common trisomies using fluorescent *in situ* hybridization (FISH). Samples can also be cultured for more in-depth analysis. Amniotic fluid or fetal blood may be analysed using molecular biology techniques if fetal viral infection is strongly suspected as the cause of IUGR. All of these sampling techniques carry risks of infection, premature rupture of membranes, and premature labour.

Retrospective tests Maternal blood testing for recent cytomegalovirus, rubella, or toxoplasmosis infection; metabolic disorders (if suspected clinically); or thrombophilias may be carried out when IUGR is detected or retrospectively. The placenta should be sent (dry) for histopathological examination and, if fetal or neonatal death occurs, permission from the parents for post-mortem examination should be sought.

The constitutionally small baby

A fetus growing parallel to the lower centiles throughout the pregnancy that anatomically normal and has normal liquor volume and umbilical arte Doppler waveform is most likely to be constitutionally small. This is particular common in the pregnancies of slim women of Asian origin, but may occur Caucasians who are also of slight build. The use of customized growth charts fe fetal ultrasound biometry has been explored, and these are utilized routinely some units. Although a fetus persistently small to palpation may precipita serial ultrasound biometry to exclude decelerating growth, no deviation fro normal antenatal or intrapartum management should be required provided r additional concerns arise.

Fetal aneuploidy

The most common aneuploidies[1] to cause fetal growth restriction are as follow in order of descending frequency: triploidy; trisomies 18, 21, and 13; and del tion of 4p. Rearrangements may also result in IUGR.

- Findings that should prompt suspicion of trisomy in IUGR include: symmetrical IUGR; normal or increased liquor volume; normal Doppler studies; structural abnormalities and soft markers (these may occasionally be a confusing effect of starvation, e.g. echogenic bowel); advanced maternal age; and biochemical or nuchal translucency screening results.
- Triploidy, which most commonly presents prior to 26 weeks gestation, may resemble IUGR of uteroplacental origin, with asymmetry in the growth restriction, reduced liquor volume, and abnormal Doppler analyses. The mothers may also develop pre-eclampsia, encouraging the assumption tha malplacentation accounts for the IUGR.
- If chromosomal abnormalities are suspected, then karyotyping should be offered with appropriate counselling, as the diagnosis of aneuploidy may influence the approach of the parents to ongoing management of the pregnancy.

Uteroplacental insufficiency

This is the most common cause of IUGR, and occurs due to abnormalities i placental development and trophoblast invasion. This may be idiopathic or du to one of a number of recognized causes. Growth restriction that is severe an of early onset may result on fetal cell hypoplasia such that, if the fetus surviv to extrauterine life, it may never exhibit full catch-up growth.[3]

Recognized causes of placental insufficiency include:

- *Connective tissue disorders* (e.g. systemic lupus erythematosis). Check history and autoantibodies, including antinuclear antibody and anti-doubl stranded DNA.
- *Pre-eclampsia*. Clinical diagnosis; see Chapter 14.
- *Diabetes*, particularly when associated with peripheral vascular disease.
- *Placental abruption*. Check for history of antepartum haemorrhage or unexplained abdominal pains.

Placental infarction or thrombosis (particularly associated with thrombophilias, especially antiphospholipid antibodies, antithrombin III deficiency or combined mutations).
Chorion amnionitis (bacterial or viral; see under 'Infection' below).
Chorionangioma may be evident on ultrasound.

erial monitoring of the IUGR pregnancy thought to be due to placental insuf-
ciency should involve regular (fortnightly) biometry. Liquor volume assess-
ient and Doppler waveform analyses (umbilical artery ± middle cerebral
rtery) may be carried out fortnightly or weekly (or more frequently), depend-
it upon the clinical situation. Delivery should occur when the risk of contin-
ed exposure to a hostile intrauterine environment appears to outweigh the
sks of prematurity.

Environmental causes of IUGR

Maternal drug usage[1]
Therapeutic drugs
IUGR may occur as a result of the ingestion of some therapeutic drugs, particularly antihypertensive drugs.

- There is a well-established link with beta-antagonists. The link with alpha/mixed receptor antagonists is less clear).
- Calcium channel blockers and methyl dopa are associated with less IUGR.
- There is some evidence that cyclosporin (in transplant patients) may be associated with growth restriction in some cases, but no good evidence of a role for corticosteroids in causation of IUGR.

However, with all these therapeutic drugs, it must be remembered that th underlying maternal disease for which the drugs are being taken may cause degree of IUGR.

Recreational drugs
By far the most common and unequivocal recreational drug use implicated i IUGR is tobacco smoking. Cigarette smoking produces a twofold relative risk o having a growth-restricted fetus. The effects are dose- and gestation-dependen with the maximum growth-restrictive effects occurring in the third trimeste although it appears that those smoking in the first trimester undergo some degre of placental adaptation if the pregnancy is not lost. Although it is the nicotin in cigarettes that is addictive, it is the carbon monoxide and cyanide that exer adverse effects on the fetus. Carbon monoxide shifts the maternal oxygen disso ciation curve to the disadvantage of the fetus, and it is preferentially taken up b fetal erythrocytes. Smokers should therefore be strongly advised to stop, an nicotine patches may be safely considered to aid their withdrawal from addiction

Alcohol to excess results in fetal alcohol syndrome (severe IUGR, central nerv ous system (CNS) involvement, and facial dysmorphism). However, the saf daily dose of alcohol has not been determined, and even moderate or low alco hol intake may be associated with IUGR or mild CNS involvement in the thir trimester. Women should probably be advised that one or two units per week i a sensible limit.

Of the illegal recreational drugs, cocaine, amphetamines, and cannabis are a known to be associated with IUGR, and there is some evidence that opiates an inhaled solvents may also restrict fetal growth. IUGR as a result of Ecstas (MDMA) abuse appears rare, provided its use is only sporadic. Management o patients using recreational drugs should be in conjunction with addiction serv ices, as sudden withdrawal of drugs of dependence may not be appropriate. Th paediatricians should be involved, with careful surveillance of the neonate, a withdrawal may be problematic.

Infection
Congenital infection with cytomegalovirus, toxoplasmosis, or rubella may resu in a number of problems, including IUGR. Serological evidence of infection i the mother may be sought and, if positive or if there are other indicators of fet infection, then invasive procedures may be used to determine fetal infection.

Asymptomatic human immunodeficiency virus (HIV) infection does not affec birthweight, but low birthweight may be encountered in advanced maternal disease

Fetal syndromes

A variety of fetal syndromes may result in growth restriction. These include skeletal deformities, which are likely to be suspected or diagnosed ultrasonographically *in utero* (osteochondrodysplasias affecting the whole skeleton—thanetophoric dysplasias or osteogenesis imperfecta; dystoces affecting single bones—hemivertibrae or limb reduction defects), or chromosome or gene abnormalities resulting in general growth reduction (autosomal recessive disorders, such as Donohue's syndrome; confined placental mosaicism; uniparental disomy; chromosome breakage syndromes, such as Fanconi's syndrome). An offer of termination may be appropriate for some of these conditions, once the parents have been fully counselled. Should the fetus prove non-viable, post mortem should be recommended, with careful, directed chromosome analysis of fetus, placenta, and parental blood wherever possible and acceptable. Genetic counselling should be offered.

References

Kingdom, J., Baker, P., and Blair, E. (2000). Definitions of intrauterine growth restriction. In *Intrauterine growth restriction, aetiology and management* (ed. J Kingdom and P. Baker), p. 1. Springer-Verlag, London.

Enkin, M., Keirse, M.J.N.C., Renfrew, M., and Neilson, J. (eds.) (1995). Assessment of fetal growth, size and well-being. In *A guide to effective care in pregnancy and childbirth*, 2nd edn, pp. 61–72. Oxford University Press, Oxford.

Weiner, C.P. (1994). Fetal growth deficiency and its evaluation. In *High risk pregnancy—management options* (ed. D.K. James, P.J. Steer, C.P. Weiner, and B. Gonik), pp. 759–70. W.B. Saunders Company, London.

Chapter 26

Prolonged pregnancy

Prolonged pregnancy is a matter of concern to women and obstetricians because of its association with fetal morbidity and mortality. This remains the most common cause of induction of labour.

Prolonged pregnancy, post-dated pregnancy, post-term, postdatism, and post-maturity are terms used to denote a pregnancy that has gone beyond 42 weeks or 294 days from the first date of the last menstrual period. These terms are used with the idea of conveying a risk situation but, in practice, prolonged pregnancy is the preferred term. Prolonged pregnancy is defined by the International Federation of Gynaecologist and Obstetricians (FIGO) as any pregnancy that exceeds 294 days from the first day of the last menstrual period in a woman with regular 28 day cycles.

The term postdatism is best avoided, and the duration of pregnancy is stated as so many days post-EDD (estimated date of delivery), e.g. 41 weeks 4 days, unless it is more than 42 weeks when it should be called prolonged pregnancy.

Incidence

The incidence of prolonged pregnancy varies from 3 to 10% or more depending on whether it is calculated in a prospective or retrospective manner. It will also vary depending on whether calculation is based on history and clinical examination alone or whether an ultrasound scan was used to calculate the gestation in the first half of the pregnancy. Naegele's rule has traditionally been used to determine the EDD.

Dates cannot be relied upon in the following circumstances.
- About 10–30% of women give a doubtful date of their LMP.
- Irregular periods.
- Recent use of combined oral contraceptive pills (COCPs).
- Conception during lactational amenorrhoea.

Perinatal mortality is increased in those with unknown dates and every effort should be made to establish the EDD in early pregnancy. Ultrasound has changed our practice. Routine early pregnancy ultrasound reduces the incidence of post-term pregnancy.

Fetal risks

Perinatal mortality and morbidity

It has long been recognized that prolonged pregnancy is associated with increased risks of perinatal mortality and morbidity. After exclusion of congenital malformations, intrapartum deaths were 4 times more common and early neonatal deaths were 3 times more common in infants born after 42 weeks of gestation. In addition to that, meconium staining of amniotic fluid and fetal distress during labour were much more common in prolonged pregnancies. Meconium aspiration is a serious problem and, when a significant amount has been aspirated, clearance of the respiratory passage and assisted ventilation may be required to treat the infant.

With the development and application of modern techniques of fetal monitoring the perinatal risk in prolonged pregnancy has been reduced.

Ultrasound is now used routinely for dating pregnancy in many units, and the prevalence of prolonged pregnancy in a well-dated population is small.

Fetal postmaturity syndrome

Postmaturity syndrome is the term used to describe post-term infants exhibiting physical signs of intrauterine malnutrition. They constitute only a small proportion of babies born after 42 weeks. It is now known that a baby born with such features can present at an earlier gestational period. Therefore the term, 'prolonged pregnancy' should be preferred to postmaturity for pregnancies beyond 42 weeks.

The following features characterize this syndrome:
- Absence of vernix caseosa.
- Absence of lanugo hair.
- Abundant scalp hair.
- Long fingernails.
- Dry, cracked desquamated skin.
- Body length increased in relation to body weight.
- Alert and apprehensive facies.
- Meconium staining of skin and mucous membranes.

This syndrome actually resembles intrauterine growth restriction (IUGR) and occurs in earlier gestations with equal frequency. Therefore the term 'postmaturity' is best avoided.

Other risks

The incidence of birth injury is higher in post-term pregnancies and is related to the higher incidence of macrosomia when compared to that in term infants. Macrosomic infants are susceptible to birth injuries such as fractures, cephalo-haematomas, and palsies.

Other neonatal complications such as hypothermia, hypoglycaemia, and poly-cythaemia are mainly due to the presence of associated growth restriction.

267

Maternal risks

- Maternal anxiety increases once the estimated date of confinement is passed.
- Maternal risks in prolonged pregnancy include increased operative delivery, haemorrhage, and psychological morbidity.

Management

The first step in the management of prolonged pregnancy is to confirm the dates and to assess the presence of any risk factors. Debate exists between the active approach of elective induction of labour at 41 weeks and the conservative approach of awaiting spontaneous onset of labour with appropriate fetal surveillance. The available evidence is reviewed here.

Confirmation of dates

Evidence should be sought from the antenatal records to confirm the dates. Clinical methods are not always accurate. Ultrasound examination in the first or early second trimester is likely to give an accurate estimation of the dates within an error margin of 1 or 2 weeks. Ultrasound dating of pregnancy in the late second or third trimester of pregnancy is not reliable. In the UK all pregnant mothers are offered a routine mid-trimester scan. Therefore, in current practice, pregnancies progressing beyond 42 weeks are very few.

Assessment of risk factors

There exists a significant but small risk of increased perinatal mortality when pregnancy is prolonged beyond 42 weeks. Therefore it is important to assess any risk factors complicating the pregnancy. Pregnancies with diabetes, pre-eclampsia, recurrent antepartum haemorrhage, and IUGR where placental insufficiency could be a potential problem should not be allowed to progress post-term.

Counselling for induction of labour or conservative approach

Women's preference is often given as reason for conservative management. With the implementation of *Changing childbirth* in the UK[1] where care of pregnant women is mainly women-centred, counselling of the woman is of paramount importance. Many women will see elective induction of labour as interference with a natural process. Therefore, appropriate facilities should exist for fetal surveillance if the conservative approach of waiting for spontaneous onset of labour is decided. In reality very few women like to wait beyond 42 weeks.

Elective induction versus conservative approach

In an uncomplicated pregnancy controversy still exists between induction of labour by 42 weeks and conservative approach of waiting for spontaneous onset of labour.

- Present evidence favours a policy of induction of labour by 42 weeks because of reduced perinatal mortality, decreased meconium staining of amniotic fluid, and a small decrease in Caesarean section compared with conservative management. This is the policy in most of the obstetric units in the UK.
- Proponents of a conservative approach argue that a conservative policy of waiting till spontaneous onset of labour is safe provided appropriate fetal surveillance is performed. However, what constitutes an appropriate method of fetal surveillance beyond 42 weeks is not clearly established. The next section details the tests used for fetal surveillance in pregnancies that go beyond 42 weeks.

Fetal surveillance

Fetal movement chart

Fetal activity in the form of fetal movements has been found to be a useful indicator of fetal health. Although inexpensive, its value in monitoring prolonged pregnancy has not been validated. Based on current data the fetal movement chart alone may not be relied upon for monitoring fetal health in prolonged pregnancy.

Cardiotocography (nonstress test)

A recording of the fetal heart rate (FHR) for a period of 20–30 min called the nonstress test has become one of the most popular methods of antenatal fetal surveillance. Definition of normal, suspicious and abnormal FHR patterns have been described by FIGO. The fetal acoustic stimulation test (FAST) where a vibroacoustic stimulus is used to elicit accelerations of FHR is a useful way to reduce the number of non-reactive traces and to shorten the testing time. Compromise to the fetus in prolonged pregnancy is generally due to oligohydramnios or reduced liquor volume. If the trace is not reactive despite stimulating the fetus or if it shows significant decelerations, then it indicates possible compromise and should be an indication for delivery.

Assessment of amniotic fluid volume

Fetal urine contributes significantly to the volume of amniotic fluid. With diminished placental function, selective perfusion of the brain and heart and reduced perfusion of other systems including the kidneys take place. This leads to reduction of fetal urine formation and thus the sequelae of oligohydramnios in severe IUGR. Thus, in prolonged pregnancy, assessing the amniotic fluid volume can help to monitor fetal compromise that is due to gradual decline in placental function. Evaluation by palpation may be deceptive whilst impression of the adequacy on ultrasonographic examination is more reliable. Amniotic fluid index is used for the assessment of liquor volume in these pregnancies. In prolonged pregnancy, an amniotic fluid index of 5 cm or less is suggestive of reduced placental function.

Other methods

More complex fetal monitoring incorporating a formal biophysical profile has been suggested for monitoring prolonged pregnancy. The role of Doppler ultrasound has been evaluated in high-risk pregnancy, e.g. IUGR or severe pre-eclampsia, but its role in prolonged pregnancy has not been properly evaluated.

Conclusions

Prolonged pregnancy remains a matter of concern for clinicians and women. The actual risk of fetal demise is small. With the use of routine ultrasound examination the incidence of prolonged pregnancy has decreased. Current evidence supports elective induction of labour by 42 weeks because of reduced perinatal mortality, decreased meconium staining of amniotic fluid and a small decrease in Caesarean section compared with conservative management. Nevertheless, some may see induction as an unnecessary intervention in a natural process of childbirth and may opt for conservative management. Fetal surveillance is necessary when a conservative approach is adopted. Surveillance should include amniotic fluid volume assessment. Special care is needed in labour and delivery to prevent meconium aspiration.

Reference

1 Department of Health (1993). *Changing childbirth, report of the Expert Maternity Group*, Cumberlege Report. HMSO, London.

Induction of labour

Induction of labour is the artificial initiation of uterine contractions prior to their spontaneous onset in an attempt to achieve progressive effacement and dilatation of the cervix and delivery of the baby. The term is usually restricted to pregnancies at gestations greater than the legal definition of fetal viability (24 weeks in the UK).

The aim of successful induction is to achieve vaginal delivery when continuation of pregnancy presents a threat to the life or well-being of the mother or her unborn child. The infant should be delivered in good condition within an acceptable time-frame and with a minimum of maternal discomfort or side-effects. In current obstetric practice induction is usually performed for obstetric or medical indications. Social induction comprises a small proportion of the total inductions.

Indications for induction of labour

In the UK the most common indication is prolonged pregnancy. There is good evidence that induction of labour should be offered routinely to all women whose pregnancies continue beyond 42 weeks gestation. Induction during this period is associated with beneficial outcome in terms of reduced Caesarean section rate; reduced operative vaginal delivery; reduced chance of fetal distress, meconium staining, and macrosomia; and reduced risk of fetal and neonatal death.

While in a few circumstances the advantages of elective delivery by induction are clear, e.g. to prevent maternal morbidity in fulminating pre-eclampsia, the advantages are less clear when it is done for fetal macrosomia. Maternal indications for induction are few as the pregnant mother is directly accessible for examination and investigation. The majority of inductions are done for fetal indications and are mainly based on epidemiological evidence. The tests available for fetal well-being also influence the induction rates.

Attention should be paid to women's views on induction, especially when the indications for induction are not strong. Many women believe that induced labour, not being natural, is more painful than spontaneous labour and that in induced labour they are not in control of what is happening to them during childbirth. Such negative attitudes may partly reflect inadequate provision of information regarding induction. Some of the common indications for induction are:

- Gestational or insulin-dependent diabetes.
- Pre-eclampsia.
- Hypertension.
- Renal disease.

Factors influencing the outcome of induced labour

Favourability or ripeness of the cervix.
Parity.
The method chosen for induction.

Failed induction is diagnosed when, in the absence of fetal distress, acute events such as abruption or cord prolapse, or failure to progress due to cephalopelvic disproportion or malposition, a woman who was induced did not deliver vaginally because the woman did not enter the active phase of labour despite adequate uterine contractions for 12 hours.

The success of induction depends largely on the state of the cervix at the beginning of induction. The parity and the method of induction, the process of prelabour cervical softening, and eventually dilatation (cervical ripening) is part of a continuum that culminates in labour. Bishop's score,[1] or a modified version of it, is used to assess the favourability of the cervix. The characteristics of the cervix and the station of the head are considered. A modified scoring system recommended in the NICE (National Institute of Clinical Excellence) guidelines[2] is given in Table 27.1.

Table 27.1 A scoring system used to assess the favourability of the cervix and the station of the head for labour[2]

	Score		
	0	1	2
Position of cervix	Posterior	Axial	Anterior
Length of cervix	2 cm	1 cm	< 0.5 cm
Dilatation of cervix	0 cm	1 cm	> 2 cm
Consistency of cervix	Firm	Soft	Soft and stretchable
Station of presenting part	−2	−1	0

Methods of cervical priming

The process of functional transformation of the cervix from a sphincteric organ acting to preserve and contain the growing fetus within the uterus to a canal that softens, shortens, and dilates to facilitate the passage of the fetus starts well before the actual labour itself. During this transformation process, a method used for cervical priming might act as a method to induce labour.

Pharmacological methods

- *Prostaglandins.* If induction is necessary, ripening with prostaglandins is useful. There are advantages to the use of prostaglandins (PG) for ripening the cervix and for induction of labour, compared with oxytocin alone (decreased need for analgesia in labour, fewer cases undelivered within 12 and 24 hours of painful contractions, decreased operative delivery). This is at the expense of increased gastrointestinal side-effects and uterine hypertonus, which occurs in up to 7% of cases. Intravaginal PGE_2 (either gel or tablets) is marginally superior to intracervical PGE_2 gel with higher successful induction rates and decreased need for oxytocin.
- *Misoprostol* is much cheaper and more easily stored than other prostaglandins. Questions still remain as to the safest and most effective dose and it is hence not recommended other than within a scientific study.
- *Oxytocin.* Regular uterine contractions achieved with intravenous (IV) infusions of oxytocin or buccal oxytocin or demoxytocin would result in cervical ripening in most cases. Control studies have shown it to be a less satisfactory method than local prostaglandin application.
- *Other topical pharmacological agents* that have been tried but are not in regular use are *oestradiol* (150–300 mg) in tylose gel, *purified porcine ovarian relaxin* (1–4 mg) in a gel applied vaginally or intracervically, and *mifepristone* an anti-progestin in a dose of 200 mg orally for 2 days, 48 hours before the formal induction.

Mechanical methods of cervical ripening

- *Hygroscopic tents*, such as natural laminaria tents or synthetic sponges impregnated with magnesium sulfate (Lamicel), into the cervical os, 12 hours before labour.
- *Foley's catheter* in the cervix with the balloon inflated with 30 mL of saline.

Since it appears that mechanical agents bring about cervical ripening through a local release of tissue prostaglandins in the cervix or the lower uterine segment, there seems little rationale for their use where topical prostaglandins are available.

Conclusion

In summary, PGE_2 intravaginal gel is currently the best agent to use. It has marginal advantages over intracervical PGE_2 gel. In primigravidae with an unfavourable cervix, an initial dose of 2 mg may be given, followed by further 1 mg doses at 6-hourly intervals to a maximum of 4 mg.

Methods of induction of labour

A wide variety of mechanical and chemical methods have been used for labour induction, namely:

Amniotomy.
Oxytocic agents (oxytocin or one of the prostaglandins).
Sweeping or stripping of the membranes (rarely as a formal method of induction).

Amniotomy

Amniotomy or artificial rupture of the membranes is one of the most irrevocable interventions in pregnancy and, more than any other procedure, calls for a firm commitment to delivery. A combination of mechanical induction by amniotomy followed by oxytocin if necessary is often used. If oxytocin infusion is commenced at the time of amniotomy rather than delayed, there are advantages of a significantly shorter induction–delivery interval, reduced operative delivery rates, and a reduction in postpartum haemorrhage. Conversely, up to 88% of women with a favourable cervix will labour within 24 hours after amniotomy alone.

Hind-water or high amniotomy with a Drew–Smythe catheter is hardly used in modern obstetrics, except for cases of polyhydramnios with a firm indication for induction. The procedure can cause damage to the fetus, placenta, or maternal genital tract and hence should be undertaken by a senior clinician.

Oxytocin

Since the introduction of oxytocin as an IV infusion in the 1940s, it has come to be the most widely used method of labour induction. The oxytocin infusion should be given via an infusion pump, and fluid load minimized. Most infusion regimens commence at low rates (1–4 mU/min) and increase titrated against contractions, arithmetically or logarithmically, at intervals of 30 minutes up to a maximum of approximately 32 mU/min. There is clear evidence that there is no benefit in using intervals of less than 30 minutes. Most but not all of the reports indicate that the use of longer intervals reduced uterine hypertonus, decreased maximum and total dose of oxytocin, and decreased the rate of Caesarean section for fetal heart rate (FHR) abnormalities. There appears to be no adverse effect on induction–delivery intervals.

Prostaglandins for induction of labour

Both prostaglandins $PGF_{2\alpha}$ and PGE_2 have been used for cervical priming as well as for labour induction. Depending on the cervical score and the dosage, prostaglandins cause cervical priming or result in induction of labour. The most widely adopted mode of administration of PGE_2 has become the vaginal route. When the cervical score is good, a single vaginal application of PGE_2, 1 mg, can induce labour and avoid the necessity for formal oxytocin–amniotomy induction in nulliparas and multiparas with a concomitant reduction in Caesarean section rates. For women with a good cervical score, amniotomy and oxytocin infusion would be the preferred method as it is less expensive and allows better control over uterine contractions than vaginal prostaglandins. For nulliparous women with a poor cervical score, vaginal prostaglandins are preferable. This could be followed by amniotomy when the cervix is favourable and oxytocin infusion if uterine contractions are inadequate or if there is poor progress of labour.

Induction of labour in special circumstances

Intrauterine fetal death

Prostaglandins PGE_2 and $PGF_{2\alpha}$ and their various analogues have been used vi
different routes for induction of labour in the presence of intrauterine death
Intra-amniotic instillation is best avoided because of the risk of sepsis an
erratic absorption through devitalized membranes. Gemeprost (Cervagem
1 mg pessaries can be used vaginally at 3-hourly intervals for a maximum o
5 doses and the course may be repeated after an interval of 24 hours in cases o
failure.

Previous Caesarean section, breech presentation, and multiple pregnancy

Although the above are considered as relative contraindications to induction o
labour, under compelling circumstances labour can be induced in such case
after careful selection.

- For women with a previous lower segment Caesarean scar, induction of
  labour with rupture of the membranes and oxytocin infusion can be
  carried out when the cervix is favourable and the pelvis appears clinically
  adequate. Use of PG has been associated with greater incidence of uterine
  rupture (25/1000) compared with those in spontaneous labour (5/1000) or
  those receiving oxytocin infusion (8/1000).
- In twin pregnancy when the first twin is in cephalic presentation and
  cervical score is favourable, induction of labour by amniotomy and
  oxytocin infusion is usually effective. A PGE_2 pessary or gel can be used for
  cervical priming in the presence of an unfavourable cervix. However, with
  twin pregnancies, an unfavourable cervical score is rare at term.
- Current evidence favours elective Caesarean section for breech presentation
  If the woman insists on vaginal breech delivery, where chances of achieving
  vaginal delivery are reasonable, labour may be induced by amniotomy and
  oxytocin infusion, especially in cases of extended breech with the
  presenting part well settled in the pelvis. Because of the significant risk of
  cord prolapse with membrane rupture in those with incomplete breech
  presentations, it is best to opt for a Caesarean section.

In these special circumstances (previous Caesarean section, twins, breech), th
rate of progress of labour especially in the active phase should be monitore
closely and early recourse to Caesarean section should be taken when th
progress is slow.

Stabilizing induction

In patients with a transverse or oblique lie with no apparent cause, especially i
multiparae, stabilizing induction at 38–40 weeks may be a valid option of man
agement. External cephalic version should allow the head to be in the lowe
segment. Artificial rupture of membranes, after excluding cord presentation
and use of oxytocin to initiate uterine contractions should stabilize the presen
tation. The accoucheur should hold the head in position till no shift is felt i
between a few uterine contractions.

Risks and complications of induction of labour

Induction of labour is a potentially hazardous obstetric intervention. There are three broad groups of risks associated with induction of labour.

- Risks associated with termination of pregnancy artificially before the spontaneous onset of labour.
- Risks associated with artificial stimulation of uterine contraction.
- Risks attributable to the specific method of labour induction.

Risks can be summarized as follows.

- Failed induction equates to Caesarean section.
- Inadvertent pre-term delivery is a risk with any induction.
- Uterine hyperstimulation could lead to fetal hypoxia and fetal death.
- In higher order multipara and in patients with a previous Caesarean section, uterine hyperstimulation could lead to uterine rupture.
- Atonic postpartum haemorrhage occurs more commonly following induced labour than with spontaneous labour and may be related to the length of labour, which is usually longer with induction. It probably occurs less commonly following prostaglandin induction compared to oxytocin induction.
- Low amniotomy may cause prolapse of the cord, especially with a high presenting part, and possible introduction of pathogenic organisms.
- Use of oxytocin, if excessive, may result in neonatal jaundice.
- Prolonged infusion of relatively high doses of oxytocin in dilute solutions can lead to maternal water intoxication, hyponatraemia, coma, and even death. Similar disturbances in neonatal biochemistry, leading to seizures, could also occur in severe cases.
- Prostaglandins may produce gastrointestinal tract side-effects. This is greater with $PGE_{2\alpha}$ and occurs less commonly with endocervical and extraamniotic administration compared to oral, intravenous, or vaginal use.
- PGE_2 may cause pyrexia due to its direct effect on thermoregulatory centres in the brain.

'The spontaneous onset of labour is a robust and effective mechanism and should be given the chance to operate. We should only induce labour when we are sure that we can do better.'[3]

References

Bishop, E.H. (1964). Pelvic scoring for elective induction. *Obstetrics and Gynecology* 24, 266–8.

National Institute of Clinical Excellence (NICE) (2001). *Induction of labour. Inherited clinical guideline D*. London. www.nice.org.uk.

Turnbull, A.C. (1976). In Obstetricians welcome reversal of trend in cases of induced labour (Nowland). *Irish Times*, 30th June 1976, p. 3.

Hydrops fetalis

Hydrops fetalis is the description given to the condition of a fetus in which fluid has accumulated in the fetal tissues or body cavities. Fluid may not be seen in all compartments but in its most severe form the fetus has ascites, pleural effusions, pericardial effusions, and soft tissue oedema. The placenta and cord may be oedematous. Hydrops is also frequently associated with polyhydramnios. Hydrops may occur at any gestation but is not usually seen till 16–18 weeks. The earlier the presentation, the worse the prognosis.

Cystic hygroma is a specific condition that falls within the definition of hydrops. It is a collection of fluid behind the fetal neck occasionally extending laterally to the sides of the neck. In its mildest form it is termed nuchal thickening, nuchal oedema, or nuchal translucency. In its most severe form, it can create a large septated sac of fluid around the fetal neck that can even extend right down the fetal body.

Causes

Fetal hydrops can be divided into 'immune' and 'non-immune' causes. Immune hydrops is due to feto-maternal blood group incompatibility and is dealt with in Chapter 13.

Causes of non-immune hydrops

There are a large number of maternal, fetal, and placental diseases that may result in hydrops.

- *Chromosomal disorders.* When hydrops presents early in gestation, chromosomal disease is the likely diagnosis. Trisomies 21 (Down syndrome) and XO (Turner's syndrome) account for 75% of disorders, but other chromosomal disorders may also exist including trisomies 18, 15, and 13; triploidy; tetraploidy; partial deletions; and rearrangements.
- *Cardiovascular disorders.* Cardiovascular disorders are the most frequent causes of hydrops in Europe. These may be either structural malformations or cardiac rhythm abnormalities. Hydrops may be associated with most major structural heart defects or cardiomyopathies, but the rhythm abnormalities are mainly due to supraventricular tachycardia or atrial flutter. Rarely, complete heart block may present with hydrops.
- *Thoracic malformations.* These mainly include:
  —Diaphragmatic hernia.
  —Pulmonary sequestration.
  —Cystic adenomatous malformation of the lung.
  —Chylothorax.
- *Urinary tract abnormalities.* Obstruction at the lower end of the urinary tract (posterior urethral valves, urethral atresia) may lead to bladder overdistension and ultimate spillage of urine into the abdominal cavity resulting in fetal ascites (rather than generalized hydrops.) In these cases, oligohydramnios is an important feature. Wilm's tumours may be associated with fetal ascites along with other rare disorders of the fetal kidney.
- *Meconium peritonitis.* Fetal ascites may result from intestinal perforation. Cystic fibrosis should be considered.
- *Skeletal dysplasias.* Many of the lethal skeletal dysplasias may be associated with hydrops.

Fetal anaemia. This is the mechanism leading to immune hydrops. However, there are other important causes of fetal anaemia:
—Massive feto-maternal haemorrhage.
—Homozygous alpha thalassaemia (most common cause of hydrops worldwide).
—Glucose-6-phosphate dehydrogenase deficiency.
—Congenital infection with Parvovirus B19.

Fetal infections. In addition to Parvovirus, other congenital infections may result in hydrops without fetal anaemia.
—Cytomegalovirus (CMV).
—Rubella.
—Varicella.
—Cocksackie virus.
—Respiratory syncytial virus.
—Herpes simplex virus.
—Hepatitis.
—Toxoplasmosis.

Monochorionic twin gestation. Hydrops may occur in the recipient twin in the twin–twin transfusion syndrome from overperfusion and congestive cardiac failure. The acardiac twin malformation may also result in the normal twin becoming a hydropic fetus.

Genetic conditions. Many syndromes associated with multiple congenital malformations are associated with hydrops. Also, many metabolic and storage disorders may present with hydrops.

Clinical presentation

When a pregnancy is complicated by fetal hydrops, the woman may complain o
- Reduced fetal movement (a severely hydropic fetus has poor activity).
- Large for dates (either due to associated polyhydramnios or a large grossly hydropic fetus).

When the fetus and placenta are grossly hydropic, the woman may present wit
severe pre-eclampsia.

Diagnosis

The diagnosis of hydrops is made by ultrasound examination of the fetu
Accumulation of fluid in the chest, peritoneal cavity, or fetal neck is easily iden
tified and soft tissue oedema can be visualized.

Ultrasound assessment

Ultrasound examination of the fetus is also important in attempting to identif
the underlying cause.
- Detailed examination of the fetal heart (including M mode) must be performed to determine structural abnormalities or rhythm defects (in particular, supraventricular tachycardia).
- Tachydysrhythmias may be intermittent. It is therefore important to check more than once.
- Careful examination of the intracranial structures and liver should be performed. Calcification may be suggestive of congenital infection (cytomegalovirus; toxoplasmosis, etc.).
- Markers of chromosomal disease may be apparent.
  —Cystic hygroma *per se* carries a 70% chance of an associated chromosomal abnormality.
  —Other markers suggestive of chromosomal disease include choroid plexu
  cysts, ventriculomegaly, facial clefting, clinodactyly, sandal gap, and shor
  femur length.
- A full skeletal survey will identity a skeletal dysplasia as the underlying cause.
- The absence of amniotic fluid may suggest an obstructive uropathy.
- The placenta, cord, and fetus must be examined to exclude vascular abnormalities (e.g. chorioangioma of the placenta).

Maternal investigations

A careful enquiry should be made into any previously affected pregnancie
inherited genetic disease or metabolic disorders, and viral illness during th
pregnancy. Investigations should include:
- Maternal blood taken for Kleihauer, haemoglobin, electrophoresis, blood group, and antibody screen.
- Viral serology (in particular, CMV, toxoplasmosis, Parvovirus B19).

etal investigations

urther management should be directed at the likely aetiology—in particular, e site of fluid accumulation may suggest the underlying cause. An invasive ocedure is usually indicated, as determination of the fetal karyotype is a basic sential. Even if a cardiac malformation or rhythm abnormality is believed to ave caused the hydrops, these malformations themselves may be associated ith a chromosomal disorder.

Invasive testing may be by amniocentesis, chorionic villous sampling (CVS), or fetal blood sampling (cordocentesis). All these invasive procedures carry a risk to the pregnancy and, as the hydropic fetus is already compromised, this risk of complications is slightly higher than normal.

—In the investigation of hydrops, fetal blood sampling is a superior procedure as, not only will a rapid and reliable karyotype be obtained, but haematological tests will also show whether fetal anaemia is the underlying disorder and whether blood transfusion is indicated (see Chapter 13).

If a metabolic condition is suspected for which the gene sequence is known, CVS for DNA extraction may be appropriate.

If a congenital infection is suspected, testing for a specific infection by polymerase chain reaction (PCR) on amniotic fluid is the most reliable test.

Management

Fetal hydrops carries a very high perinatal mortality (81–95%). The mortality increases with decreasing gestational age at diagnosis. Treatment should be directed at the cause.

In utero treatment

- Fetal anaemia is one of the more treatable conditions whether the anaemia is due to maternal–fetal blood group incompatibility, viral infection, or haemorrhage. Intrauterine blood transfusions are relatively safe, whereby blood is transfused directly into the umbilical vein (intravascular transfusion) or peritoneal cavity (intraperitoneal transfusion).
- Idiopathic tachydysrhythmias may respond to maternal administration of cardiac dysrhythmic agents (e.g. digoxin, verapamil, propranolol, flecainide adenosine).
- Isolated pleural effusions may be due to a benign condition (e.g. chylothorax), but prognosis is impaired because of fetal lung compression. *In utero* drainage and/or insertion of a pleuro-amniotic shunt may dramatically improve the outcome.
- If a lethal condition is diagnosed (e.g. chromosomal, skeletal dysplasia), the parents should be counselled and offered the option of termination of pregnancy.
- If maternal complications exist (e.g. pre-eclampsia), delivery of the fetus may be necessary for maternal health.

Prognosis

In general, the prognosis for fetal hydrops is poor. Fetal mortality has been reported as between 81 and 87%, and as high as 95% in cases diagnosed before 24 weeks gestation. If the diagnosis is uncertain, and a reasonable gestation has been reached, delivery may be considered to enable further investigation and treatment in the neonatal period.

recommended further reading

Machin, G.A. (1997). Hydrops, cystic hygroma, pericardial effusions and fetal ascites. In *Potter's pathology of the fetus and infant* (ed. E.Gilbert-Barness), pp. 163–81. Mosby Year Books, St. Louis.

Jones, D.C. (1995). Non-immune fetal hydrops: diagnosis and obstetrical management. *Seminars in Perinatalology* **19**, 447–61.

Nicolini, U. (1999). Fetal hydrops and tumours. In *Fetal medicine: basic science and clinical practice* (ed. C.H. Rodeck and M.J. Whittle), pp. 737–54. Churchill Livingstone, Edinburgh.

Sebire, N.J. and Nicolaides, K.H. (1996). Thoracoamniotic shunting for fetal pleural effusions. In *The fetus as a patient* (ed. F.A. Chervanak and A. Kurjak), pp. 317–26. The Parthenon Publishing Group Ltd, New York.

McCoy, M.C., Katz, V.I., Gould, N., and Kuller, J.A. (1995). Non immune hydrops after 20 weeks gestation: review of 10 years experience with suggestions for management. *Obstetrics and Gynaecology* **85**, 578–82.

Chapter 29

Oligohydramnios and polyhydramnios

The fetus is surrounded by amniotic fluid everywhere except at its attachment with the umbilical cord. Underlying fetal or maternal conditions may alter the volume of fluid. Oligohydramnios and polyhydramnios are conditions associated with reduced and excessive liquor volume, respectively.

Origin, composition, and volume of the amniotic fluid

The precise origin of amniotic fluid still remains unresolved. It is largely derived from fetal urine and fetal lung secretions, although an additional contribution to the amniotic fluid comes from amniotic membrane secretions. There is continual exchange of fluid, most of which is swallowed and re-excreted by the fetus, and to a lesser extent it is exchanged through transfer of fluid to the mother through the membranes.

The composition of amniotic fluid is heterogeneous consisting of protein (albumins and globulins), lipids (phospholipids, cholesterol, and lecithin), carbohydrates (predominantly glucose), inorganic salts, and cells derived from fetal epithelium, amniotic membrane, and dermal fibroblasts. This latter cell type grows well in culture and is frequently used for karyotyping.

The volume of the amniotic fluid varies according to the gestational age of the fetus and is summarized in Fig. 29.1. The amniotic fluid index (AFI) is a qualitative ultrasonic assessment of liquor volume that is a summation of the deepest vertical pool depth in each of four quadrants surrounding the fetus.

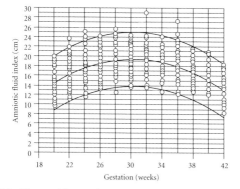

Fig. 29.1 Ultrasound four-quadrant assessment of amniotic fluid (AFI) according to gestation. (Reprinted from Magowan, B. Oligohydramnios. In *Pocketbook of obstetrics and gynaecology*, 1st edn (ed. B. Magowan), p. 50. © 1996 permission of the publishers Churchill Livingstone, Edinburgh.)

Oligohydramnios

Oligohydramnios is commonly defined as an AFI of less than the 5th centile f the gestational age, though it has in the past also been defined as the depth the deepest vertical pool—being less than or equal to 3 cm. The aetiology oligohydramnios is summarized in Table 29.1. An explanation for the reducti in liquor volume can be ascertained in over 85% of cases and therefore a ca ful history, thorough examination, and appropriate investigations are mand tory. The sequelae and management of oligohydramnios are dependent up the cause.

Important causes and management

- *Pre-labour rupture of membranes* (PROM) occurs in up to 15% of pregnancies and is defined as occurring prior to the onset of labour. The majority of patients are beyond 36 weeks, though an important minority present at an earlier gestational age. In most cases the clinical history is diagnostic and is confirmed by visualizing pooling of liquor in the vagina. Management of term and preterm PROM is discussed in Chapters 22 and 23. When oligohydramnios occurs early in pregnancy it can be associated with pulmonary hypoplasia and skeletal deformities.

- *Pre-eclampsia* is a complex disease of uncertain aetiology characterized by hypertension and proteinuria. It can affect any organ and may produce thrombosis in the placental vasculature. Consequent to this thrombosis, asymmetrical intrauterine growth restriction (IUGR) can occur. This may often be associated with oligohydramnios. The management of pre-eclampsia depends upon the severity of illness and the gestational age of the fetus. Pre-eclampsia is discussed in Chapter 14.

- *Fetal abnormalities.* As previously mentioned, there is a continual exchang of amniotic fluid, most of which is swallowed and subsequently re-excrete by the fetus. Renal tract abnormalities as listed in Table 29.1 prevent re-excretion and are therefore associated with oligohydramnios. The diagnosis of renal tract abnormalities is made by ultrasound, although visualizing the renal system may be difficult in view of associated anhydramnios and consequent lack of acoustic window. Karyotyping of the fetus may be useful. The management of a fetus with renal tract abnormalities or Potter's syndrome is difficult and must include the input of fetal medicine specialities and neonatologists.

- *Prolonged pregnancy* can be associated with poor placental function. This can lead to redistribution of blood with selective perfusion for fetal brain and heart and reduced perfusion to the kidneys. As a consequence of diminished urine production oligohydramnios occurs. Measurement of liquor volume forms an important part of assessing fetal well-being in prolonged pregnancy. Management options for prolonged pregnancy are discussed in the Chapter 26.

290

Conclusions

Oligohydramnios can signify underlying fetal compromise. Detailed histo clinical examination, and ultrasound assessment of the fetus are necessary determine the cause. Severe oligohydramnios occurring at early gestation associated with poor fetal prognosis. This is mainly due to deformities, prem turity, and underlying pulmonary hypoplasia. Reduced liquor volume is asso ated with fetal heart rate abnormalities. The risk of hypoxia increases duri labour and passage of meconium is common. Labour should be regarded high risk and continuous fetal monitoring should be employed.

ble 29.1 Causes of oligohydramnios

ıtrogenic
mniocentesis
1aternal
re-eclampsia
re-labour rupture of membranes (PROM)
etal
ıfections
evere IUGR
enal tract anomalies
Renal agenesis
Renal dysplasia
Ureteric or urethral obstruction
Polycystic kidneys
ongenital abnormalities
lacental
ost-maturity/prolonged pregnancy
hrombosis

Polyhydramnios

Polyhydramnios is defined as an AFI above the 95th centile for gestational a
or the depth of the deepest vertical pool equal to or greater than 8 cm.

The causes of polyhydramnios are listed in Table 29.2, though in most cases th
aetiology is unknown. It is diagnosed on the basis of a history of increasin
abdominal distension beyond gestational age that is often accompanied b
maternal discomfort, difficulty in palpating fetal parts, a symphyseal func
height greater than the gestational age, and fluid thrill elicited on percussio
Measurement of the amniotic fluid by ultrasound confirms the diagnosis.

Risks and management

Polyhydramnios predisposes to preterm labour, malpresentation, cord prolaps
and placental abruption following rupture of membranes and postpartu
haemorrhage. Therefore diagnosis is important for anticipation of the ensui
risks and management is largely dependent upon the degree of polyhydramnio

When polyhydramnios is suspected clinically an ultrasound examinatio
should be carried out to quantify the degree of polyhydramnios and exclude a
fetal structural abnormality. A glucose tolerance test is useful in detecting gest
tional diabetes mellitus. Further management depends on the cause.

A severe degree of polyhydramnios gives rise to maternal discomfort and
extreme cases can cause respiratory embarrassment. Hospital admission may
indicated in such severe cases.

- If there is a threat of preterm delivery, maternal steroids should be
  administered to reduce the risk of respiratory distress syndrome.
- Indomethacin is used for medical amnioreduction but carries the risk of
  fetal anuria and therefore should not be used for a prolonged period of
  time.
- Serial amnioreduction by amniocentesis is another therapeutic option. Th
  is commonly used in twin-to-twin transfusion syndrome to relieve the
  pressure on the placental bed.
- Selective feticide of the growth-restricted twin and severing the vascular
  anastomosis by laser are some other invasive approaches to manage severe
  polyhydramnios in twin-to-twin transfusion. They all carry considerable
  risks and should be performed in centres with the established expertise.

Conclusions

Severe polyhydramnios is rare and usually signifies some fetal abnormality
multiple pregnancy. A mild degree of polyhydramnios is often idiopathic and
usually managed expectantly. Increased vigilance is required during labour
the risks of cord prolapse, abruption, malpresentation, and postpartum haer
orrhage are high.

ble 29.2 Causes of polyhydramnios

Idiopathic

Maternal

Diabetes mellitus

Fetal

Multiple pregnancy
  Twin to twin transfusion
  (Recipient twin)

Obstructive defects

Gastrointestinal abnormalities
  Oesophageal/duodenal atresia
  Tracheo-oesophageal fistula
  Small intestine/colonic obstruction

Facial tumour

Anencephaly

Myotonic dystrophy

Non-obstructive defects

Macrosomia

Neural tube defects

Infections, e.g. Parvovirus

Placental

Angioma

Tumours

Chapter 30

Antenatal fetal surveillance

This chapter is a brief summary of the methods available for antenatal surveillance of the fetus.

Symphyseal fundal height

Symphyseal–fundal height measurement provides a useful screening method for detection of the baby that is small or large for gestation, and provides the mainstay of antenatal surveillance.[1] In the third trimester this measurement (in centimetres) should approximate to the number of weeks of the gestation. The variation is ±2 cm from 20–35 weeks, ±3 cm from 36–38 weeks, and ±4 cm after that due to engagement of the head and reduction in liquor volume. The inter and intraobserver variation is not that great, but the measurement precludes the accurate differentiation of growth restriction from the constitutionally small baby. It is recommended that further investigation be instigated if the fundal height differs by more than expected for that gestation. The sensitivity of this screening method is further limited in the presence of multiple pregnancy, maternal obesity, or polyhydramnios. Its specificity is limited by ethnic origin. For example, women of Asian origin will commonly deliver healthy small babies. The use of customized growth charts for plotting fundal height has not been fully explored.[2]

Fetal movement chart

The presence of fetal movement is a sign of fetal well-being and occurs in a cyclical pattern. A reduction or cessation in fetal movements may occur prior to fetal demise and may predate death by a number of days in some instances.[3] Any marked decrease in movements or change in pattern may be significant and requires consideration and investigation. This should include a full assessment of the pregnancy, utilizing clinical examination and ultrasound scanning (including fetal biometry and liquor volume and, if necessary, biophysical profile and umbilical artery Doppler). Cardiotocograph (CTG) appears to be the main modality in many centres because of its ready availability. CTG alone may provide false reassurance, as the CTG carries no intermediate or long-term predictive value. Studies have demonstrated poorer fetal outcome in populations where single CTG alone is used to determine fetal well-being following reported reduction in movements, as opposed to management based on additional parameters.

In high-risk pregnancies (previous poor obstetric outcome; maternal medical disorders, such as endocrine diseases, thrombophilias, or drug dependence; pregnancies complicated by pre-eclampsia or antepartum haemorrhage (APH); and those where a subjective reduction in movements has already been reported, the use of fetal movement charts (defining normality as 10 movements per day) may be of some benefit. However, their use as a routine screening tool in low-risk pregnancies has demonstrated no benefits in improved obstetric outcome, and a high false-positive rate leads to increased testing and intervention.[4]

Cardiotocography

The cardiotocograph (CTG) provides a means of monitoring fluctuations in fetal heart rate (FHR) over time and correlating this with any uterine activity. From 32 weeks, the fetal cardiograph may be categorized as normal, suspicious, or pathological and interpreted in accordance with the clinical situation.

A normal antenatal (non-stress) CTG should demonstrate a FHR with a baseline between 110 and 160 beats/minute with short-term variability around that baseline of between 5 and 25 beats/minute. At least two accelerations should occur within each 20 minutes (an acceleration being defined as a rise of at least 15 beats lasting for at least 15 seconds). There should be no decelerations from the baseline (a deceleration being defined as the converse of an acceleration).

A suspicious CTG, in which the baseline is up to 10 beats outside the normal parameters, the baseline variability is < 5 beats/minute, or accelerations are reduced or absent, should be continued, as fetal activity is cyclical and the abnormalities may simply constitute a normal fetal resting trace, which may occur for up to 40 minutes. If the pattern continues then further assessment will be required.

A baseline more than 10 beats/minute outside the normal range, variability less than 5 beats/minute, or the presence of decelerations constitute a suspicious (one feature is not normal) or abnormal (if two features are not normal) CTG and, depending on the situation, will usually require additional testing by other modalities or delivery of the fetus.

Prior to 32 weeks gestation, interpretation of the antenatal CTG may be much more difficult. Incomplete development of the autonomic nervous system does not allow the predictable responses of the FHR to movement or stress that characterize the CTG of the more mature fetus.

The CTG provides a useful means of excluding current fetal hypoxia and acute compromise. The CTG may not be reactive (show no accelerations) for reasons other than hypoxia, e.g. anaemia, infection, medication, cerebral haemorrhage, maternal metabolic disturbance, and chromosomal or congenital malformation. It is part of the assessment following reported reduced fetal movements and is also employed in the assessment of many complications of pregnancy, namely, antepartum haemorrhage (APH), hypertensive disorders, and intrauterine growth restriction (IUGR). It is rare to find an abnormal CTG in the presence of normal fetal movements. The intermediate and long-term prognostic value of the CTG is poor and, if a normal CTG is extrapolated to provide this information, false reassurance may be gained and inadequate investigation of fetal well-being will occur as a result.[5]

Ultrasound assessment of fetal growth

A fetus considered at risk of IUGR from maternal medical or obstetric history or thought to be small or large for gestational age clinically may be more accurately assessed by ultrasonic biometry.[6] Various growth charts are used, all based upon cross-sectional (rather than longitudinal) population studies, indicating the centiles for the UK population. The majority of centres will chart abdominal and head circumference, biparietal diameter, and femur length on charts with the 5th, 50th, and 95th centiles for gestation defined. Some centres also plot amniotic fluid index (AFI). However, the interpretation of fetal measurements is rarely straightforward, particularly when based upon a single scan, and over interpretation frequently leads to unnecessary intervention.

- Dating of the pregnancy may be inaccurate and lead to the false diagnosis of a small baby.
- Precision of measurement is limited and may be further hampered by fetal position, maternal obesity, or oligohydramnios.
- A baby that appears small for gestational age may be constitutionally so and not subject to any pathological process, as the majority of centres use growth charts that are not customized for maternal size or ethnicity.

Serial growth scans are more useful in the detection of a fetus with growth restriction. Such growth restriction may be due to a number of possible causes and determination of the cause may be essential to determine the optimal management of the pregnancy.

- For example, chromosomal abnormalities such as trisomies (e.g. trisomy 18) or triploidies may result in symmetrical growth restriction, where all parameters may show progressive descent through the centiles of the growth chart, sometimes from early in the pregnancy.
- In contrast, growth restriction due to placental insufficiency may demonstrate an asymmetrical pattern, with sparing of head measurements at the expense of abdominal circumference and liquor volume, and is more commonly manifest in the third trimester. Placental insufficiency may be idiopathic or related to an underlying problem, such as pre-eclampsia, maternal thrombophilia, or recurrent placental abruption.
- Other fetuses may demonstrate growth restriction that fits neither of these patterns and is caused by specific factors such as maternal alcohol or recreational drug abuse (particularly heroin, cocaine, and cannabis) or infection in utero (e.g. cytomegalovirus (CMV)).

The serial measurement of amniotic fluid volume, while contributing to fetal biophysical assessment and providing a useful indicator in fetal urinary tract disorders, has not been adequately independently evaluated in trials.

Serial ultrasonic growth assessment in the low-risk pregnancy leads to increased intervention in the absence of any improvement in perinatal outcome.

etal biophysical profile

ve parameters have been used together in an attempt to provide an assessment
f fetal well-being that surpasses the CTG alone.[7] These are:

Amniotic fluid volume.

Fetal tone.

Fetal movements.

Fetal breathing movements.

The CTG.

ach parameter is given a score of zero or 2. The lower the score, the further
om normality the variable. A score of eight or above would be considered nor-
al. A properly performed biophysical profile assessment involves the evalua-
on of each parameter over a 20-minute period, and requires the time of a
killed obstetric sonographer. It has not been demonstrated by randomized con-
olled trial to provide any improvement in fetal outcome, although it is better
: *predicting* outcome based on prospective descriptive studies involving large
umbers. The randomized studies performed so far have involved relatively
nall numbers.[8]

he most important predictive parameter of perinatal deaths is liquor volume,
nd it has been suggested that this is as effective when used alone. This is com-
nonly expressed as the amniotic fluid index (AFI, the sum of four pool depths,
erived from the deepest pool in each quadrant).

Doppler ultrasonography

The Doppler waveform of a number of fetal and maternal vessels may be used to gain information about the well-being of the pregnancy.[9] The Doppler signal indicates the directional velocity of flow of a liquid. Analysis of the difference between velocity of flow in the umbilical artery in fetal systole and diastole allows the calculation of the resistance or pulsatility indices.

- Decreasing umbilical artery diastolic flow velocity is an indicator of increased placental resistance and hence of developing placental insufficiency.
- In the high-risk pregnancy, use of umbilical artery Doppler has been demonstrated to reduce perinatal mortality by permitting timely delivery.[1] Doppler waveform changes may precede fetal demise by at least a week, permitting expediting of delivery and giving time to introduce steroids in the preterm infant.
- The incidence of intrapartum signs of fetal compromise or of perinatal morbidity are not altered by the antenatal use of Doppler.
- Umbilical artery Doppler is of no demonstrated benefit as a screening tool in the low-risk population, as the waveform may vary with time and result in false-positive results, leading to unnecessary intervention.[11]

The hypoxic infant with reduced end diastolic flow in the umbilical artery may demonstrate brain-sparing compensation with increased flow in the middle cerebral artery throughout the cardiac cycle, and particularly in diastole. The maternal uterine artery may demonstrate notching between the systolic and diastolic component, indicative of increased placental bed resistance secondary to poor spiral artery remodelling in response to trophoblast invasion. Such pathophysiological change is thought to be pivotal in the development of pre-eclampsia and growth restriction later in the pregnancy.[12] The presence of uterine artery waveform notching in those with a previous history of IUGR or pre-eclampsia is a strong predictor of recurrence, with absence of this sign in these women providing 98% reassurance for this pregnancy. However, the test appears to provide a poor screening tool in the low-risk population.[13]

Biochemical testing

A number of biochemical markers have been related to fetal compromise. The overlap of normal and abnormal ranges for most markers renders them poor screening tools, and most markers are no longer utilized in clinical practice. Two previously commonly used such markers were oestriol and human placental lactogen (HPL).

Maternal serum alpha-feto protein (MSAFP) is routinely measured in most centres during the second trimester as a screening test for fetal abnormality (specifically, neural tube defects, abdominal wall defects, gastrointestinal tract obstruction) and, in conjunction with beta human chorionic gonadotrophin (β-hCG), as part of screening for fetal aneuploidy. Raised maternal MSAFP may be due to increased placental permeability or to feto-maternal haemorrhage and, in the absence of fetal structural abnormality, is statistically significantly associated with poor obstetric outcome, particularly IUGR, low birth weight, increased perinatal mortality, preterm labour, and pre-eclampsia. Increasing the MSAFP concentration by one multiple of the mean approximately doubles the risk of a pregnancy complication. However, the sensitivity of MSAFP as a predictor of obstetric complications remains too low to justify its use as a screening tool outside of its use as an adjunct to the detection of congenital abnormality.[14]

Summary

The low-risk pregnant population has long been well served by the use of simple clinical surveillance in antenatal care. More sophisticated methods of surveillance do not improve overall outcome in this group.

The suspicion by abdominal examination or by reported reduction in fetal movement, or the advent of other risk factors (such as APH or raised MSAFP) that indicate that the fetus may be compromised, requires the use of appropriate testing to ascertain fetal well-being. The use of ultrasound scanning, with or without Doppler studies or biophysical profile, can improve the perinatal mortality rate when used to investigate this group, if appropriate action is taken based on the results of these tests. Pregnancies considered to be high risk will require the tailoring of antenatal surveillance from the above techniques, and the consequent improvements in outcome are well documented in clinical trials.

30 Antenatal fetal surveillance

References

1 Lindhard, A., Nielsen, P.V., Mouritsen, L.A., Zachariassen, A., Sorensen, H.U., and Roseno, H. (1990). The implications of introducing the symphyseal–fundal height measurement: a prospective randomized controlled trial. *British Journal of Obstetrics and Gynaecology* **97**, 675–80.

2 Gardosi, J. and Francis, A. (1999). Controlled trial of fundal height measurement plotted on customized antenatal growth charts. *British Journal of Obstetrics and Gynaecology* **106**, 309–17.

3 CESDI (1998). *Confidential Enquiry into Stillbirths and Deaths in Infancy* (*CESDI*) *Fifth Annual Report*. Maternal and Child Health Research Consortium, London.

4 Grant, A., Elbourne, D., Valentin, L., and Alexander, S. (1989). Routine formal fetal movement counting and risk of antepartum late death in normally formed singletons. *Lancet* **ii**, 345–9.

5 Altman, D., Hytten, F., Grant, A., and Elbourne, D. (1995). Non-stress cardiotocography. In *A guide to effective care in pregnancy and childbirth* (ed. M. Enkin, M. Keirse, M. Renfrew, and J. Neilson), pp. 63–4. Oxford University Press, Oxford.

6 Warsof, S.L., Cooper, D.J., Little, D., and Campbell, S. (1986). Routine ultrasound screening for antenatal detection of intrauterine growth retardation. *Obstetrics and Gynecology* **67**, 33–9.

7 Manning, F.A. (1990). The fetal biophysical profile score: current status. *Obstetrics and Gynecology Clinics of North America* **17**, 147–62.

8 Altman, D., Hytten, F., Grant, A., and Elbourne, D. (1995). Fetal biophysical profile. In *A guide to effective care in pregnancy and childbirth* (ed. M. Enkin, M. Keirse, M. Renfrew, and J. Neilson), p. 68. Oxford University Press, Oxford.

9 Reed, K.L. (1997). Doppler—the fetal circulation. *Clinical Obstetrics and Gynecology* **40**, 750–4.

10 Fong, K.W., Ohlsson, A., Hannah, M.E., *et al.* (1999). Prediction of perinatal outcome in fetuses suspected to have intrauterine growth restriction: Doppler US study of fetal cerebral, renal and umbilical arteries. *Radiology* **213**, 681–9.

11 Goffinet, F., Paris-Llado, J., Nisand, I., and Breart, G. (1997). Umbilical artery Doppler velocimetry in unselected and low risk pregnancies: a review of randomized controlled trials. *British Journal of Obstetrics and Gynaecology* **104**, 425–30.

12 Yoshimura, S., Masuzaki, H., Miura, K., Gotoh, H., and Ishimaru, T. (1998). Fetal blood flow redistribution in term intrauterine growth retardation (IUGR) and post-natal growth. *International Journal of Gynaecology and Obstetrics* **60**, 3–8.

13 Bewley, S., Cooper, D., and Campbell, S. (1991). Doppler investigation of uteroplacental blood flow resistance in the second trimester: a screening study for pre-eclampsia and intrauterine growth retardation. *British Journal of Obstetrics and Gynaecology* **98**, 871–9.

14 Pahal, G.S., Acharya, G., and Jauniaux, E. (2000). Biochemical markers of fetoplacental growth restriction. In *Intrauterine growth restriction* (ed. J. Kingdom and P.N. Baker), pp. 239–56. Springer Verlag, London.

303

Labour

Labour is the process whereby the products of conception are delivered from the uterus after the 24th week of gestation. Although it is difficult to time the onset of labour it can be defined as that point at which uterine contractions become regular and cervical effacement and dilatation begin. For scientific studies the observed lengths of the various stages of labour following admission to hospital are considered. Labour is characterized by:

- The spontaneous onset of uterine contractions which increase in frequency, duration, and strength with progress of time.
- The time taken for cervical effacement (shortening of the cervix) and dilatation which is slow until 3 cm (latent phase) followed by a rate of cervical dilatation of 1 cm/hour (active phase) till full dilatation of the cervix (10 cm) is the *first stage of labour.*
- The process of labour is usually accompanied by rupture of membranes with leakage of amniotic fluid, which should normally be clear.
- Once the cervix is fully dilated, *second stage* is diagnosed. Descent of the presenting part through the birth canal is more during this stage. If the woman has an epidural *in situ* then it is often common practice to wait for a further hour (passive second stage) to allow descent of the head before commencing pushing in time with contraction.
- Birth of the baby is expected after approximately 1 hour of bearing down efforts in a primigravid woman, while a considerably shorter second stage is anticipated in a multiparous woman.
- The *third stage* is from delivery of the baby to delivery of the placenta and membranes and is usually about 30 minutes.
- The normal blood loss associated with placental separation is usually less than 500 mL. Blood loss more than this amount is termed a postpartum haemorrhage (PPH).

The mechanism of labour

The head usually engages in the transverse position and the passage of the head and trunk follows a well-defined pattern through the pelvis (Fig. 31.1). Not all the diameters of the fetal head can pass through a normal pelvis. The process of labour therefore involves the adaptation of the fetal head to the various segments of the pelvis

The normal process of movement of the head in labour for a normal vertex presentation involves the following sequence.

1 *Descent* with increased flexion as the head enters the cavity. The sagittal suture lies in the transverse diameter of the brim.
2 *Internal rotation* occurs at the level of the ischial spines due to the grooved gutter of the levator ani muscles. Flexion produces a small diameter of presentation changing to the suboccipito-bragmatic diameter from the occipito-frontal diameter.
3 Distension of the perineum with crowning is followed by extension of the head as it comes out of the vulva.
4 *Restitution.* The head rotates back for the occiput to be in line with the spine
5 *External rotation.* The shoulders rotate when they reach the levators until the bi-acromial diameter is anteroposterior. Accordingly, the head externally rotates by the same amount.
6 Delivery of the posterior shoulder occurs by lateral flexion of the trunk anteriorly.
7 Delivery of the anterior shoulder occurs by lateral flexion of the trunk posteriorly.
8 Delivery of the buttocks and legs follows the delivery of body.

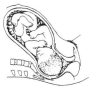

(1)
1st stage of labour. The cervix dilates. After full dilatation the head flexes further and descends further into the pelvis.

(2)
During the early second stage the head rotates at the level of the ischial spine so the occiput lies in the anterior part of pelvis. In late second stage the head broaches the vulval ring (crowning) and the perineum stretches over the head.

(3)
The head is born. The shoulders still lie transversely in the midpelvis.

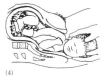

(4)
Birth of the anterior shoulder. The shoulders rotate to lie in the anteroposterior diameter of the pelvic outlet. The head rotates externally, 'restitute, to its direction at onset of labour. Downward and backward traction of the head by the birth attendant aids delivery of the anterior shoulder.

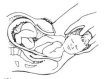

(5)
Birth of the postrior shoulder is aided by lifting the head upwards whilst maintaining traction.

g. 31.1 Mechanism of labour and delivery. (Reproduced from Collier, J., ▸ngmore, M., and Brown, T.D. (eds.). *Oxford handbook of clinical specialties,* ⁁ edn, p. 83, © 1999, by permission of the publisher Oxford University Press.)

Assessment of progress of labour

The first stage

Braxton–Hicks contractions are non-painful contractions (15 mm Hg pressure) of the uterus that occur from 30 weeks gestation and are more common after 36 weeks. Contractions in labour are painful and contraction pressure gradually increases, as well as the frequency and duration

The minimum acceptable rate is 1 cm/hour. The active first stage usually takes up to 8–12 hours in a primipara and 6–8 hours in a multipara.

- During the first stage maternal pulse, blood pressure (BP), and temperature are checked half-hourly.
- The contractions are assessed every 30 minutes to record the frequency (every 10 minutes) and duration in seconds.
- Vaginal examination is carried out every 4 hours to assess the rate of cervical dilatation and the position and station of the head (measured in cm above the ischial spines). Note is also made of the degree of the caput and moulding and the state of the liquor.
- Maternal urine is tested 4-hourly for ketones and protein. An IV infusion 10% dextrose saline is set up if the mother becomes ketotic.
- The fetal heart rate (FHR) is monitored by auscultation every 15 minutes if it is not being continuously monitored electronically. The FHR before, during, and immediately after a contraction is noted.

Failure to progress in the first stage

Delay in the first stage of labour is identified when progress in the 'active phase' falls to the right of the action line drawn parallel and 1–2 hours to the right of the alert line drawn at a rate of 1 cm/hour from the admission cervical dilatation (Fig. 31.2). If the labour was slow from the early active phase, it is termed primary dysfunctional labour and, if the rate of progress was slow after adequate progress previously, then it is termed secondary arrest of labour. In some cases the labour may be prolonged in the latent phase. The causes of poor progress in the first stage are inefficient uterine activity (power), malposition or malpresentation, cephalopelvic disproportion (passenger), inadequate pelvis (passage), or a combination of the three. Rare causes include pelvic tumours.

The management relies on careful assessment and appropriate corrective action

- Assessment begins with a review of the history and patient records; abdominal palpation for lie, presentation, and station (as fifths of head palpable above the brim); fetal size; and frequency and duration of contractions.
- The fetal condition needs to be assessed by reviewing the FHR recording or cardiotocograph (CTG) and the colour and quantity of liquor if membranes have been ruptured. Maternal hydration and analgesia should be reviewed.
- A vaginal assessment should identify the presentation and, if vertex, the amount of caput and moulding and the position. The station of the leading bony skull and the degree of flexion should be noted along with the assessment of the bony pelvic adequacy.

PARTOGRAPH

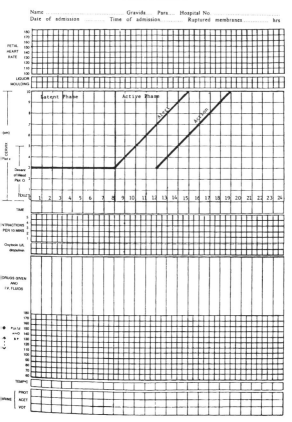

Fig. 31.2 Partogram.

Assessment of progress of labour (*continued*)

In grand multiparous women and in women with a uterine scar, an experience obstetrician should review the case prior to commencement of oxytocin.

- The management options are delivery by lower segment Caesarean section (LSCS) if there is obvious cephalo-pelvic disproportion (CPD) or fetal distress.
- If uterine activity is inadequate with no contraindications for augmentation, oxytocin infusion titration to achieve optimal contractions (4 in 10 minutes, each lasting > 40 seconds) for 3 to 4 hours should be followed by further reassessment to confirm that adequate progress is bein made after the contractions were augmented.

The second stage

The second stage is the time from complete cervical dilatation until the baby born. The physiological second stage commences when the mother has a des to bear down when the cervix is fully dilated. She uses her abdominal musc with the Valsalva manoeuvre to deliver the baby.

- With the attendant scrubbed, gowned, and gloved, the mother is placed in either the supine (with the head of the bed tilted upwards), left lateral, or lithotomy position. Some women prefer to deliver in the squatting positic
- As the head is pushed down with each contraction, it distends the perineu and the anus. The anus is covered with a pad and the descent of the occip controlled with the left hand, the head being kept well flexed until crowne when it is allowed to extend. This way perineal distension is minimized ar precipitated delivery is prevented.
- Once the head is delivered, the eyes and nasal pharynx are cleaned.
- If the perineum appears to be tearing extensively, an episiotomy is performed, and the incision is made mediolaterally from the fourchette after infiltrating the perineum with a local anaesthetic.
- With the next contraction the head is gently pulled towards the perineum until the anterior shoulder is delivered under the subpubic arch.
- Gentle traction downwards and anteriorly helps to deliver the posterior shoulder and the remainder of the trunk.

Normal time for second stage is 60 minutes in a nullipara and 30 minutes in multipara.

In the management of the second stage of labour, if the woman has an epidu *in situ* and the FHR pattern is normal, 1 hour may be allowed for the preser ing part to descend with uterine contractions. During this hour it is importa to ensure that good contractions are present and, if there are any concer regarding the FHR, delivery could be expedited by judicious instrumental vag nal delivery.

- In a nulliparous woman if, after an hour of effective expulsive efforts, delivery is not imminent and there has been no significant progress, then the situation needs to be reassessed with a view to an assisted instrumenta delivery.
- In a multiparous woman, delivery is generally expected within 30–45 minut of effective expulsive efforts and failure to achieve this should raise suspicio of malposition, malpresentation, or disproportion.

tting the cord between clamps after pulsations stop allows more blood to
e baby. Holding the baby 20 cm below the introitus and delaying clamping
r 30 seconds results in higher haematocrit levels. It reduces transfusion and
ygen supplement requirements in premature babies. The condition of the
by is assessed at 1 and 5 minutes using the Apgar scoring system and the baby
nded to the mother.

he third stage

he third stage is the duration from delivery of the baby to delivery of the
acenta.

The mother is turned on to her back if she is not already in the supine
position. A dish is placed under the cord and at the introitus to collect any
blood loss. The left hand is placed on the abdomen over the uterine fundus.
Routine use of syntometrine (ergometrine maleate 0.5 mg IM + oxytocin
5 IU IM) as the anterior shoulder of the baby is born has decreased third
stage time (to about 5 minutes), and has also decreased the incidence of
PPH. One should be sure to exclude multiple pregnancy with such practice.
As the uterus contracts to a 20-week size after the baby is born, the placenta
separates from the uterus through the spongy layer of the decidua basalis.
At this point the uterus will be felt to become more firm and globular, the
cord will lengthen, and there will be trickle of fresh blood.
Cord traction is applied with the right hand, whilst supporting the fundus
with the left hand (Brandt–Andrew's technique).

ssisted delivery of the placenta is usually completed within 5 minutes of deliv-
y. The placenta and membranes are checked for missing cotyledons and to see
the membranes are complete. The blood loss is recorded.

ost complications of the third stage, such as PPH, uterine inversion, or vulval
perineal haematoma, occur in the first 2 hours after delivery. Usually the
omen are kept in the delivery unit for these 2 hours to observe their pulse, BP,
mperature, uterine size and contractions, fresh bleeding per vaginum, or
inful swelling of the vulva or perineum. Effort is also taken to support the
other in breastfeeding the baby, to clean and weigh the baby, and to clean the
other and to offer her some refreshments. If there were no complications dur-
g the 2 hours, she is transferred to the postnatal ward. Some are allowed home
ter a further 3 to 4 hours of observation. Relaxation of the uterus may lead to
emorrhage. In situations where the uterus is overstretched, as in multiple
egnancy, big babies, polyhydramnios, or in prolonged labour or placenta
aevia, a syntocinon infusion, e.g. 40 units in 500 mL of saline, is set up as an
infusion over 3–4 hours to reduce this complication.

Fetal surveillance in labour

Labour has been defined as the most dangerous journey made by anyone and such the fetus needs all the help it can get to complete this journey successfu Each fetus enters labour with different resources and reserves and hence a different capacity to withstand the stress of labour. It is estimated that only 10% cerebral palsy (CP) is due to intrapartum events, the rest being attributed antenatal events but, given the relatively short duration of labour compared the antenatal period, the 'risk per unit time' is greatest in labour. The blood su ply to the placental pool is restricted with each contraction and this is furth aggravated by voluntary bearing down efforts in the second stage. A fetus the fore that was coping well in the antenatal period but has no extra reserve cap ity may decompensate in labour. Intrapartum surveillance therefore shou begin with a review of antenatal risk factors that affect the reserves and the fore the capacity with which each fetus enters labour.

Electronic fetal monitoring (EFM)

When EFM was introduced it was expected to dramatically reduce perina morbidity and cerebral palsy (CP). However, it has resulted in increased inte vention and operative delivery rates without marked reduction in CP. The re son for this is that CTG is very sensitive but not specific in detecting fe hypoxia. Additional tests such as fetal scalp blood sampling in labour required to improve the specificity. Interest is also growing in the use of fe electrocardiographic (ECG) ST waveform analysis and pulse oximetry adjuncts to improve the positive predictive value of CTG.

Recently, guidelines on EFM have been issued by NICE (National Institute Clinical Excellence) and the RCOG (Royal College of Obstetricians a Gynaecologists). The options for intrapartum surveillance are intermittent au cultation and continuous EFM. It is recommended that on admission in labo an admission assessment is made to identify fetal or maternal risk factors th would suggest EFM.

- *Maternal risk factors* include previous Caesarean section, pre-eclampsia, post-term pregnancy, prolonged rupture of membranes, induced labour, diabetes, antepartum haemorrhage, and other maternal medical conditio
- *Fetal risk factors* include IUGR, prematurity, oligohydramnios, abnormal Doppler velocimetry, multiple pregnancy, meconium-stained liquor, and breech presentation.
- Although low risk on admission, *intrapartum risk factors* may develop suc as the need for oxytocin augmentation, epidural analgesia, intrapartum vaginal bleeding, pyrexia, and fresh meconium staining of liquor or abnormal FHR on intermittent auscultation. If none of the above apply, t woman may be suitable for intermittent auscultation which should be performed for a full minute after a contraction at least every 15 minutes i the first stage and every 5 minutes or after every other contraction in the second stage.

Definitions of terms used in EFM

- *Baseline rate* is the mean level of the FHR when this is stable and accelerations and decelerations have been excluded.
- A *bradycardia* is a baseline FHR of less than 110 beats/min (100–110 beats/min is termed moderate baseline bradycardia and, provided other parameters are normal, it is considered normal). A baseline below 100 beats/min should raise the possibility of hypoxia or other pathology (beware of maternal heart rate being recorded as the FHR).
- A *tachycardia* is a baseline FHR of more than 160 beats/min. A baseline of 160–180 beats/min is termed moderate baseline tachycardia and, provided other features are normal, is regarded as not indicative of hypoxia.
- An *acceleration* is a transient rise in FHR by at least 15 beats over the baseline lasting for 15 seconds or more (Fig. 31.3).
- A *deceleration* is a reduction in the baseline of 15 beats or more for more than 15 seconds.

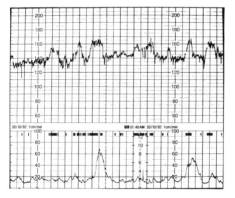

Fig. 31.3 A CTG trace showing normal baseline rate accelerations and normal baseline variability.

Fetal surveillance in labour (*continued*)

—Decelerations can be uniform in appearance and timing and are defined as early when associated with head compression (Fig. 31.4).

—If synchronous with a contraction and late, decelerations are associated with uteroplacental insufficiency (Fig. 31.5). There is at least a 15 second time lag between the peak of the contraction and the nadir of the deceleration.

—The majority of decelerations, however, are variable and are associated with cord compression (Fig. 31.6), which can be subdivided into typical and atypical. Suspicious features associated with variable decelerations are a duration of greater than 60 seconds with a loss of more than 60 beats from the baseline, slow recovery to baseline, a combined variable and a late deceleration component, and a rising baseline rate.

- *Baseline variability* is the degree to which the baseline varies, i.e. the bandwidth of the baseline after exclusion of accelerations and decelerations. A variability of 0–5 beats/min is defined as silent, 5–25 beats/min as normal, and greater than 25 beats/min as saltatory.

The CTG is classified as normal, suspicious, or pathological on the basis of the following criteria.

- *Normal.* All four features are reassuring.
- *Suspicious.* No more than one non-reassuring feature when analysing the CTG.
- *Pathological.* Two or more non-reassuring features or one or more abnormal features.

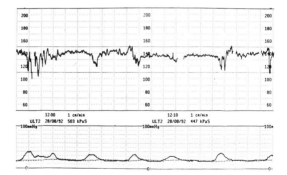

Fig. 31.4 CTG with early decelerations.

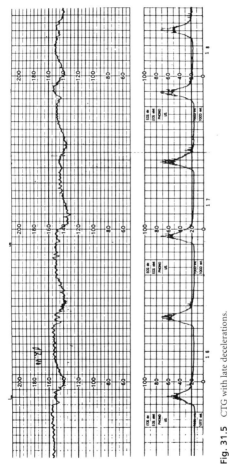

Fig. 31.5 CTG with late decelerations.

Fetal surveillance in labour (*continued*)

Reassuring, non-reassuring, and abnormal features include the following.

- *Reassuring features.* Baseline rate of 110–160 beats/min, baseline variability greater than 5 beats/min, no deceleration, and 2 accelerations per 20 minutes. (The absence of accelerations in an otherwise normal CTG is of uncertain significance.)
- *Non-reassuring features.* Baseline 100–109 or 161–180 beats/min, variability less than 5 beats/min for more than 40 but no more than 90 minutes, early decelerations, uncomplicated variable deceleration, or a single prolonged deceleration of up to 3 minutes.
- *Abnormal features.* Baseline rate of less than 100 beats/min or greater than 180 beats/min, sinusoidal pattern for more than 10 minutes, baseline variability of less than 5 beats/min for more than 90 minutes, atypical variable decelerations, late decelerations, and a single prolonged deceleration for more than 3 minutes duration.

Action with non-reassuring CTGs

Where abnormal or non-reassuring features are encountered on the CTG, it i important to search for and correct any causes such as uterine hyperstimulation hypotension, maternal dehydration/temperature, and the need for pain relief. no remediable cause is found, in some situations a fetal scalp blood sample ma be appropriate to determine fetal acid–base status. A scalp blood pH less tha 7.20 should prompt arrangements for immediate delivery, a pH of 7.20–7.2 should lead to a repeat of fetal blood sampling (FBS) in 30–45 minutes t determine the trend in relation to progress of labour, whilst a pH greater tha 7.25 should be repeated with persistent CTG abnormality.

The assessment of CTGs should always be done in the context of the clinical pic ture. A normal baseline rate does not exclude hypoxia and the change in base line may indicate gradually developing hypoxia. Good baseline variability is a indicator of adequate oxygenation of the autonomic system and, in conjunctio with a reactive CTG, is an indicator of good fetal health. A CTG trace with n accelerations, baseline variability <5 beats/min, and shallow deceleration (eve < 15 beats) may indicate the possibility of longstanding hypoxia. With pro longed decelerations lasting > 90 seconds and reaching < 80 beats/min wit short-term recovery (< 30 seconds) to the baseline, the fetus may get hypoxi within a short period of time (< 60 min). Hypoxia may develop rapidly whe the FHR remains < 80 beats/min for > 10 min (prolonged bradycardia). A ris ing baseline with loss of variability and/or slow recovery of prolonged decelera tions indicates the need for scalp blood pH or delivery and, in the active secon stage, is an indication for assisted delivery if spontaneous delivery is not imm nent. If the CTG is abnormal without decelerations in labour, the possibility c infection, drugs, cerebral haemorrhage, and congenital/chromosomal malfor mation should be considered.

It is important to always remember that the true monitors of fetal well-being ar the attending obstetricians and midwives, and the EFM equipment is merely recording device.

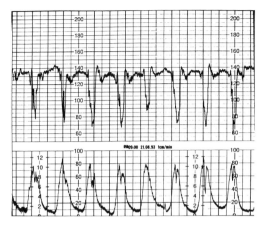

Fig. 31.6 CTG with variable decelerations.

Meconium-stained liquor

There are two principal reasons why meconium is passed. One is a function of fetal maturity, but it may also indicate possible fetal compromise. The incidence of meconium staining of the liquor increases from 36 to 42 weeks reaching around 20% at this stage. It can thus be a marker of maturation of the central nervous system and the gastrointestinal system. Passage of meconium in the preterm fetus, however, is rare and should raise the possibility of intrauterine infection such as listeriosis.

Traditionally three grades of meconium are described.
- Grade 1 meconium (light) is diluted by a large volume of amniotic fluid that is lightly stained by meconium.
- Grade 2 (moderate) meconium is a reasonable amount of amniotic fluid with a heavy suspension of meconium.
- Grade 3 meconium (thick meconium) suggests the presence of meconium in small amounts of amniotic fluid.
  —If no amniotic fluid is obtained at artificial rupture of membranes, one should consider this as being in the same risk category as grade 3 meconium and the fetal condition should be observed closely.

The significance of meconium varies with presentation. Thus where there is a breech presentation in the late first or second stage the passage of meconium is likely to be due to mechanical causes and therefore less sinister than in a cephalic presentation or with a breech presentation in early labour with a high presenting part.

The presence of scanty fluid with thick meconium is suggestive of oligohydramnios and, if there are added CTG abnormalities in early labour, delivery by Caesarean section may be preferable.

Meconium aspiration syndrome (MAS) has an incidence of 1 per 1000 births in Europe. Meconium can be aspirated *in utero* or after birth. Although fetuses do not normally draw amniotic fluid into the airway, they gasp when asphyxiated. Therefore the coexistence of asphyxia and acidosis may precipitate meconium aspiration. Asphyxia causes added damage to the lungs and therefore further complicates management of MAS. Meconium creates a ball valve effect in the airways caused by its chemical irritant properties. Aggressive tracheal toilet at delivery helps to reduce the load but will not significantly impact on cases with pre-existing *in utero* aspiration. It has clearly been documented that meconium aspiration does happen *in utero* and this is precipitated by gasping of the fetus as a result of hypoxia/acidosis. Hence it is imperative to avoid any scenario that may lead to hypoxia/acidosis.

Pain relief in labour

Undoubtedly labour is a painful process and adequate provision of analgesia is important. The request for analgesia in childbirth varies in different cultures and is also influenced by the previous obstetric experience of the woman, the course of labour, and its anticipated duration. Professionals are expected to provide expert advice about analgesia but the final decision rests with the woman.

Non-pharmacological means

Relaxation techniques including lying in warm water and breathing exercises do not relieve pain as such but may help the woman cope with or manage her pain better. Homeopathy, acupuncture, and hypnosis, although used occasionally, have not been demonstrated to alter objective assessments of pain or the need for conventional analgesia.

Transcutaneous electrical nerve stimulation (TENS) works on the principle of blocking pain fibres in the posterior ganglia by stimulation of the small afferent fibres. Low-intensity continuous stimulation is applied to the dermatomes associated with pain. It is a safe form of analgesia and is often found useful in the very early stages of labour. It may postpone the need for stronger analgesia but will not often be adequate throughout the course of labour.

Pharmacological means

Nitrous oxide (entonox)

This is self-administered premixed nitrous oxide and oxygen in the ratio 1:1. It has a quick onset of action and is short-lasting. The main side-effects are transient lightheadedness and nausea. Appropriate use of entonox can be highly effective and is safe for mother and baby.

Narcotic agents

- Pethidine is a synthetic analgesic and antispasmodic and is very useful in labour. It can cause nausea in 20% of women and, therefore, it is best co-administered with an anti-emetic. It is used in doses of 50–150 mg IM or 50–100 mg IV. If given within 2 hours of delivery it is important to be aware of the possibility of neonatal respiratory depression.
- Morphine is an alkaloid of opium and is a stronger analgesic without antispasmodic properties. It is used in IM doses of 10 mg and is also associated with side-effects of nausea and vomiting. Hence it is co-administered with an anti-emetic. There is a risk of neonatal respiratory depression with a delivery within 2 hours of the previous dose.
- Diamorphine is a very powerful opiate and particularly useful for the anxious mother with a prolonged labour. It is used in doses of 5–10 mg IM and may cause neonatal respiratory depression for 3–4 hours after the last dose.

The main advantages of IM narcotic analgesia are the ease of administration and reasonably rapid action with a relatively low incidence of side-effects. The main disadvantages in addition to nausea and vomiting are that they may be inadequate in terms of analgesia for up to 40% of women and may cause confusion and inability to cooperate and delay in gastric emptying.

pudendal nerve block/local anaesthesia

Pudendal nerve block involves blocking the pudendal nerve with 10 mL xylocaine 0.5–1% about 1–2 cm medial and below as it courses around the ischial spine. It is usually performed transvaginally but can be performed through the perineum. This form of anaesthesia is sufficient for outlet forceps and vacuum deliveries along with repair of episiotomies and tears. Local infiltration of the vulva, vagina, labia, and perineum are useful for cutting episiotomies and prior to repair of tears and episiotomies.

regional anaesthesia

This is a form of analgesia that relies on blocking nerve roots at their point of outflow to prevent reception and transmission of painful impulses.

Epidural block. An epidural cannula is inserted into the peridural fat at the L2–3, L3–4, or L4–5 interspace and, after confirming that no blood or cerebrospinal fluid (CSF) can be aspirated, bupivicaine 1% or marcain 0.25–0.5% is administered after an initial test dose.

—Epidural anaesthesia can be administered as intermittent top-up boluses every 2–3 hours as required or as a continuous infusion and it aims to block the nerve root T11–S4.

—Contraindications to the use of epidural analgesia are the lack of experienced personnel to site and monitor the epidural, infection at the injection site or systemic sepsis, coagulation defects or bleeding diathesis, anticoagulation, shock and hypovolaemia, bony abnormalities of the spinal column, and idiosyncratic reactions to local anaesthetics.

—In addition to pain relief in labour, operative deliveries can be performed under epidural anaesthesia.

Spinal block. A fine-gauge spinal needle is inserted into the subarachnoid space and a small volume of 'heavy' local anaesthetic ± opiate is administered at the level of L3–4 after which the spinal needle is withdrawn. The main use of spinal anaesthesia in obstetrics is for operative deliveries and repairs of extensive genital tract trauma (i.e. 3rd/4th degree tears or extensive vaginal lacerations). It is also used for Caesarean sections.

Caudal block. This is a form of localized epidural through the sacral hiatus and gives good anaesthesia for operative deliveries but is effective in only 80% of cases.

The complications of regional anaesthesia are discussed in Chapter 35.

Episiotomy and tears

An episiotomy is a surgical incision of the perineum made to increase the diameter of the vulval outlet during childbirth (Fig. 31.7). Episiotomy is cut at the judgement/discretion of the attending professional with the woman's consent. The popularity of episiotomy has waxed and waned over the years from a high of 90% in primigravidas in the 1970s to the World Health Organization (WHO) recommendation for an episiotomy rate of 10% in normal deliveries.

Indications for an episiotomy
- Where perineal tearing appears inevitable.
- In association with most forceps deliveries.
- To expedite a spontaneous delivery where there are concerns about the FHR.
- Failure to progress late in the second stage due to perineal rigidity.
- During a breech delivery.
- Previous perineal reconstructive surgery.
- Previous pelvic floor surgery.

Types of episiotomy
- *Midline episiotomy* is a vertical cut from the fourchette towards the anus (more common in the US). The principal problem associated with midline episiotomies is the high incidence of associated third- and fourth-degree tears—hence its unpopularity in the UK. Midline episiotomies are associated with less bleeding, better healing, and less pain in the puerperium and are easier to repair, but this must be set against the higher incidence of third- and fourth-degree tears.
- *Mediolateral episiotomy* (standard in the UK) starts in the midline in the fourchette and is directed laterally to avoid the anal sphincter.

An episiotomy should be performed at the correct time. Too early an incision increases blood loss. Adequate analgesia should be used—regional block topped up or local infiltration. Sharp straight scissors should be used to make a single cut rather than repeated small extensions that would invariably result in a zigzag incision. Repair should be performed as soon as possible after delivery.

Side-effects of episiotomies/tears
- *Pain.* This can be reduced by prompt, careful, and expert repair.
- *Bleeding.* This can be kept to a minimum by timely episiotomy and early repair. If a large vessel is bleeding this can be tied off or artery forceps applied to it while waiting to commence repair.
- *Breakdown* is often a consequence of infection, bad technique, or inappropriate suture material. Management depends on the merits of the case.
- *Dyspareunia.*

Perineal tears
- First-degree tears involve the skin only.
- Second-degree tears involve perineal muscles (most episiotomies fall into this group).
- A third-degree tear is a perineal tear leading to partial or complete disruption of the anal sphincter.
- The fourth-degree tear is the same as the third-degree tear with involvement of the anal epithelium.

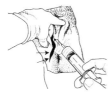

(1)
Swab the vulva towards the perineum. Infiltrate with 1% lignocaine ➤ (arrows).

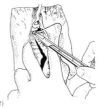

(2)
Place tampon with attached tape in upper vagina. Insert 1st suture above apex of vaginal cut (not too deep as underlying rectal mucosa nearby).

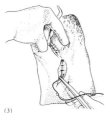

(3)
Bring together vaginal edges with continuous stitches placed 1 cm apart. Knot at introitus under the skin. Appose divided levator animuscles with 2 or 3 interrupted sutures.

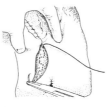

(4)
Close perineal skin (subcuticular) continuous stitch is shown here).

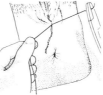

(5)
When stitching is finished, remove tampon and examine vagina (to check for retained swabs). Do a PR to check that apical sutures have not penetrated rectum.

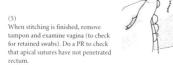

g. 31.7 Steps in repairing an episiotomy. (Reproduced from Collier, J., ongmore, M., and Brown, T.D. (eds.) *Oxford handbook of clinical specialties*, h edn, p. 147, © 1999, by permission of the publisher Oxford University Press.)

Episiotomy and tears (*continued*)

Principles of perineal repair
- Adequate exposure and lighting.
- Adequate analgesia.
- Identification and securing the apex. Failure to do so at onset of repair will result in continuous bleeding or the development of a paravaginal haematoma.
- Absorbable synthetic suture material.
- Good anatomical approximation.
- Deep perineal tissues can be sutured with interrupted stitches.
- The vaginal wall is approximated with continuous locking sutures to achieve better haemostasis and approximation and prevent vaginal shortening.
- The perineal skin may be closed by interrupted mattress sutures but subcuticular suture is associated with less pain in the immediate postpartum period.
- On completion of repair, a vaginal examination should be done to confirm haemostasis, check alignment, and to remove the tampon and any accumulated blood clots. A rectal examination also needs to be performed to exclude accidental suture involvement of the rectum.
- Instruments, swabs, and needle numbers should be checked, detailed documentation with estimated blood loss needs to be recorded, and analgesia needs to be prescribed.

Complications
- Immediate: bleeding, distorted anatomy, pain, suture through rectum.
- Delayed: haematoma, infection, scarring, dyspareunia, fistula formation, scar endometriosis.

Third- and fourth-degree tears
The important feature here is recognition and reconstitution of the disrupted muscle and/or epithelium. Two methods of repair are the end to end or the overlapping method. This procedure needs to be done with adequate lighting, assistance, and appropriate instruments and suture material, which are all more accessible in the theatre setting. All patients need to routinely receive laxative, stool softener, and antibiotic. Due to the significant risk of incontinence of faeces and flatus these women should be seen for follow-up in the hospital setting to check on symptoms.

Postpartum haemorrhage (PPH)

- Primary PPH is traditionally defined as the loss of more than 500 mL of blood from the genital tract in the first 24 hours after delivery or any loss less than 500 mL if associated with haemodynamic changes in the mother.
- If the loss occurs between 24 hours and 6 weeks post-delivery it is defined as secondary PPH.
- PPH occurs in 2–11% of deliveries but in most situations when blood loss is estimated visually it is underestimated.
- Quantitative measurements of blood loss increase the PPH rate to 20% but life-threatening haemorrhage occurs in approximately 1 per 1000 deliveries.
- Primary PPH is one of the major causes of maternal deaths in the triennial Confidential Enquiry into Maternal Deaths in the United Kingdom, with the majority of deaths occurring after Caesarean sections.
- Worldwide over 125 000 women die of PPH each year.

The main causes of primary PPH are uterine atony, retained placenta or placental fragments, and lower genital tract trauma along with coagulopathy, which compounds the problem. Uterine inversion and uterine rupture are less common causes. Of cases of PPH, 90% are due to uterine atony.

Management of primary PPH

The two main aspects of management of PPH, which should be performed simultaneously, are resuscitation of the patient and identifying the specific cause of PPH in order to institute immediate appropriate management.

Resuscitation

Resuscitation involves fluid replacement, investigations, and monitoring. All appropriate staff should be alerted and made available. Essential staff include an experienced obstetrician, anaesthetist, midwives, theatre practitioners, blood bank/haematologist, as well as portering staff to ferry samples and blood products to and from the labs.

- As a minimum two large cannulae (size 14 gauge) should be inserted with colloid (haemaccel, gelofusine) running through one line and with crystalloid (Hartmann's, 0.9% saline, etc.) through the other until blood becomes available. When transfusing under such conditions, blood is preferable, using a compression cuff and blood warmer. It is preferable not to transfuse more than 2000 mL of crystalloids, 1500 mL of colloid, and 2 units of uncross-matched group-specific blood while awaiting cross-matched blood.
- The aim of fluid replacement should be to replace all previous loss in the first hour, followed by maintenance fluids to replace continuing loss and maintain normal vital parameters of pulse, blood pressure, and respiration.
- If coagulopathy develops, liaison with a medical haematologist is imperative to obtain fresh frozen plasma (FFP), cryoprecipitate, and platelets.

Monitoring of the patient's condition is vital. This should include:
- Continuous oximetry.
- Pulse and blood pressure measurement every 15 minutes.
- Indwelling urinary catheter and hourly urine output measurements.
- Central venous pressure (CVP).
- An arterial line if indicated.

The information should be recorded on intensive therapy unit (ITU) style charts to allow easy assessment of any change in the patient's condition.

The primary cycle of investigations should include full blood count (FBC), cross-match of 6 units blood, coagulation screen, and estimation of fibrin degradation products. Other investigations may be required such as chest X-ray if a CVP line is inserted and arterial gases if oxygen saturation falls on oximetry. Electrolytes, urea, and creatinine should be measured to monitor serum levels, which may be deranged with intravenous fluids, blood transfusion, and diminished renal function secondary to acute hypotension. The primary cycle of investigations should be repeated as deemed necessary, probably at least ½-hourly until the patient's condition is stabilized.

Subsequent care in a high-dependency unit (HDU) or intensive care unit (ICU) setting should be considered if massive transfusion (> 12 units), respiratory problems, persistent oliguria, or persistent coagulopathy are encountered.

Establishing a cause

Establishing a cause should be done in parallel to stabilization. Assessment should be in theatre if required, to identify and remove retained placental tissue or repair lower genital tract soft tissue trauma.

- If uterine atony appears to be the underlying problem, the bladder needs to be emptied and uterine contractions rubbed up, whilst pharmacological means (oxytocics) are employed to contract the uterus.
- Whilst an infusion of oxytocin (40 IU oxytocin in 0.9% sodium chloride) is being prepared, a bolus of 250 μg of ergometrine should be administered IV. If the bleeding persists a bolus dose of intravenous oxytocin (10 IU) should be administered and bimanual compression applied.
- If the haemorrhage continues, 15-methylprostaglandin F2a (Haemobate) 250 μg IM can be administered either into the thigh/gluteal muscle or directly into the myometrium and can be repeated up to three more times at 15 minute intervals.
- For PPH unresponsive to oxytocin and/or ergometrine or when ergometrine is contraindicated, misoprostol administered rectally may have a role. Sustained uterine contractions can be produced within 3 minutes of a rectal dose of 800 μg of misoprostol.
- If bleeding still remains refractory and other potential causes (retained products, soft tissue trauma, coagulation disorder) have been excluded, a number of surgical options are described for dealing with intractable haemorrhage and a senior obstetrician/consultant should be available on site by this stage.

Surgical management of primary PPH

Surgical management of postpartum haemorrhage has traditionally relied on hysterectomy and ligation of internal iliac arteries. Over the last few years a number of new and simpler techniques (which also preserve fertility) have come to be used before resorting to complex and risky major surgical procedures.

- Undersuturing the placental bed. Where postpartum haemorrhage follows a placenta praevia or low-lying placenta, the large sinuses that are responsible for the bleeding must be undersewn.

327

Postpartum haemorrhage (PPH) (*continued*)

- The 'tamponade test'. Where coagulopathy has been excluded or corrected, but intractable haemorrhage remains a problem despite all pharmacological means, the 'tamponade test' provides a means of selecting those patients that require further surgery.
  —A Sengstaken–Blakemore tube or Rusch balloon catheter can be inserted into the uterine cavity and the balloon filled with 100–500 mL warm saline. The warm saline speeds up the rate of the clotting cascade. If no or minimal bleeding is observed, the test is considered successful and a laparotomy could be avoided.
- Uterine 'compression sutures': B-Lynch suture and modifications. The B-Lynch suturing technique involves a pair of vertical brace sutures around the uterus essentially to appose the anterior and posterior walls and to apply continuing compression. The brace sutures probably work by direct application of pressure on the placental bed bleeding and also by reducing blood flow to the uterus.
- Uterine artery ligation. The uterus receives 90% of its blood supply from the uterine arteries and uterine artery ligation therefore has a role in the management of PPH.
- Utero-ovarian artery anastomosis ligation. The utero-ovarian anastomosis can be ligated after identifying an avascular area in the meso-ovarium.
- Internal iliac artery ligation. Internal iliac artery ligation may help control uterine and vaginal bleeding as the vagina is supplied by the vaginal branch of the internal iliac artery. Bilateral internal iliac artery ligation results in 85% reduction in pulse pressure in the arteries distal to the ligation and blood flow by 50% in the distal vessel, turning an arterial pressure system into one with pressures approaching those in the venous system and more amenable to haemostasis via clot formation. The success rate of the procedure in achieving its target is reported to be around 40%.
- Arterial embolization. This procedure is usually available in a small number of tertiary centres with appropriately trained interventional radiologists. Access is usually gained via the femoral artery. The catheter is advanced above the bifurcation of the aorta and the bleeding point is identified by contrast injection. The feeder artery is catheterized and embolized with absorbable gelatine sponge, which is usually resorbed in about 10 days.
- Hysterectomy. Hysterectomy is the last resort in the management of PPH due to uterine causes. In most instances a subtotal hysterectomy, which is quicker, simpler, safer, and associated with less blood loss, is adequate. Total hysterectomy is needed in cases where bleeding is in the lower segment such as in cases with placenta praevia with accreta and tears in the lower segment. Hysterectomy is reserved when all other avenues available have been exhausted, where bleeding continues, in a severely shocked patient or where further delay may compromise the patient, and in cases of coagulopathy where no replacement blood products are available.

Other causes of PPH

Injuries to the genital tract

Bleeding from soft tissue injuries in the genital tract (cervical and vaginal lacerations) can be torrential leading to cardiovascular compromise if appropriate resuscitative measures are not carried out while the bleeding is being brought under control. Optimal repair of genital tract lacerations requires correct positioning of the patient, satisfactory analgesia/anaesthesia, adequate lighting and exposure, along with appropriate assistance and instruments such as retractors and long needle holders. These prerequisites often mean that the patient requires transfer to an obstetric theatre. While this is being organized, blood loss can be reduced by vaginal packing or, if a bleeding source is identifiable, this can be clamped with artery forceps.

Disseminated intravascular coagulopathy (DIC)

DIC may compound all the above causes of obstetric haemorrhage and it is not until the deranged coagulation is corrected that postpartum haemorrhage can be effectively controlled whatever other measures are required and employed. DIC may be a result of abruptio placentae, sepsis, massive blood loss or transfusion, severe pre-eclampsia, or amniotic fluid embolism. Dealing with the underlying pathology (emptying the uterus in sepsis or abruption) may prevent the onset or progression of DIC.

Uncontrolled bleeding without clot formation may result from consumption of platelets, fibrinogen, and coagulation factors (in the DIC process or during bleeding) or from elevated levels of fibrinogen degradation products (FDPs). Unless FDP levels are very high, the presence of minimum levels of clotting factors will serve to arrest bleeding. The D-dimer component is the most commonly used parameter to assess FDP levels as it is specific for fibrin breakdown. Levels are under 200 ng/mL normally but often exceed 2000 ng/mL in cases of DIC.

In situations of massive obstetric haemorrhage it is essential to involve a senior medical haematologist, who will advise the appropriate investigations and provide the appropriate blood products to correct coagulation disturbances.

Blood products used in the correction of deranged coagulation include:

- Cryoprecipitate. Each unit is approximately 200 mL in volume and contains the equivalent of 0.2 g of fibrinogen and 80 units of factor VIII. Contains no platelets. The usual requirement is 10–15 units.
- Fresh frozen plasma (FFP). Each unit is approximately 200 mL in volume and contains 0.4 g of fibrinogen and all clotting factors. The usual requirement is 5 units.
- Platelet concentrate. Each unit is approximately 60 mL in volume and contains a minimum of 5.5×10^{10}/L. The usual requirement is 5–6 units.

329

Retained placenta

Failure to expel the placenta within 30 minutes of delivery of the baby is defined as retained placenta. Where there is no significant bleeding, an hour is commonly allowed before manual removal is performed. Varying degrees of success have been reported when 10 IU of oxytocin is milked up the umbilical vein to enhance expulsion of the placenta. An infusion of oxytocin (40 IU oxytocin in 500 mL 0.9% saline at a rate of 125 mL/hour) is set up to maintain uterine contraction and manual removal of the placenta in theatre is organized. The procedure requires an effective regional block (functioning epidural or spinal) or general anaesthesia.

Blood needs to be sent for haemoglobin estimation, group and screen, or cross-match.
- At the onset of the procedure a broad-spectrum antibiotic such as coamoxiclav or a combination of ampicillin and metronidazole should be administered intravenously.
- During the procedure, the external hand should steady the uterus by pressing on the fundus, to facilitate removal of the placenta and reduce the risk of perforating the uterus.
- The aim is to identify the plane between the placenta and uterine wall and, using the fingers in a side to side shearing motion, to separate and remove the placenta.
- Once the placenta has been removed, the placenta and membranes should be inspected, the uterine cavity checked and confirmed as empty, and the oxytocin infusion continued to maintain uterine contractions.

Morbidly adherent placenta

Attachment of the placental villi to the myometrium due to absence of the decidua basalis or imperfect development of the fibrinoid layer is known as placenta accreta, while invasion of the myometrium and penetration through to the peritoneum are known as placenta increta and percreta, respectively.

The risk of morbid adherence of the placenta increases with repeated surgical terminations of pregnancy, Caesarean sections, and myomectomy.
- In most instances of morbidly adherent placenta, especially with heavy bleeding, the treatment is immediate blood replacement and recourse to hysterectomy.
- If bleeding is minimal and not of concern then a conservative approach of leaving the placenta *in situ* with no further treatment may be adopted. This is an option only if adequate facilities for monitoring and management of the patient are available.
- An alternative course of action involves no attempt at placental separation and the administration of cytotoxic agents such as methotrexate in addition to antibiotics and follow-up with serial serum β-hCG (beta-human chorionic gonadotrophin) measurements and ultrasound scans.

Uterine inversion

Complete inversion of the uterus is usually due to mismanagement of the third stage either by excessive cord traction on a fundally implanted placenta that has not yet separated or secondary to fundal pressure erroneously thought to aid placental expulsion. Uterine inversion, however, may also occur spontaneously with an atonic uterus and sudden increase in intraabdominal pressure (coughing/sneezing). Although often associated with massive haemorrhage, the shock is disproportionate to the blood loss and probably partly neurogenic due to traction on the uterine supports.

If diagnosed within a short time following inversion the best course of action is immediate replacement by pushing up on the fundus with the palm of the hand and fingers in the direction of the long axis of the vagina. If this is not successful or diagnosis is delayed, assistance should be summoned and resuscitation with intravenous fluids and blood as appropriate commenced. If the placenta is still attached, it should be left *in situ* (unless there is partial separation and bleeding) till the set up is ready for reduction. When the patient is haemodynamically stable, correction of the uterine inversion is performed followed by removal of placenta unless removal first facilitates reduction. The rationale for this course of action is to minimize further haemorrhage.

Before attempting replacement of the uterine fundus, a tocolytic ritodrine 6 mg, terbutaline 0.25 mg, or glyceryl trinitrate 100 to 200 μg may be administered IV for uterine relaxation. The replacement is attempted manually as described above or by the hydrostatic method. The latter (known as the O'Sullivan method) involves replacing the inverted uterus in the vagina and rapid infusion of 2 or more litres of warm saline into the vagina with one hand sealing the labia. This leads to ballooning of the vaginal fornices, exerts an even hydrostatic pressure that gradually forces open the constricting cervix and pushes upwards the rim of inverted uterine wall, thus reducing the inverted uterus. If the placenta is intact this can be removed and an oxytocin infusion commenced after the uterus has been restored to its normal configuration. Removal of placenta just prior to reduction may make the procedure easy.

In the rare circumstance where manual and hydrostatic methods of restoring the uterus are not successful, possibly due to a dense constriction ring, laparotomy may be required. At laparotomy, traction is placed on the round ligaments with Allis forceps and an assistant pushes from below. The process may be aided by placement of a suture in the fundus to use for traction. Occasionally, where the constriction ring still prohibits repositioning, the Haultain technique of making a vertical incision in the posterior cervico-isthmic portion of the constriction ring to expose and restore the fundus to its normal configuration can be used. Operative procedures should be the last resort as in most cases persistent pressure from below to reduce the uterus under an anaesthetic yields good results.

Chapter 32

Instrumental deliveries (forceps/ventouse)

Forceps delivery

Forceps consist of a pair of fenestrated blades with a handle connected to the blades by a shank. They are designed with a cephalic curve that fits around the fetal head and a pelvic curve that fits the pelvis. They are mainly used for traction. The Kielland's forceps have a reduced pelvic curve, making them suitable for rotation of the fetal head in cases of malpresentation (only in experienced hands).

Conditions for use

On abdominal examination, the fetus should not be too large, suggestive of possible disproportion, and the head should be one-fifth or less palpable above the pelvic brim. There should be good uterine contractions. The bladder should be empty. On vaginal examination, the cervix must be fully dilated with ruptured membranes and a vertex presentation with no excess caput or moulding. The position of the vertex should be known (e.g. left occipitoanterior (LOA), left occipitotransverse (LOT), etc.), the station should be below +1, and there should be descent of the head with contraction and bearing down effort.

Adequate analgesia must be achieved before application of forceps using one of the following.

- Local analgesia: pudendal block, and perineal infiltration (not suitable for Kielland's).
- An existing epidural block, usually with a top-up.
- Spinal anaesthesia.

Consent should be obtained from the mother explaining the indication for the instrumental delivery, the steps in the procedure, and the advantages and disadvantages.

Indications for use

- Forceps may be used when there is delay in the second stage as a result of poor maternal expulsive efforts or due to malposition or minor disproportion. Often it may be related to the absence of the urge to bear down with epidural anaesthesia and inadequate uterine activity due to absent Ferguson reflex (reflex release of oxytocin with distension of vagina).
- Forceps may also be used when there is fetal distress or a prolapsed cord or eclampsia in the second stage of labour.
- They are also used to prevent undue maternal effort in women with cardiac and respiratory diseases and in severe pre-eclampsia.
- They can also be applied to the after-coming head in a breech presentation and may also be used to extract the fetal head at Caesarean section.
- They have also been used to assist a face presentation in mento-anterior position.

Techniques

- The mother is placed in the lithotomy position with her bottom just over the edge of the delivery bed.
- The vulva and perineum are cleansed and the mother catheterized.
- The position of the fetal head is identified. Moulding may make this difficult. The inverted Y shape described by the occipital bone on the parietal bone identifies the posterior fontanelle. The overriding of the parietal bones on the frontal bones identifies the anterior fontanelle. There are four sutures that delineate the anterior fontanelle.

32 Instrumental deliveries (forceps/ventouse)

- If in doubt one must feel for the fetal ear and check in which direction the ear flicks to identify the direction of the occiput.
- The pudendal block is inserted and the site of episiotomy is infiltrated with up to 20 mL of 1% lignocaine hydrochloride (plain), if the mother has no epidural.
- For occipitoanterior positions the Neville Barnes forceps or the Simpson's forceps (similar to Neville Barnes but with no axis traction handle) can be used.

The blades are assembled to check that they fit, with the pelvic curve pointing upwards. The handle that lies on the left hand is the left blade and is inserted first (to the mother's left side), negotiating the pelvic and cephalic curve with a curved movement of the blade between the fetal head and the accoucheur's hand kept along the left vaginal wall. The right blade is inserted in a similar manner. If the blades were applied correctly, the handles should lock easily. Traction in the direction of the pelvic curve must not be excessive. Traction is synchronized with contractions and maternal bearing down efforts, guiding the head downwards initially. An episiotomy is usually needed when the head is at the vulva. The direction of traction is changed to up and out as the head passes out of the vulva.

Kielland's forceps

Before Kielland's forceps are used, it is essential to identify abdominally the side of the baby's back. The forceps are applied with the 'knobs' facing towards the baby's occiput. The anterior or posterior blade may be applied first directly depending on the preference of the obstetrician. The anterior blade usually is positioned by the 'wandering method' (first placed over the face and then moved to lie on the side of the fetal head) and the posterior blade directly. The blades are locked and asynclitism corrected by sliding the blades on each other into position. If the asynclitism was correct, the sagittal suture of the fetus will lie equidistant from the two blades of the forceps. If the blades cannot be locked easily the application of the forceps should be checked and reapplied if necessary.

An abnormal position (e.g. occipitotransverse) is corrected by rotating the handles of the forceps blades and directing the fetal occiput to the anterior position to emerge underneath the symphysis pubis. The head is flexed at the same time. An excessive twisting force should not be used. Rotational forceps and vacuum deliveries are best done by an experienced person or under supervision.

Complications of forceps

- *Maternal trauma.* Labial and vaginal and perineal tears are not uncommon and rarely third- and fourth-degree tears.
- *Fetal trauma.* Fetal facial bruising, VII nerve paralysis (usually resolves), and skin abrasions are seen on and off and, rarely, cephalhaematomas and fracture of the skull.

335

Ventouse delivery

An alternative to forceps delivery is the application of a suction cup to the fetal scalp and extraction by traction. The Ventouse, or vacuum extractor is associated with less maternal trauma than forceps and is becoming popular in the UK. It may be used in preference to rotational forceps because, as traction is applied with the cup over the fetal occiput, spontaneous rotation to occipitoanterior position occurs during delivery. It can be used through a partially dilated cervix (advanced cervical dilatation) in a multipara, but should not be used if the head is above the ischial spine. It is best to leave such deliveries to someone with good experience. Ventouse should be avoided in preterm (< 34 weeks) babies, face presentations, and in those with bleeding disorders.

A silicon or metal cup should be applied on the 'flexion point' (just in front of the occiput on the midline) and a suction force of up to 0.2 kg/cm^2 is created initially. The rim of the cup is checked to make sure that there is no maternal tissue caught inadvertently under the suction cup. The pressure is then increased to 0.8 kg/cm^2 and traction exerted with uterine contractions and maternal bearing down effort. The baby's scalp is often sucked up to form a 'chignon', which resolves in 2 days. There is increased rate of fetal cephalhaematoma and neonatal jaundice. A posterior cup (metal or rigid cup) should be the choice for occipitotransverse or posterior positions to enable one to apply the vacuum over the 'flexion point'. The flexion point is on the midline along the sagittal suture and is 3 to 4 cm anterior to the posterior fontanelle.

The use of the vacuum extractor rather than forceps for assisted vaginal delivery appears to reduce maternal mobidity. Cephalhaematoma and retinal haemorrhage are more common with vacuum (Cochrane) although no long-term ill effects are attributed to these complications. Follow-up studies show no consistent trend to physical or cognitive impairment from low outlet instrumental deliveries.

Trial of instrumental delivery

At times it is difficult to assess whether instrumental delivery could be carried out safely or whether to opt for a Caesarean section. If fetal distress is present, Caesarean section may be a better option, as further delay may compromise the baby. Such procedures should be done in the theatre under good epidural or spinal anaesthesia and with the theatre team, anaesthetist, and paediatrician present. The intent is to abandon instrumental vaginal delivery (IVD) should there be any difficulties and to proceed to Caesarean section immediately. This should have been explicitly explained to the mother and her partner and appropriate consent obtained prior to the procedure, which should be undertaken by a senior person.

32 Instrumental deliveries (forceps/ventouse)

Chapter 33

Malpresentations in labour (face, brow, shoulder)

Malpresentation is said to occur when the fetus is not presenting by the vertex. The vertex is a diamond-shaped area defined by the parietal eminences, the anterior fontanelle, and the posterior fontanelle. Breech, brow, face, and shoulder presentations fall into this category.

Breech presentation is the most common malpresentation (3–4% at term). The appropriate clinical management of breech presentation antenatally and in labour is discussed in Chapter 19.

Brow presentation

The incidence is 1:1500 deliveries. It may be associated with a contracted pelvis or a very large baby. The engaging diameter is the mentovertical (13 cm). In normal-sized baby, if the presentation does not correct itself in labour, delivery is by Caesarean section Occasionally a brow may extend to become a face and delivers spontaneously if it is mentoanterior. To ensure this happens the mother should have a vaginal examination every 2 hours to identify satisfactory progress. Failure to progress is an indication of disproportion due to the presenting diameter and syntocinon augmentation should not be used.

- *Diagnosis and management.* The head remains high and does not engage and is therefore easily palpable. On vaginal examination the forehead is palpable and with additional vigilance the brow is palpable between the bridge of the nose and supraorbital ridges. The mentovertical diameter that is presented is 13.5 cm and safe delivery is by Caesarean section.

Face presentation

This occurs in approximately 1:500 deliveries. Of these, 15% are due to congenital abnormalities such as anencephaly, a tumour in the neck such as a thyroid goitre, or shortened fetal neck muscles. Most occur by chance as the head extends rather than flexes as it emerges. The diameters of the face are the biparietal diameter (9.5 cm) and submentobragmatic (9.5 cm).

- *Diagnosis and management.* Abdominally the fetal spine feels S-shaped, the uterus is ovoid without fullness in the flanks, and there is a deep groove between the occiput and the back. On early vaginal examination the nose and eyes may be felt but later this may not be easy because of oedema. Most engage in the transverse (submentobragmatic diameter = 9.5 cm). 90% rotate so that the chin lies behind the symphysis pubis (mentoanterior), and the head can be born by flexion. If the chin rotates posteriorly (mentoposterior), then there is a large area of skull comprising the vertex and occiput that cannot follow the face under the mother's symphysis pubis. Delivery is then required by Caesarean section.

Shoulder presentation

This occurs in 1:400 deliveries and usually in multiparous women. If labour starts when the lie is transverse, it is clear that vaginal delivery cannot occur unless the fetus is very small or macerated. Placenta praevia, fibroids, ovarian cysts, fetal malformations, multiple pregnancy, and abnormal uterus should be excluded. The transverse lie may evolve into a shoulder presentation and, as the cervix dilates, the arm may prolapse.

- *Diagnosis and management.* If the shoulder is presenting no attempt should be made to replace or apply traction to the arm. Unless the lie can be corrected before the situation occurs, the only appropriate method of delivery is by Caesarean section. Uterine relaxants such as 0.25 mg terbutaline in 5 mL saline may be given IV to relax the uterus to accomplish the delivery through a lower segment transverse incision. It may be necessary to perform a classical Caesarean section with a vertical incision in the upper segment if the membranes have ruptured and the uterus has been contracting as there will be considerable difficulty delivering the baby through a lower segment incision.

Caesarean section

Caesarean section (CS) is the process whereby the child is removed from the uterus by direct incision through the abdominal wall and the uterus. The incidence is between 10 and 20% and is still rising. It has an associated maternal mortality of 0.33 per 1000.

Types of Caesarean sections

There are two main uterine incisions for Caesarean sections.

Lower uterine segment incision
This is the most commonly performed procedure. The bladder is reflected from the lower segment and a transverse incision is made. The presenting part is then delivered through the lower segment. The lower segment muscle wound is closed in two layers. In comparison to the classical incision, surgery is much easier, is associated with less blood loss, and heals better, and the chance of uterine and intraabdominal infection rate is low (because of the peritoneal cover). Uterine rupture in subsequent spontaneous labour is about 5/1000, with the use of oxytocin it is 8/1000, and with prostaglandins for induction of labour it is 25/1000.

Classical Caesarean section
In this procedure a vertical incision is made in the upper segment of the uterus and the child is delivered through this incision. This is not widely used because it has a much higher morbidity postoperatively and a much higher incidence of subsequent rupture of the scar. The indications for this type of incision include
• Transverse lie of the fetus with ruptured membranes and liquor draining.
• Structural abnormality makes lower segment approach difficult.
• Constriction ring present due to neglected labour.
• Fibroids in the lower segment.
• Anterior placenta praevia with abnormally vascular lower segment.
• The mother is dead and rapid delivery is desired.
• Very preterm fetus (especially breech presentation) where the lower segment is poorly formed.

Caesarean hysterectomy
Caesarean section and hysterectomy are sometimes performed at the same time, e.g. where there is uterine rupture, placenta accreta, uncontrollable postpartum haemorrhage, and in cases of cervical malignant disease.

Indications for Caesarean section

Caesarean section can be performed either as an emergency or as an elective procedure. Indications for elective Caesarean section include known cephalo-pelvic disproportion, placenta praevia, some malpresentations (e.g. brow presentation), history of suburethral repair, vesicovaginal fistula repair, and maternal infections, e.g. herpes, HIV. In the case of a repeat section it is important to localize the placenta on ultrasound to exclude placenta praevia as this is slightly more common in women with a scar, and more likely to be complicated by placenta accreta—hence the risk of massive haemorrhage and the possibility of needing a hysterectomy.

Emergency Caesarean section may be needed because of antenatal complications, e.g. severe pre-eclampsia, abruptio placentae (baby still alive). The need for emergency Caesarean section may become apparent during labour when there is fetal distress in the first stage of labour, failure to progress in the first stage of labour, prolapsed cord, (if fetus is alive), obstructed labour, or disproportion becoming evident during labour and after failed induction.

- *Fetal indications.* On occasion Caesarean section is carried out almost entirely in the interest of the fetus, e.g. severe intrauterine growth restriction (IUGR), preterm fetus that needs delivery presents by the breech, although the evidence for the latter practice is not strong. Postmortem Caesarean section occasionally may be performed to save the life of the baby if it is still alive. In this case a classical type of operation may be indicated to extract a child with the utmost speed.

- *Maternal indications.* Caesarean section may be performed on account of previous surgery, e.g. a previous hysterotomy or myomectomy. Previous myomectomy does not constitute an absolute indication for Caesarean section. If a vaginal delivery is allowed in these circumstances great care must be taken during labour to look out for signs of imminent rupture of the uterus.

Elective and emergency Caesarean sections

Timing of elective Caesarean section

When Caesarean section is carried out in the maternal interests there is usually little choice in the timing of the procedure. When the fetal interest is paramount, timing of the operation is influenced by two main factors: fetal maturity and fetal condition. Elective Caesarean sections are usually performed after 39 weeks gestation, although in special cases they can be done before that time. Clinical knowledge and experience are important in making the decision about when the infant is at less risk in the nursery, compared to within the uterus.

Before an emergency section

- Explain to the mother and her partner about the need for an emergency CS and obtain their consent.
- Activate the anaesthetist, theatre staff, porters, and paediatrician.
- Have the mother breathe 100% oxygen if there is fetal distress.
- Neutralize gastric contents with 20 mL of 0.3 sodium citrate and promote gastric emptying with metoclopramide 10 mg IV (ranitidine 150 mg, an H2 agonist, is given for elective sections 2 hours before surgery).
- Consider pre-operative emptying of the stomach (e.g. if prolonged labour or if the patient had a meal recently or if opiate was given). These measures are necessary to minimize risk of postoperative aspiration (Mendelson's syndrome).
- Transfer to theatre. Set up an IV infusion with a 14 cannula and take blood for Hb% and cross-match, e.g. 2 units (4 units if anterior placenta praevia or placental abruption).
- Catheterize the bladder.
- Tilt the mother to left lateral position by 15° on operating table using a wedge.
- Pneumatic inflatable boots are used for the legs to reduce incidence of deep vein thrombosis (DVT).
- Use pulse oximetry, peri- and postoperatively.
- Use prophylactic antibiotics to reduce the incidence of infection.
- Inform the paediatrician if the mother has had opiates in the last 4 hours. Halothane is not used for obstetric procedures because uterine muscle relaxation increases bleeding.

Other anaesthetic problems include vomiting on induction and light anaesthesia causing awareness, although the woman is paralysed. Most CS are now performed under spinal/epidural anaesthesia. It is important to have an experienced anaesthetist in order to reduce maternal morbidity.

Complications of Caesarean section

The immediate complications are those of haemorrhage, primary or secondary, that may lead to shock and the complications of anaesthesia. There may be damage to the bladder, ureters, or colon, a vesico-uterine fistula, or retained placental tissue and bleeding (this should be rare as the uterine cavity should be inspected and cleaned during Caesarean section).

After a Caesarean section, all excess blood should be removed from the peritoneal cavity and the ovaries and tubes inspected. Rhesus-negative mothers should have anti-D and a Kleihauer test to determine the dose of anti-D if the baby is found to be rhesus-positive. The mother should be mobilized early.

Prophylaxis against thromboembolism

Low risk

Women with no risk factors undergoing elective Caesarean section in an uncomplicated pregnancy require only early mobilization and good hydration.

Moderate risk

- Age over 35 years.
- Obesity over 80 kg.
- Para 4+.
- Pre-eclampsia.
- Emergency section in labour.
- Gross varicose veins.
- Current infection.
- More than 4 days of prior immobility.
- Major concurrent illness (heart diesease, nephritic syndrome, cancer).

These women require heparin prophylaxis (e.g. heparin 7500 IU SC (subcutaneous) bd (twice daily); enoxaparin 40 mg SC od (once daily); dalteparin 5000 IU SC od) and/or mechanical methods (physiotherapy before and after surgery, pneumatic boots during surgery, graded elastic stockings postoperatively, early mobilization).

High risk

These women should all receive heparin until 5 days postoperatively or until fully mobilized. The use of leg stockings confers additional benefit. Those at high risk include the following.

- Any women with three risk factors under the 'Moderate risk' heading.
- Extended surgery, e.g. Caesarean hysterectomy.
- Family or past history of thromboembolism or thrombophilia.
- Paralysed lower limbs.
- Women with anti-phospholipid antibody (cardiolipin antibody or lupus anticoagulant).

Women who have had thromboembolism in pregnancy should receive thromboprophylaxis as mentioned above for 6 weeks postpartum.

Obstetric analgesia and anaesthesia

The role of the anaesthetist in an obstetric unit is to administer safe analgesia and anaesthesia and to be part of the multidisciplinary team concerned in the management of the sick parturient. This chapter deals with analgesia and anaesthesia, where the help of an anaesthetist is required. Other forms of pain relief are discussed in Chapter 31.

Analgesia

Adequate pain relief in labour is not available to the majority of women in the world. Anaesthetists are usually not involved in pain management unless an epidural is requested/required. Epidural anaesthesia for pain relief has been discussed in Chapter 31. More details related to epidural anaesthesia are discussed here.

Advantages of epidurals
- Epidurals are the most effective method of providing pain relief in labour.
- A good working epidural can be topped up for an instrumental delivery if required.
- Epidurals can be converted to provide anaesthesia for an operative delivery or for the removal of a retained placenta.
- Epidurals can be used as an adjuvant in the control of blood pressure in pre-eclamptic women.
- Epidural opiates (diamorphine or morphine) provide good postoperative pain relief for many hours.
- Epidural analgesia allows a woman to be clear-headed and thus to be in control of her labour.

Disadvantages of epidurals
- Epidurals are invasive procedures with side-effects and complications.
- Women with epidurals *in situ* require close monitoring ideally with a one-to-one midwife.

Side-effects and complications of epidurals
- The blood pressure may drop (from blockade of sympathetic nerves).
- The block may be unilateral or patchy.
- Motor nerves as well as sensory nerves may be blocked (with loss of mobility).
- There is a less than 1% possibility of a dural tap by the needle or catheter.
- Approximately 60% of women who have had a dural tap develop a severe headache, which may require an epidermal blood patch as treatment.
- Loss of sensation of a full bladder can lead to retention, breakthrough pain, and the need for catheterization for a period of time.
- Neuropathy. The majority of postpartum neuropathies occur in women who have not had any anaesthetic intervention. But there is an incidence of nerve damage both of the cord and of peripheral nerves due to incorrect drug administration, direct trauma from the needle tip, or from infarction during a hypotensive episode.
- Meningitis bacterial and chemical.
- Epidural abscess.
- Epidural haematoma.
- Short-term backache. (It is now established that women who have had epidurals for labour are no more likely to suffer long-term backache than those women who did not have epidurals for labour.)

35 Obstetric analgesia and anaesthesia

Consent issues

The pros and cons of epidurals cannot realistically be discussed with a woman who is in the throes of labour, especially if she has already had pethidine and is breathing entonox. It is often difficult for the anaesthetist to ensure that the woman has adequate understanding to give valid consent. Ideally, anaesthetists should be involved antenatally in the discussion of pain relief in labour.

Performing an epidural

- Consent must be obtained.
- Blood should be taken for coagulation studies in potentially at risk patients.
- A large-bore intravenous (IV) cannula for administration of fluids should be established (to counteract any fall in blood pressure).
- The woman may be lying on her side or sitting but the back should be curved to open up the intervertebral spaces.
- Using an aseptic technique the anaesthetist infiltrates local anaesthetic into the skin over L2/3 or L3/4 (if a combined spinal epidural technique is being used then the space should be L3/4 to avoid the possibility of the spinal needle damaging the spinal cord which usually ends at L1 level). The average epidural space is approximately 4 to 5 cm deep. The Tuohy needle is marked at 1 cm intervals to allow depth to be gauged.
- The epidural space is identified using a loss of resistance technique to saline or air.
- The epidural catheter is threaded through the needle and the needle withdrawn.
- Local anaesthetic, usually bupivacaine, is often initially given in a test dose to ensure that the epidural catheter has not inadvertently entered the subarachnoid space giving a consequent drop in blood pressure.
- A bolus dose is then given and the epidural is run either on bolus top-up doses 1–2 hourly as required or more effectively as a continuous infusion. Some anaesthetists offer women a patient-controlled epidural with or without a continuous infusion. Mobility can be encouraged.
- Blood pressure readings must be taken at 5 minute intervals for 20 minutes after each top-up and at half hour intervals once established.
- The level of block height must be monitored by testing the dermatome level to which the block has spread using cold or touch sensation. Motor power is tested by the ability to lift the leg and bend the knee.
- Blood pressure, block height, and motor block must be documented.

With low-dose epidural infusions, good analgesia can be established particularly when small doses of opiate (usually fentanyl) are added. The incidence of instrumental delivery (ventouse or forceps) was greater in women who had large volumes of high-concentration bupivacaine, which caused increased motor block. With low-dose weak concentration there is no higher risk of instrumental delivery except when the epidural has been running for a long time and there is some motor block combined with maternal fatigue.

Anaesthesia

Emergency
Epidurals
Conversion of a working epidural from analgesia to anaesthesia is the anaesthetic of choice for a labouring woman who requires instrumental or operative delivery. The indication for Caesarean section (e.g. a cord prolapse or sudden massive obstetric haemorrhage) may mean there is no time to top up the epidural adequately and a general anaesthetic will be required.

When epidurals are in place:
- Ephedrine should be available at all times to counteract any fall in blood pressure.

Facilities and drugs should always be ready for rapid conversion to general anaesthesia:
- If the block progresses too high.
- If the woman experiences pain and requests a general anaesthetic.
- If the surgery is complicated and may proceed to Caesarean hysterectomy.

NB. To put a woman to sleep against her wishes constitutes assault. Prior discussion about the possibility should obviate potential complaint.

Spinals
When there is no epidural *in situ* and a woman requires an emergency Caesarean section there is usually time for the anaesthetist to give a spinal anaesthetic.

Elective
A woman having an elective Caesarean section has the choice of general or regional anaesthesia (Regional anaesthesia can either be epidural, spinal, or combined spinal epidural (CSE).)

Regional anaesthesia is:
- Safer for mother.
- Safer for baby.
- Allows immediate bonding.
- Allows birth partner to be present.
- Allows better management of postoperative pain especially when opiates are used.

Epidurals
Disadvantages of epidurals:
- Can take up to three-quarters of an hour to establish a good block *de novo*.
- May be unilateral.
- Fewer cases can be performed on a list.
- There is a higher conversion level to general anaesthetic.

Advantages of epidurals:
- Can be topped up during surgery if the operation is taking a long time.
- Catheter may be left in for postoperative pain management.

35 Obstetric analgesia and anaesthesia

Spinals

Disadvantages of spinals:
- May wear off if surgery is prolonged.
- Less control of fall of blood pressure.
- May cause more nausea and vomiting.
- More likely to cause nerve damage.

Advantages of spinals:
- Technically easier to perform.
- Definite end point (cerebral spinal fluid (CSF)).
- Less likely to be unilateral.
- Give a good dense block within a few minutes.

Combined spinal epidurals

These are usually performed by the 'needle though needle' technique, i.e. the spinal needle is passed through the Tuohy needle into the CSF, but can be performed by two separate injections.

Disadvantages:
- Technically more difficult.
- Higher risk of chemical and bacterial meningitis.
- Spinal may be unilateral if performed in the lateral position and there is difficulty threading the epidural catheter.

Advantages:
- Have the advantages of both epidurals and spinal.

The majority of elective Caesarean sections are performed under spinal anaesthesia in the UK.

General anaesthesia

General anaesthesia is indicated when:
- The mother requests to be asleep.
- Regional anaesthesia is contraindicated:
  —In the presence of coagulopathies.
  —In a patient who is anticoagulated.
  —Where there is local infection at the injection site.
  —When there is systemic bacteraemia or septicaemia.
  —In certain cases of back injury or previous back surgery.
  —In certain cardiac diseases.
  —Where there is allergy to local anaesthetic.

There are some relative contraindications to regional procedures, e.g. certain neurological diseases, but antenatal discussion should provide information on the basis of which the woman can decide whether she wishes to be awake or asleep.

Dangers of general anaesthesia:
- Risk of difficult intubation (especially in pre-eclampsia).
- Risk of inhalation of gastric content (Mendelson's syndrome).
- General anaesthetics cross the placenta and can depress the baby.
- There is delayed bonding of mother and baby.

Anaesthesia (*continued*)

There is a decrease in lower oesophageal tone, which increases the risk of passive reflux. All pregnant women having a general anaesthetic for whatever reason from 20 weeks onwards will have a rapid sequence induction (pre oxygenation and cricoid pressure).

In obstetric units there should be good communication between midwives, obstetricians, and anaesthetists as it is important for the successful management of women with known pre-existing medical problems. There should be a plan as to the management and mode of delivery of these women which should be documented in the antenatal notes.

Physiological changes of pregnancy affecting anaesthesia

The obstetric patient presents the ananaesthetist with particular challenges. The physiological changes that occur in a woman during pregnancy add to the potential risk of anaesthesia.

- *Changes in blood volume.*
  - —There is an increase in plasma volume (40–50%).
  - —There is an increase in red cell volume (15–20%).
  - —There is consequently 'physiological anaemia of pregnancy'.
  - —Clotting factors increase for protection at the time of delivery such that the woman is in a hypercoaguable state.
- *Cardiovascular changes.*
  - —There is an increase in cardiac output (30–40%).
  - —There is an increase in heart rate (15–20 beats/minute).
  - —There is downregulation of alpha and beta receptors.
  - —There is a profound effect on venous return when the large gravid uterus compresses the inferior vena cava and also the aorta (aortacaval compression or supine hypotension syndrome).

  A pregnant woman must never lie flat on her back. Care must be taken especially when she is being transferred on to a trolley or operating table. Her hips should be tilted to one side using a wedge or pillow. The operating table should be in left lateral tilt.
- *Respiratory effects.*
  - —An increase in minute volume (40%).
  - —An increase in respiratory rate (15%).
  - —A decrease in functional residual capacity.
  - —A decrease in expiratory reserve volume.
  - —A decrease in residual volume.
  - —Increased oxygen consumption and decreased functional residual capacity mean that women develop hypoxaemia very rapidly. Anaesthetists must pre-oxygenate for a longer time before induction of general anaesthesia.
  - —There is a decrease in minimum alveolar concentration (MAC) that increases susceptibility to inhalation anaesthetic agents.

35 Obstetric analgesia and anaesthesia

Gastrointestinal effects: In order that the fetus can grow, maternal nutrition must provide the placenta with adequate nutrients.

—To maximize absorption, particularly of iron gastrointestinal motility is decreased.
—There is an increased secretion of gastric acid stimulated by the hormone gastrin towards term.
—Gastric pH is low and there is delayed gastric emptying.
—The lower oesophageal tone is lowered and hence re-flux of acid gastric content can occur.
—Inhalation of gastric contents in pregnancy was first described by Mendelson (Mendelson's syndrome or acid aspiration syndrome).
—*Antacid prophylaxes*. H2 receptor antagonists (ranitidine), which make gastric secretion less acidic, and sodium citrate, which neutralizes acid already in the stomach, should be prescribed. Women should be given ranitidine six-hourly during labour.

Weight gain.
—The average parturient gains approximately 27 kg in weight.
—This weight gain can cause difficulty when lifting patients.
—Difficulty with venous access.
—Potential intubation difficulties (every pregnant woman is given a rapid sequence induction for general anaesthesia).

Large patient.
—Large pendulous breasts hinder laryngoscope movements.
—Oedema especially in pre-eclamptic patients when there is often laryngeal oedema.
—High oxygen demand leading to rapid desaturation.
—Potential of inhalation of gastric contents increased.

Resuscitation

Cardiac arrest during pregnancy is rare.

Causes:
—Cardiac disease, especially after delivery when there is an increase in blood volume by autotransfusion from involution of the uterus.
—Cocaine abuse, now the most common cause of cardiac arrest at term in the USA.
—Haemorrhage.
—Iatrogenic: anaphylaxis, general anaesthesia (e.g. failed intubation), and regional anaesthesia (inadvertent intravenous injection of local anaesthetic; inadvertent total spinal from subarachnoid injection of local anaesthetic).

Management:
—ABC (airway, breathing, and circulation) as for all cardiac arrests.
—Plus left lateral tilt (it is impossible to resuscitate a woman when the venous return to the heart is blocked).
—Cricoid pressure (if enough personnel available).
—Immediate delivery of the baby (the chances of successful resuscitation of the mother are small but are increased by the delivery of the baby).

Chapter 36

Neonatal resuscitation

Anticipating problems is the key to effective resuscitation. Call the paediatrician in good time for deliveries where problems may occur, e.g.

- Preterm deliveries < 35 weeks completed gestation.
- Emergency Caesarean section deliveries.
- Breech birth.
- Fetal distress.
- Thick meconium.
- Expected major fetal abnormality.
- Concern for other reasons, e.g. maternal drug addiction.

Term infants requiring resuscitation often respond to simple measures: dry and warm; clear the airway; mild stimulation. An inverted pyramid (Fig. 36.1) illustrates the relative frequencies and priorities of neonatal resuscitation.

Practical aspects of resuscitation

Before delivery
Check resuscitaire and equipment:
- Heater on.
- Oxygen supply connected.
- Pressure valves set at 25–30 cm H_2O.
- Laryngoscope illuminating effectively.
- Suction device functioning and suction catheters available.
- Endotracheal tubes (ETT) available.
- Emergency resuscitation box available.

At delivery
This section assumes there is no meconium-stained liquor. Resuscitation of the infant with meconium-stained liquor is discussed later (in the eponymous section).

- Start clock.
- Transfer baby to resuscitaire.
- Dry baby and wrap in warm towel/gauze.
- Assess condition:
  —*Breathing.* Assess rate and quality.
  —*Heart rate.* Listen to the apex beat with a stethoscope. Palpate the brachial or femoral pulse or palpate the base of the umbilical cord.
  —*Colour.* Look at the trunk, lips, and tongue. Note if the baby is centrally pink, cyanosed, or pale. Peripheral cyanosis is common and by itself does not indicate hypoxaemia.

Condition of the newborn infant at birth

After assessing breathing, heart rate, and colour, the baby can usually be placed in one of four broad categories.
1 Healthy. Pink; crying lustily; heart rate >100 beats/minute.
   —*Action.* Dry and give to mother.

Primary apnoea. Cyanosed; heart rate > 100 beats/minute; some respiratory effort, tone, and response to stimulation.

—*Action.* Gentle stimulation and facial oxygen. This baby is likely to begin to breathe spontaneously—a short wait of not more than 1 minute is acceptable. Stimulate by: rubbing with a dry towel; gentle oral or nasal suction; oxygen to the face. If no response by 1 minute use bag and mask ventilation.

Terminal apnoea. Pale; heart rate < 60 beats/minute; floppy and apnoeic.

—*Action.* Bag and mask ventilation immediately. This baby will not breathe without help. If not improving quickly, intubation and cardiac compressions will be required.

Fresh stillbirth. Apnoeic; pale; floppy; no heart rate.

—*Action.* Full cardiopulmonary resuscitation immediately (follow ABC set out in the next section).

—Assist breathing: positive pressure ventilation via ETT (or with bag and mask until skilled help for intubation available).

—Give cardiac compressions (this will be of no benefit unless effective ventilation is established).

Assess (support): temperature (warm and dry)

Airway (position and suctioning)

Breathing (stimulate to cry)

Circulation (heart rate and colour)

Always needed

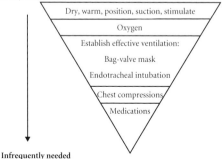

Dry, warm, position, suction, stimulate

Oxygen

Establish effective ventilation:

Bag-valve mask

Endotracheal intubation

Chest compressions

Medications

Infrequently needed

Fig. 36.1 An inverted pyramid illustrating the relative frequencies and priorities of neonatal resuscitation.

ABC of resuscitation

The 'ABC' stands for attention to airway, breathing, and circulation. To these should be added temperature control.

Temperature control
Keep the baby dry and warm. This reduces the risk of hypoglycaemia and acidosis and minimizes oxygen consumption.

Airway
- Position baby face upwards with head in the neutral position.
- Use soft suction catheters and a negative pressure of 5–10 kPa to gently clear airway. Avoid deep pharyngeal suction as vagal stimulation can cause bradycardia or laryngospasm.

Breathing
Bag and mask ventilation
Indications for use:
- Shallow irregular respiration with heart rate < 100 beats/minute and falling.
- Apnoea.

Choose a mask big enough to cover the face from the bridge of the nose to below the mouth. Connect the bag to an O_2 supply. Without a reservoir bag you will only be able to deliver about 40–50% O_2. The bag usually has a blow-off valve that operates at 30–40 cm H_2O. If a greater inflation pressure is necessary put your finger on top of the valve to override it. Squeeze bag to achieve adequate chest expansion and establish a rate of 30–40 breaths/minute.

On some resuscitaires it is also possible to give effective ventilation via a T-piece system connected to the O_2 outlet. Ensure blow-off valve on resuscitaire is set at the correct pressure. The hole on the connector is occluded with your finger to allow the pressure to build up and ventilation is delivered by releasing and re-occluding the hole on the connector at the desired rate (Fig. 36.2).

Tracheal intubation
- Indications for use:
  —Primary apnoea that does not respond promptly to bag and mask ventilation.
  —Terminal apnoea or asystole.
- For small babies use size 2.5 mm ETT.
- For term babies use 3.0–3.5 mm ETT.

Hold the first inflation for 2 or 3 seconds to allow proper expansion of the lungs and establish a functional residual capacity. After the first few breaths establish a rate of 30–40 breaths/minute with inspiratory times of approximately 0.5–1. If there is poor chest movement the pressure can be increased sequentially up to 40 cm of water.

Following intubation check for:
- Bilateral chest movement.
- Breath sounds bilateral and equal on auscultation.
- Absence of breath sounds over the stomach.

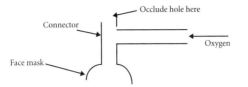

Fig. 36.2 Diagram showing procedure for giving effective ventilation via a T-piece system connected to the O_2 outlet on a suitable resuscitaire.

Circulation

Cardiac compression

- Indication for use: heart rate < 60 beats/minute despite effective ventilation.

Cardiac compression may be performed in one of two ways.
1. Encircle chest with both hands so that fingers lie behind the baby and thumbs are opposed over the mid-sternum.
2. Place two fingers over sternum 1 cm below the internipple line.

Depress sternum at a rate of 120 compressions/minute to a depth of 1–2 cm. Give three chest compressions for every inhalation.

Drugs

The use of drugs is indicated if adequate ventilation with 100% oxygen and effective chest compressions have failed to increase the heart rate above 60 beats/minute.
- Adrenaline is the most important drug. It can be given either intravenously (via umbilical venous catheter) or down the endotracheal tube.
  —*Doses.* 10 µg/kg (0.1 mL/kg, 1 in 10 000) intravenously or 20 µg/kg via ETT. Adrenaline 10–30 µg/kg is given every 3–5 minutes if there is no response.
- Sodium bicarbonate is indicated if the heart rate remains < 60 beats/minute despite good ventilation, chest compressions, and intravenous adrenaline.
  —*Dose.* 1 mmol/kg intravenously (use 2 mL/kg of 4.2% solution (= 0.5 mmol/mL)).
- Volume expanders are indicated if there is no response to resuscitation, especially if any evidence of hypovolaemia. Use 0.9% saline or 4.5% human albumin solution.
  —*Dose.* 10–20 mL/kg over 5–10 minutes. O rhesus-negative blood is given when significant acute blood loss is suspected.
- Dextrose 10% is given intravenously at 2–3 mL/kg.
- Naloxone is only indicated for persisting apnoea related to maternal opiate analgesia in an otherwise well baby. It does not improve cardiac performance and should not be given to an asphyxiated baby or a baby whose heart rate is < 60 beats/minute or if mother is opiate-dependent.
  —*Dose.* 100 µg/kg intramuscular (IM).

Resuscitation of the infant with meconium-stained liquor

When thick meconium is present at delivery:
• Aspirate the mouth and nostrils with a wide-bore suction catheter when th head is delivered.
• Following delivery move the baby quickly to the resuscitaire.

For a pink and vigorous baby,
• Continue suction of oropharynx if meconium is still present.
• Intubation is not usually required.

If the baby shows depression of respiratory effort,
• Suck out pharynx before the baby is either encouraged to breathe or given artificial respiratory support.
• If there is meconium in the mouth, visualize larynx and the vocal cords with laryngoscope.
• If there is meconium at the level of or below the vocal cords, intubate and apply suction. Remove ETT slowly, re-intubate with a clean tube, and repeat the procedure. This can be continued for up to 2 minutes in an infant with a good heart rate. Where the heart rate is < 60 beats/minute full resuscitation should be commenced at 1 minute, even if all the meconium has not been removed.

Actions in the event of poor initial response to resuscitation

1 Check for technical fault.
   —Is oxygen connected?
   —Is ETT in the trachea? If in doubt remove ETT and replace.
   —Is ETT down one bronchus? If in doubt remove ETT and replace.
   —Is ETT blocked? If in doubt remove ETT and replace.
   —Check that blow-off valve is set at 30 cm H_2O
   —Check flow rate of oxygen at 5–8 L/minute.
2 Does the baby have lung pathology, e.g.
   —Pneumothorax.
   —Diaphragmatic hernia.
   —Hypoplastic lungs.
   —Hydrops.
3 If the baby has good chest movement has there been
   —Fetal haemorrhage? Consider plasma or O rhesus-negative blood 20–30 mL/kg via umbilical vein.
   —Severe asphyxia?

Resuscitation of the preterm infant

Preterm babies are likely to be deficient in surfactant and may require relative higher inflation pressures than term babies. Start resuscitation with a pressure of 20–25 cm water but increase if this does not produce satisfactory chest wall movement.

When should resuscitation be stopped

If signs of life were present shortly before delivery it is justifiable to carry out full cardiopulmonary resuscitation on a fresh stillbirth. Published data, however, suggest that if there are still no signs of life by 15 minutes then very few babies will survive. If there is no response to full resuscitation, the decision to discontinue should be made by the most senior paediatrician available.

Recommended further reading

Joint Working Party of the Royal College of Paediatrics and Child Health and the Royal College of Obstetricians and Gynaecologists (1997). *Resuscitation of babies at birth.* Royal College of Paediatrics and Child Health and the Royal College of Obstetricians and Gynaecologists, London.

Advanced Life Support Group (2000). *Advanced paediatric life support*, 3rd edn. BMJ Books, London.

Chameides, L. and Hazinski, M.F. (eds.) (1997). *Pediatric advanced life support.* American Heart Association Incorporated, Washington, DC.

Hamilton, P. (1999). Care of the newborn in the delivery room. *British Medical Journal* 318, 1403–6.

Care in the puerperium

The puerperium is the time when the mother's body is returning to its pre
pregnant state. Most of the physical changes are complete by 6 weeks. The puer
perium is also a time for psychological adjustment—the mother's joy at the
arrival of the new baby may be tempered by anxiety about her child's welfare
and her ability to cope and these anxieties may be compounded if she is tired
after labour or if there were medical complications during labour. Although the
puerperium is a time of great importance for mother and baby, it is an aspect of
maternity care that has received little attention.

Physiological changes to the uterus and lower genitourinary tract in the puerperium

Involution of the uterus and renal system

The postpartum uterus, which weighs about 1 kg, returns to its pre-pregnancy
weight of around 80 g. Postdelivery, the uterine fundus lies just below the
umbilicus but by 2 weeks it can no longer be felt above the symphysis. This
process of involution involves autolysis of muscle cells, with absorption of the
protein into the circulation and excretion with the urine.

- The most common causes of delayed involution include full bladder, loaded
  rectum, uterine infection, retained placental fragments or membranes,
  fibroids, or possible broad ligament haematoma.
- By the end of the second week the cervical internal os is closed and unable
  to admit a finger, while the stretched, smooth, and oedematous vaginal
  walls regain their ruggae by the 3rd week postnatally.
- If lactation is suppressed the uterine cavity is covered by new endometrium
  by 3 weeks and the first menstruation occurs by 6 weeks. In breastfeeding
  mothers, ovarian activity is suppressed and resumption of menstruation
  may be delayed for many months.
- During the first few days, the bladder and the urethra may show evidence
  of minor trauma sustained at delivery but this resolves rapidly. Within
  2–3 weeks the calyceal dilatation and hydorureter become less evident
  although complete return to normality takes 6–8 weeks.

Lochia

This bloodstained uterine discharge consists of blood and necrotic superficial
decidua. During the first few days the lochia is red, then it gradually changes to
pink, and by the end of the second week it becomes serous.

- Persistent red lochia may be associated with infection or retained products.
- Uterine tenderness with pyrexia and offensive lochia is highly suggestive
  of intrauterine infection and justifies immediate treatment with broad-
  spectrum antibiotics and, if there are retained products, evacuation of
  the uterus with antibotic cover.

Problems in the puerperium

Thrombosis and thromboembolism

Thromboembolism accounted for the largest proportion of direct maternal deaths in the 1997–99 triennial Confidential Enquiry Into Maternal Death (CEMD) report.[1] Over half the cases of death were in the puerperium, and the majority were following Caesarean section. It is therefore essential to adhere to thromboprophylaxis guidelines and to have a high index of suspicion in women who have recently given birth when they present with signs or symptoms that raise the possibility of thromboembolic disease and to investigate them appropriately.

Perineal pain/discomfort

Perineal discomfort is the most common problem encountered postnatally, occurring in 42% of women after spontaneous delivery and persisting after the first 2 months in 8–10%. The figures following assisted vaginal deliveries are 8 and 30%, respectively. Perineal pain is worse following instrumental delivery, episiotomy, or spontaneous tears. Treatments such as local cooling and topical applications of local anaesthetic provide short-term relief, with longer relief being provided by nonsteroidal anti-inflammatory drugs (NSAIDs) such as diclofenac suppositories. It is important to exclude infection as a result of bacterial contamination. If there are signs of infection this needs to be aggressively treated with antibiotics and drainage of any collection of pus. Where an episiotomy or tear repair breaks down, resuturing is contraindicated in the presence of infection and healing by secondary intention should be allowed.

Bladder dysfunction

- Voiding difficulties and urinary retention may occur after delivery especially if regional anaesthesia has been used. Loss of bladder sensation with epidural or spinal anaesthetic may lead to overstretching of the detrusor muscle dampening bladder sensation with subsequent voiding difficulties.
- Difficult instrumental delivery and multiple or extended vulvovaginal lacerations may cause pain and periurethral oedema that may impede voiding.
- Other sources of pain, such as prolapsed haemorrhoids, abdominal wound pain, or even faecal impaction, may all contribute to voiding difficulties.
- In general, after a Caesarean section under regional anaesthesia, an indwelling catheter is left for 12–24 hours to avoid bladder overdistension and it may be advisable to use this approach where a difficult instrumental delivery with extensive perineal repair has been performed.
- If there is any difficulty voiding it is always good practice to send a specimen of urine for culture and sensitivity to exclude underlying infection.
- Incontinence early in puerperium should be investigated to exclude the rare possibility of a fistula.
- Urinary tract infection (UTI) is not uncommon in the puerperium with 3–5% reporting a UTI in the first year after delivery and a further 5% reporting urinary frequency for the first time after delivery. The increased incidence of UTIs may be due to bladder stasis, voiding difficulties, and catheterization in labour. Management involves the appropriate use of antibiotics.

Bowel function

Constipation is common in pregnancy and remains so in the puerperium. The problem of constipation may further be exacerbated by the fear of defecation due to pain of prolapsed haemorrhoids (affecting 18% of women), anal fissure, or the sutured perineum. The importance of avoiding straining at defecation is greatest where there has been a third- or fourth-degree tear repair. Hence such women should have stool softeners prescribed routinely.

It is now becoming clear that the trauma to the anal sphincter is greater than previously thought with 35% of primiparas having occult anal sphincter trauma on anal endosonography, but only 13% admitting to bowel symptoms by 6 weeks postpartum. Both direct trauma and nerve damage following assisted vaginal delivery or spontaneous vaginal delivery contribute to this. Incontinence of flatus or faeces is reported in 4% of women after delivery. Furthermore, 20–50% of women who had primary third- and fourth-degree repairs may suffer some degree of faecal or flatus incontinence. Thus, follow-up in the hospital setting should be arranged as a routine after third- or fourth-degree tear repairs. It is essential that such women are encouraged to come forward for proper investigation and treatment.

Postnatal depression and tiredness

0–15% of women experience postnatal depression within the first year after delivery. Tiredness is the most commonly reported problem postdelivery, affecting 42% of women while in hospital and rising to 54% at 2 months. Extreme exhaustion lasting at least 6 weeks is reported in 12% but may well represent depression.

Breast problems

Two-thirds of women who start breastfeeding report problems. These problems (nipple pain, engorgement, cracks, and bleeding) are preventable or surmountable with advice regarding positioning of the baby's mouth coupled with sympathetic supportive counselling. In cases of mastitis, feeding should continue to overcome the blocked duct, while a breast abscess will need incision and drainage. Both conditions may need a course of antibiotics.

Secondary postpartum haemorrhage (PPH)

The most common presentation is at 7–14 days and is generally due to retained placental tissue. The differential diagnosis includes endometritis, hormonal contraception, bleeding disorders, and choriocarcinoma. Management is according to the underlying cause but, if bleeding is heavy, resuscitation of the patient is the priority followed by examination in theatre and curettage of the uterus under antibiotic cover.

Traumatic neuritis

This may present with footdrop, paraesthesia, hypoaesthesia, sciatic pain, and muscle wasting in one or both lower limbs following delivery. The mechanism is as yet not fully elucidated but may be associated with herniation of the lumbosacral discs at L4–5 due to exaggerated lithotomy and instrumental delivery. The management entails bed rest, physiotherapy, and spinal/orthopaedic opinion with appropriate imaging.

Problems in the puerperium (*continued*)

Peroneal neuritis may result from compression of the peroneal nerve betwee the head of the fibula and the lithotomy pole and presents as footdro Treatment is supportive with physiotherapy.

Diastasis of the symphysis pubis

Incidence is around 0.1% after spontaneous delivery. It may be associated wi a forceps delivery, a rapid second stage, or exaggerated flexion and abduction maternal thighs such as in McRobert's manoeuvre. The symptoms are of pa over the symphysis, which is exaggerated by weight-bearing. The clinical sig are a waddling gait, tenderness over the joint, and, occasionally, a palpable inte pubic gap. Management is supportive with bed rest, physiotherapy, analges and anti-inflammatory drugs, and a pelvic support brace.

Reference
Confidential Enquiry into Maternal Deaths (CEMD) (2001). *Why mothers die, 1997–1999. The confidential enquiries into maternal deaths in the United Kingdom.* RCOG, London.

Chapter 38

Puerperal pyrexia

Puerperal pyrexia is defined as a maternal temperature of more than 38°C on more than one occasion in the first 14 days after delivery.

Aetiology

- 90% of infections are genital or urinary tract in origin. Genital tract infections are commonly due to *E.coli*, *Streptococcus A* or *B*, or *Clostridium*. Urinary tract infections are predominantly due to *E.coli*, *Proteus*, or *Klebsiella*.
- Other causes are mastitis (usually staphylococcal), infected perineal or Caesarean section wounds, chest infections, and infected pelvic haematomas.
- Venous thrombosis may be associated with pyrexia as may breast engorgement without infection.
- Uterine infections are more likely following prolonged rupture of the membranes and after instrumental delivery.

Diagnosis

History
- Check for prolonged rupture of membranes, intrapartum pyrexia, prolonged labour, operative delivery, and any difficulty with the delivery of the placenta.
- Ask about associated symptoms of offensive or unusually heavy lochia and abdominal, breast, or wound pain.
- Ask about any previous treatment and allergies.
- Perineal infections usually present around the second day after delivery.

Examination
- Check the patient's general condition, pulse, and blood pressure.
- Check the breasts for any areas of tenderness and erythema and listen to the chest.
- Inspect abdominal wound for swelling or associated cellulitis.
- Check the fundal height and tenderness of the uterus.
- Perform a gentle pelvic examination and check the appearance of the perineum.
- Assess for tenderness of the uterus on bimanual examination and look for evidence of swelling in the adnexa. Endometritis is associated with lower abdominal pain, offensive liquor, and a tender uterus on bimanual vaginal examination.
- Check legs for signs of superficial thrombophlebitis or deep vein thrombosis.

Investigations
- Send a midstream urine sample for culture.
- Take swabs for bacterial culture and for *Chlamydia* from the cervix and lochia.
- Take sample of sputum or any discharge from wounds or nipples for culture.
- Take blood for full blood count (FBC) and cultures.

Management

itial therapy depends on diagnosis, allergies, and whether the patient is breast-
eeding (avoid tetracyclines if breastfeeding). For suspected pelvic infections
art with Amoxil 500 mg three times a day (erythromycin if allergic to peni-
llin) and metronidazole 400 mg three times a day or Augmentin 675 mg three
ne a day. Substitute flucloxacillin 250 mg three times a day for Amoxil for
ound or breast infections. Encourage the patient to continue milk expression
prevent blockage of the milk ducts and breast engorgement. Trimethoprim
)0 mg twice a day is a suitable alternative for urinary tract infections.
Intravenous therapy should be used if the patient is vomiting, systemically
unwell, or you suspect pyelonephritis.
If the patient fails to respond to initial therapy review the results of the initial
cultures, assess her clinically, and arrange a pelvic ultrasound scan to
exclude pelvic collection. If there is a wound or a pelvic or breast abscess, it
may need draining. Otherwise, change antibiotics according to sensitivities
or, if these are not available, consider adding gentamicin or a third-
generation cephalosporin.

arly involvement of microbiologists is invaluable in severely ill patients and
ose who fail to respond to treatment. If group B haemolytic *Streptococcus*,
hlamydia, or *Neisseria gonorrhea* are cultured inform the pediatricians if the
atient is still in hospital or the patient's GP if she has been discharged home so
at the baby can be tested for infection. Early surgical referral is essential if
ere is any evidence of rapidly evolving cellulitis with necrosis of the overlying
in and breast infection not responding to treatment with antibiotics.

Chapter 39

Breastfeeding

Breastfeeding is the healthiest way to feed a baby and has important health benefits for both mother and baby. The World Health Organization/UNICEF Baby Friendly Hospital Initiative summarizes the practices necessary to support breastfeeding in the hospital and community.

In order to make an informed decision about how to feed a baby it is vital that information is available to women before they give birth.

Benefits

- Protects baby against:
  —Gastroenteritis.
  —Urinary tract infections.
  —Ear infections.
  —Chest infections.
- Reduces the risk of accidental scalding/burns.
- Reduces risk of allergies and juvenile-onset diabetes.
- Babies have better mental, teeth, and jaw development.
- Protects mother against:
  —Pre-menopausal breast cancer.
  —Ovarian cancer.
  —Osteoporosis.
- Contraceptive effect, if exclusively breastfeeding.
- Reduces risk of postpartum haemorrhage (PPH) and aids uterine involution.

Disadvantages of formula

Formula-fed infants are disadvantaged because of constituents of the formula, production problems that lead to excesses or deficiencies in substances, and accidental contamination. Immunologically, formula cannot compete with breastmilk.

Steps to success

- *Skin to skin contact after delivery.* Encourage contact within 30 minutes of birth. This helps to keep the baby warm and to stabilize the baby's heart rate and breathing. It calms the baby, promotes bonding, and can help to start off breastfeeding.
- *Initiating the first breastfeed.* Encourage babies to breastfeed soon after they are born. Babies can be weighed and have a neonatal check before initiating skin to skin contact and feeding.
- *Rooming in.* Baby stays with mother all the time. This builds the mother's confidence in caring for the baby and helps her learn feeding signals, and how to comfort the baby.
- *Demand feeding.* Healthy, term babies can feed whenever they want, for as long as they want. This helps in establishing and maintaining a good milk supply.
- *Help and support.* Midwives, infant-feeding advisors, health visitors, and breastfeeding counsellors are available for support. Peer support groups can also be vital in increasing the number of women who continue to breastfeed. It is important not to give conflicting advice. Positively supporting the mother's efforts is vital even when advising change.

Importance of good positioning and attachment.
—In the mother this prevents sore nipples, breast engorgement, poor milk supply, blocked ducts, and mastitis.
—In the baby this prevents a hungry baby, an unsettled baby, low weight gain, and prolonged feeding.

Dummies and teats whilst breastfeeding. Avoid using until breastfeeding is established. This helps to prevent a poor supply of breastmilk and nipple–teat confusion.

Initiating breastfeeding

Remember, breastfeeding is natural *but* it is not always instinctive. Some babies need to learn how and some learn faster than others. Before feeding, women should make themselves comfortable—a chair may be more practical than sitting on a bed. A pillow to help support baby may be required. Initially, it may be better to undress the baby down to its nappy to prevent overheating.

Holding the baby

The mother can hold the baby in a number of positions for feeding. One way is to hold the baby horizontally, head opposite the nipple, turned completely on its side with legs under the arm. The baby's bottom is brought close with the elbow and the baby's neck and shoulder are supported between spread-out fingers and thumb. The baby's head should fall back gently between the V shape the finger and thumb create, which helps raise the baby's chin off its chest so that its mouth can be opened wide.

Attaching baby to the breast

- Cup breast underneath with the hand, the little finger touching the ribs and the thumb resting on edge of areola in a 'C' shape.
- Fingers are then kept away from areola and nipple. The nipple should be lined up with baby's nose and not be aimed centrally into the mouth. The baby will smell the milk and open its mouth wide.
- The baby should be brought to the breast and the bottom lip should make contact with the areola, well away from the base of the nipple. The mother thumb quickly slides or rolls forward the nipple under the palate.
- Once a good feeding rhythm is established, the hand should be slowly released from the breast and brought to rest under the baby. The baby should be held firm and close as if gently 'squashing' him or her.
- A drawing sensation is felt on initial attachment; thereafter no pain should be felt. The baby initially suckles quickly to facilitate the let-down reflex, and then nutritive feeding is established with a rhythmical slow suck–swallow pattern.

Early days

Healthy term babies may not feed very much in the first 48 hours. Colostrum (first milk) is high-density and low-volume: neonate's immature kidneys cannot cope with large volumes of fluid without metabolic stress. Despite the small quantity, colostrum provides sufficient fluid and nutrients for healthy term babies. A busy feeding period usually follows and soon passes. Frequent feeds according to the baby's demands will reduce the risk of engorgement and maintain milk supply. Breastmilk changes to meet the needs of the baby as he or she grows and matures.

Expressing breastmilk

This is an essential skill that enables a mother to know where her milk reservoirs are. Expressed milk on the nipple can tease the baby to open his or her mouth and can help relieve engorgement or blocked ducts.

Gently massage the breast and stimulate the nipple to encourage the let-down reflex.

1 Position the thumb and the first two fingers about 2.5–3.5 cm behind the nipple. Place the thumb above the nipple and the fingers below in a 'C shape'. The fingers are positioned so that the milk reservoirs lie beneath them.

2 Push straight into the chest wall—avoid spreading the fingers apart. For large breasts first lift and then push into the chest wall.

3 Roll thumb and fingers forward as if making thumb and finger prints at the same time. The rolling motion of the thumb and fingers compresses and empties the milk reservoirs without hurting sensitive breast tissue.

4 Repeat rhythmically to drain the reservoirs, i.e. position, push, roll, release. Position, push, roll, and release.

5 Rotate the thumb and finger position to milk the other reservoirs. Use both hands on each breast for more effective expressing.

Problems associated with breastfeeding

Women who experience any problems with breastfeeding should have access to trained staff and voluntary breastfeeding counsellors.

- *Sore and cracked nipples* should not occur if the baby is correctly attached at the breast. Expressed breastmilk can be helpful during the healing phase.
- *Nipple sensitivity* is usually transient. It is due to enhanced lactational hormones, prolactin, and oxytocin. On examination there is usually no obvious nipple damage, only occasional redness, and the mother needs reassurance that this will resolve.
- *Breast fullness (engorgement)*. Breasts can become full when the milk comes in. This should not occur if the baby is demand feeding and attached correctly to the breast. If breasts become red and painful, it is resolved by correctly attaching the baby to the breast and should quickly improve if this could lead on to non infective mastitis. Simple analgesia may be helpful, ice packs or hot flannels should be used with caution.
- *Mastitis (non Infective)* is characterised by a pinky red flushing over the breast, which may or may not be associated with lumpy areas and flue like symptoms. It is caused by a build up of breastmilk which has not been effectively removed from the breast. Antibiotics are not usually required, correct positioning and attachment is essential. Hand expressing to improve quality of attachment before feeding or after feeding may be beneficial. Symptoms should subside quickly and usually resolve within 24 hours. If non-infective mastitis is incorrectly managed this may lead to Infective mastitis.
- *Mastitis (Infective)* is characterised by a red lumpy area of breast, usually wedge shaped, pyrexia, pain and flu like symptoms. It may be caused by a blocked duct, infection, poor attachment or bra pressure. It is important to find the cause of mastitis as this can lead to abscess formation if left untreated. Breastfeeding should continue, breastfeeding from the infected breast first is recommended to facilitate effective milk removal, but if breastfeeding at the affected breast is too painful, milk should be expressed to facilitate milk removal and maintain the milk supply. If symptoms do not improve, treatment with antibiotics will be necessary, breastfeeding should continue as above.
- *Breast abscess* is a possible complication of infective mastitis which is poorly managed and is most likely to occur when breastfeeding is stopped abruptly. Breastfeeding should continue, breastfeeding from the infected breast can continue, but if breastfeeding at the affected breast is too painful milk should be expressed to facilitate milk removal and maintain the milk supply. Symptoms include elevated temperature, red swollen area and possible discharge from the affected area. It is important that medical opinion is sought and that antibiotics are administered. Severe abscesses require drainage and breastfeeding may cease if symptoms do not resolve.
- There are, on rare occasions, a number of situations where infants cannot feed, or should not be breastfed, e.g. when mother is on certain medications. Specialised advice from pharmacist should be sought.

Inborn errors of metabolism with implications for breastfeeding

Some congenital and hereditary disorders, characterized by specific enzyme deficiencies, severely limit the use of certain milk components. Some of these disorders usually present as mild failure to thrive until the baby is weaned when the symptoms suddenly worsen, whereas others are alleviated by breastfeeding.

● *Galactosaemia.* There are two main forms of this disease. One is characterized by a deficiency of galactokinase in which infants who are fed breastmilk, or any lactose-containing preparation can develop cataracts. The other form is even more serious, due to a deficiency of galactose-1 phosphate uridyl transferase. The resulting metabolite accumulates in the blood causing considerable damage. Symptoms include diarrhoea, vomiting, hepatomegaly, jaundice, and splenomegaly. If lactose is not excluded from the diet then cataracts, hepatic cirrhosis, and mental retardation result.

● *Phenylketonuria* is characterized by defective metabolism in the amino acid phenylalanine hydroxylase. This can result in moderate to severe mental retardation. Routine screening can diagnose this and the condition can be avoided by providing a low-phenylalanine diet. Fortunately, breastmilk contains a low concentration of this amino acid, lower than that of cow's milk. Babies suffering from phenylketonuria may be breastfed while their phenylalanine levels are monitored. Breast milk can then be supplemented or replaced by special low-phenylalanine formula if the concentrations reach dangerous levels.
  —Incidence: 1–20 per 100 000 population.

● *Maple-syrup urine disease.* This rare disease is due to a defect in the metabolism of the branch-chain amino acids valine, leucine, and isoleucine. It is characterized by the urine's typical maple-syrup colour, refusal of food, vomiting, metabolic acidosis, and progressive neurological and mental retardation. Special synthetic formulas have been developed for feeding such infants, although outcomes are usually poor.
  —Incidence: 0.5 per 100 000 population.

Obstetric emergencies

Maternal collapse

The causes of maternal collapse are numerous and may be related to pregnan or they may be incidental causes that may have been aggravated by pregnan The management needs to concentrate on resuscitation of the patient wh simultaneously working out the diagnosis to institute appropriate treatment

Obstetric causes
- Postpartum haemorrhage (PPH) is by far the most common cause and is discussed separately.

- Eclampsia.
- Amniotic fluid embolism.
- Uterine inversion.
- Uterine rupture.
- Intraabdominal bleeding such as broad ligament haematoma.
- Unrecognized genital tract haematoma (especially if not associated with external trauma).

Incidental causes
- Massive thromboembolism.
- Ruptured hepatic, splenic, or aortic aneurysm.
- Ruptured liver or spleen.
- Myocardial infarction.
- Cardiac cause, e.g. arrhythmia or cardiac failure.
- Cerebrovascular accident.
- Subarachnoid haemorrhage.
- Anaphylactic shock.
- Septic shock.
- Metabolic/endocrine cause.
- Abuse of medication/substance abuse.

Management
Resuscitation is the first priority. This involves securing an airway (A), ensuri ventilation if necessary by bag and mask or intubation and administration 100% oxygen (B), and maintaining the circulation if necessary by external ca diac massage (C). Assistance from an experienced obstetrician and anaesthet should be summoned and theatres forewarned that there may be a need f urgent laparotomy. The direction of initial investigations will be dictated symptoms and signs and events leading up to the collapse from the midwife from the patient if she is alert/conscious.

A full clinical examination including a neurological assessment should be mad In general, adequate intravenous (IV) access by two large-bore cannulae always useful for administration of fluids to support the circulation as well drugs required in the resuscitation process.
- Baseline blood (full blood count (FBC), cross-match specimen, coagulatio screen, electrolytes, blood glucose, and liver function) tests should be performed.
- Monitoring of pulse, blood pressure, oxygen saturation, and urine output needs to be instituted and the need for invasive monitoring addressed.
- If a cardiorespiratory cause is suspected, chest X-ray, arterial gases, electrocardiography (ECG), FBC, and electrolytes will be required.

Alteration in conscious state in the absence of cardiorespiratory signs raises the possibility of a neurological lesion (cerebrovascular accident, subarachnoid haemorrhage (SAH), previously undiagnosed space-occupying lesion (SOL)) but may also suggest a metabolic or endocrine problem.

Where a neurological cause is suspected, imaging of the brain would be the investigation of choice.

here there is no excessive external bleeding or any other cause to account for e maternal collapse, the possibility of massive internal haemorrhage should be nsidered. This may be a consequence of a ruptured uterus due to a previous ur, ruptured viscous such as liver or spleen, or a ruptured splenic, hepatic, or rtic aneurysm. Intraperitoneal bleeding will cause peritonism and circulatory anges out of proportion to external signs. Abdominal girth may be noted to increasing and an abdominal ultrasound will reveal free fluid in the peri-neal cavity. If the maternal collapse is due to massive internal bleeding an hergency laparotomy will be required to bring it under control, possibly th the involvement of other disciplines such as general surgical colleagues, th postoperative care requiring a high dependency/intensive treatment unit tting.

he possibility of occult genital tract haematoma should also be remembered as certain situations there may be no external trauma with a supralevator ematoma presenting with shock and maternal collapse. Clinical examination this situation may reveal a mass in either iliac fossa or a mass in the vaginal rnix displacing the uterus. The management of other obstetric causes such as lampsia, massive PPH, uterine inversion, and amniotic fluid embolism is dis-ssed in other chapters.

he general principles of management are to resuscitate and stabilize maternal ndition, organize initial investigations on the basis of the working diagnoses, volve senior members of the clinical team, and obtain assistance from other levant disciplines whilst ensuring adequate documentation of events and anagement. Conditions that lead to maternal collapse are discussed in other apters.

Shoulder dystocia

Difficulty in the delivery of the shoulder after delivery of the head is shoulder dystocia. This is due to the anterior shoulder being impacted against the symphysis pubis or the posterior shoulder being impacted against the sacral promontory. Usually it is the anterior impaction and, rarely, it could be both anterior and posterior impaction.

This occurs in approximately 1:200 deliveries. When it occurs shoulder dystocia is an acute obstetric emergency that necessitates prompt, skilful intervention in order to prevent serious fetal trauma or death. Anticipation and step-wise management are the keys to a successful outcome.

Associations

Macrosomia appears to be one of the most important factors associated with shoulder dystocia, which, even in the presence of significant risk factors, remains largely unpredictable. Shoulder dystocia occurs in 9% of babies > 4000 g, 15% > 4500 g, and 40% above 5700 g. However, 50% of the cases of shoulder dystocia occur in babies who weigh less than 4000 g.

Anticipation—antenatal associations

- Multiparity, pre-pregnancy heavy maternal weight, previous large babies, past history of shoulder dystocia.
- Excessive weight gain in pregnancy.
- Diabetes—established or gestational.
- Symphyseal fundal height larger than dates/clinically large baby.
- Post-term pregnancies.
- Ultrasound biometry showing growth > 90th centile (more so with asymmetrical macrosomia).

Anticipation—intrapartum associations

- Prolonged labour, especially protracted late first stage with loosely applied cervix.
- Prolonged second stage of labour.
- Midpelvic instrumental vaginal delivery.
- Head delivered and shoulder does not emerge with next bearing down effort.
- Unable to feel the neck of the baby—turtle neck sign.
- 'Rosy fat cheeks', suggesting a big baby (diabetic mother).

Immediate assistance should be sought as soon as the diagnosis is suspected made.

Diagnosis

Shoulder dystocia is diagnosed when the fetal head retracts or recoils against the maternal perineum, (turtle neck sign) and external rotation is not accomplished. This results in the inability to deliver the shoulders after the head has been delivered.

Management

Place the mother in McRobert's position, so that her legs are slightly abducted and hyperflexed at 45° to the maternal abdomen. This position flattens the sacral promontory and increases the pelvic outlet.

Adequate episiotomy to help with manipulations.

Firm directed suprapubic pressure (this reduces the bi-acromial diameter).

Gentle traction on the fetal head towards the longitudinal axis of the fetus (extreme downward traction causes cervical cord injuries).

If this fails to release the anterior shoulder, attempt to rotate the body of the baby so that the posterior shoulder moves anteriorly (Wood's manoeuvre) so that the bi-acromial diameter enters the larger oblique inlet diameter of the pelvis.

If there is no rotation possible, deliver the posterior arm and shoulder by inserting the fingers into the restricted space available in the back of the baby's chest in order to flex the posterior arm at the elbow and then bring it down. Once the posterior arm has been brought down, there is more space and the anterior shoulder slips behind the symphysis pubis effecting the delivery.

Cutting or fracture of the clavicle or a symphysiotomy may be a last resort. Replacement of the fetal head followed by Caesarean section is a good alternative.

Delivery on all fours may make delivery of an impacted shoulder easier.

If the baby dies prior to delivery, cutting through both clavicles (cleidotomy) with strong scissors may assist delivery.

A paediatrician and anaesthetist should be on standby for assistance needed with the mother and baby. Check the baby for possible damage, e.g. Erb's palsy or fractured clavicle.

The couple should have been warned about the possibility of dystocia and the steps that would be undertaken if shoulder dystocia was anticipated. After the delivery, the procedure and the outcome should be explained to the couple.

Should there be difficulty or nerve damage or asphyxia, a postnatal visit should be arranged to counsel the couple, especially regarding future pregnancies and the appropriate management.

Cord prolapse

The cord is said to be presenting when it lies below the presenting part in an intact bag of membranes and prolapses when the membranes rupture. Cord prolapse is an obstetric emergency because of the risk of cord compression and/or occlusion of the umbilical arteries going into spasm causing fetal asphyxia. Delivery must be effected as quickly as possible. There is an increased incidence of cord prolapse with malpresentations, such as a flexed breech or shoulder presentation, high head, premature or small fetus, unduly long cord, or polyhydramnios. Cord prolapse is a possible risk when artificially rupturing the membranes with a poorly applied presenting part. It is less likely to occur in spontaneous rupture of the membranes in labour as the presenting part may be fixed to the brim with uterine contractions.

Diagnosis

A loop of cord is felt in the vagina, or may be seen at the vulva. It is good practice that a woman at high risk of cord prolapse is examined vaginally as soon possible after rupture of the membranes, whether she is having contractions or not, in order to exclude a diagnosis of prolapse of the cord. The loop of cord should be felt to see if pulsations are present, and the fetal heart should be auscultated at the same time (pulsations may be absent and the fetus may still be alive) and at times an ultrasound examination would be useful. The degree of cervical dilatation should be noted.

Management

The aim is to prevent the presenting part from occluding the cord. This may be effected by displacing the presenting part by putting a hand in the vagina and pushing the presenting part to avoid pressure on the cord, especially during contractions. Alternatively, the woman may be placed either in a knee–elbow position (kneeling so rump is higher than head). Infusion of 500 mL warm saline into the bladder through a size 16 catheter may be an alternative. The cord is kept in the vagina to keep it warm and moist to prevent the arteries going into spasm.

Attempts to replace the cord are usually unsuccessful and may also produce spasm of the cord vessels. If the cervix is fully dilated and the presenting part sufficiently low in the pelvis, immediate delivery with the forceps (if cephalic) is performed. If there is a breech presentation and the presenting part is high in the pelvis, Caesarean section may be preferable to breech extraction (except if it is in a second twin). For other malpresentations that would require correction before vaginal delivery is possible, Caesarean section is best if the fetus is still alive. There are few other emergencies where speed is so vital.

If it is certain that the fetus is dead, labour is left to continue until eventual vaginal delivery takes place. In an impacted transverse lie at term, a Caesarean section may be needed (even with a dead fetus) to avoid uterine rupture.

Home birth

Current evidence suggests that, for any given cohort of low-risk women and their babies, outcomes attributed to birth at home are at least as good as for birth in hospital. Positive outcomes are both clinical and psychological. Some women with risk factors will also do well at home. There will need to be a discussion on a case-by-case basis. Anyone considering a home birth should be strongly advised to discuss this request with her community midwife as soon as possible.

Providing information

Information should be tailored to the particular woman and her baby. Factors to be discussed include:
- The woman's clinical history.
- The progress of her current pregnancy.
- Her plans and expectations for labour and birth, and those of her partner.
- Available midwifery expertise in the community.
- Availability to the family of transport.
- Time needed to travel to the nearest acute unit at all times of day and night.
- Access to a telephone.
- Available family and community support.

Information should be given in an unbiased, non-threatening, and sensitive manner. It should take into account medical, obstetric, and psychiatric history and social factors.

Explanations need to be specific, concise, realistic, and tailored to the individual situation. Statements based on relative risk should *not* be used since these are known to be very misleading (e.g. 'the risk of perinatal death when the pregnancy is continued beyond 41 weeks gestation is 7:3000 compared to 1:3000 when labour is induced' and *not* 'the risk is seven times greater').

Establishing risks and benefits

The theoretical risk of a problem in pregnancy does not automatically rule out an initial home birth booking. In the event of the risk materializing, the booking can be changed. Conversely, if the risk involves consultant input in the early stages but is then resolved (e.g. screening for fetal abnormality), the booking can be changed to home once the risk is ruled out.

In discussing risk, a distinction should be made between the following:
- Any actual condition with a high imminent risk to mother or baby (e.g. insulin dependent diabetes; major degree placenta praevia, or severe pre-eclampsia).
- Any actual condition or history of a condition with a low risk of acute adverse event in labour, or with a non-imminent risk of recurrence (e.g. nulliparity, maternal age over 35, or previous forceps for failure to progress).
- History of a risk that is minimized before labour (e.g. previous history of congenital fetal abnormality when all screening tests in this pregnancy do not signify risk).

As the pregnancy progresses, the lead professional concerned should offer the woman and her partner the opportunity to review the choice of place of birth, whether hospital or home.

In some unusual cases, such as a baby with a lethal congenital abnormality or a known intrauterine death, where there are no anticipated maternal complications, a woman and her family may seek a home birth. They should be informed of the likely maternal risks in their particular case. If they choose a home birth, the decision should be respected and facilitated with sensitivity.

Legal issues

- The fetus has very limited legal rights, and decisions about safety cannot be made for the fetus against the wishes of a mentally competent mother.
- Even where mental incompetence is suspected, intervention cannot take place against her expressed wishes without the ratification of a court order.
- This does not preclude care given in an emergency, where there is no explicit advance directive and no opportunity to obtain consent.
- The legal position on the right of access to a home birth within the UK National Health Service (NHS) is currently unclear.

General points

- Consider the risk that the refusal of support for a home birth may lead to the woman giving birth at home unattended.
- Decisions should not be governed by the attitude of the professionals. Obvious disapproval causes anxiety and conflict.
- Only the woman and her family can make the final assessment of the relative risks and benefits to them and their baby. Although you may not actually support the mother's decision, you should respect her considered choice.
- Copies of any letters relating to the choice of home birth should be sent both to the GP and the community midwife. All discussions should be recorded in both the handheld and the hospital notes.

Recommended further reading

1 Campbell, R. and Macfarlane, A. (1994) *Where to be born? The debate and the evidence*, 2nd edn. National Perinatal Epidemiology Unit, Oxford.

2 Chamberlain, G., Wraight, A., and Crowley, P. (eds.) (1997). *Home births*. Parthenon Publishing Group, Carnforth.

Chapter 42

Management of massive obstetric haemorrhage

Massive obstetric haemorrhage is defined as blood loss of more than 1500 mL or greater than 25% of the circulating blood volume. Haemorrhage is the third most common cause of direct maternal mortality, accounting for 6.5% of all maternal deaths. Of cases 50% are due to postpartum haemorrhage (PPH), 25% due to placenta praevia, and 25% due to placental abruption.

Normal response to blood loss

Normal blood flow to the uterus at term is 500 mL/minute. After delivery of the placenta, blood flow from the placental bed is controlled mainly by myometrial contraction and the formation of a fibrin clot over the placental bed. The higher plasma volume and red cell mass of the pregnant woman compensate for the blood loss associated with parturition.

The response to *excess blood loss* (10–15% of circulating volume) is to maintain blood flow to critical organs by a combination of increasing cardiac output and reducing the effective vascular volume. These changes are mediated through a combination of neural and hormonal mechanisms. Increased cardiac output occurs mainly as a result of an increase in heart rate with some increase in stroke volume. Endovascular volume is reduced by peripheral vasoconstriction. Blood flow to skin, skeletal muscle, gut, and kidney is reduced while cerebral and myocardial perfusion are preserved.

Pathological response to blood loss

Fear, anxiety, and pain may lead to a counterproductive increase in blood pressure whilst the release of endorphins counters the beneficial effects of increased sympathetic tone. Table 42.1 gives the clinical signs and symptoms associated with blood loss.

- *Cellular/microvascular level changes.* As tissue perfusion is reduced, anaerobic respiration leads to the release of lactic acid. When cellular adenosine triphosphate (ATP) production is insufficient to maintain membrane integrity there is an influx of sodium, calcium, and water into the cells and the release of potassium into the circulation and cell death. Lysosomal contents from autolysis are then released into the circulation and locally acting vasodilators such as 5-HT overcome centrally mediated vasoconstriction and trigger disseminated intravascular coagulation (DIC).
- *Tissue level changes.* Endothelial breakdown allows bacteria and toxins to enter the circulation. Impaired hepatic function cannot clear these and this stimulates the development of defects in the clotting mechanism, allowing further blood loss.

Table 42.1 Clinical signs and symptoms

% Blood loss	Heart rate	Systolic blood pressure	Tissue perfusion
10–15	Increased	Normal	Postural hypotension
15–30	Increased +	Normal	Peripheral vasoconstriction
30–40	Increased ++	70–80	Pallor, restlessness, oliguria
40 +	Increased ++	50	Collapse, anuria, air hunger

Management

The aim is to control the blood loss and restore oxygen-carrying volume to the tissues. For the treatment of specific causes of blood loss see Chapter 20 on antepartum haemorrhage and the section of Chapter 31 covering postpartum haemorrhage.

Immediate treatment

1 Summon help. This should include the obstetric registrar if not already present, anaesthetist, additional midwives, theatre staff, porters, blood transfusion, and the haematologist on-call.
2 Set up two large-bore intravenous (IV) lines (16 g or larger).
3 Take 30 mL of blood for cross-matching (minimum 6 units), full blood count (FBC), and clotting studies.
4 Replace circulating volume with crystalloids (Hartmann's, dextrose saline, or 0.9% sodium chloride solution) or a plasma expander (Haemaccel, Gelofusin). Crystalloids lack oncotic pressure and will tend to move into the extravascular space so they should not be overused. However, an initial fluid challenge of up to 2 L in a young woman is unlikely to cause pulmonary oedema unless there are other causes of endothelial damage such as pre-eclampsia.
5 Commence oxygen by face mask.
6 Catheterize to check urinary output.
7 Give blood as soon as possible. Restoration of normovolaemia is the first priority. If the bleeding is controlled and the blood pressure stable after IV fluids, transfusion can be delayed until cross-matched blood is available. If a more urgent transfusion is required, ABO and rhesus D compatible blood should be given. The use of uncross-matched O-negative blood is usually only indicated where the estimated blood loss exceeds 40% of circulating volume. Blood should be given using a suitable compression cuff and a blood warmer once more than two units have been given. Blood filters are unnecessary and slow transfusion.

If more than 40% (6 units) of blood volume have been lost

- Give additional colloid (and possibly human serum albumin) with further packed cells.
- In consultation with the on-call haematologist replace clotting factors, fresh frozen plasma cryoprecipitate, and platelets as indicated. Repeat platelet count and coagulation studies.
- Give additional calcium if indicated by serum biochemistry using 10% calcium chloride.
- Site central venous and arterial lines.

Once the bleeding is controlled

- Monitor pulse, blood pressure, central venous pressure, blood gases, electrolytes, and urinary output.
- Repeat the coagulation profile as requested by haematology.
- Consider transfer to an intensive treatment unit (ITU) in consultation with the consultant anaesthetist and obstetrician on-call.

Early involvement of senior is staff essential, especially where there is ongoing bleeding or evidence of deranged clotting.

Amniotic fluid embolism

This is a rare event estimated to occur in 1 in 20 000–80 000 deliveries. It was one of the major causes of maternal deaths in the UK in the triennium 1997–99. In those who develop amniotic fluid embolism, maternal mortality is around 60–70%. Maternal morbidity is significant and the fetus fares little better. The onset is rapid and death ensues quickly in many cases. The aetiology remains obscure and management of the condition is mainly supportive.

Pathophysiology

There are similarities between the clinical aspects of amniotic fluid embolism (AFE) and anaphylactic and septic shock suggesting a similar pathophysiology. The name 'anaphylactoid syndrome of pregnancy' has therefore been suggested. This may involve an anaphylactoid response involving the non-immunological release of endogenous mediators such as arachidonic acid metabolites. Another view of the development of AFE is that it is an immunoglobulin-mediated anaphylactic reaction. There is not enough evidence to support or refute either mechanism.

- Hypotension is an essential factor of AFE and is due to poor ventricular function.
- The hypoxia that is the other feature of the syndrome has a secondary effect leading to the neurological sequalae often seen in survivors of AFE.
- If the initial insult is passed the patient may die from massive haemorrhage as a result of profound coagulopathy.

Clinical presentation

AFE may occur in the antenatal period or in a woman in labour or who has just undergone vaginal delivery, Caesarean section, or termination of pregnancy. It has even occurred up to 48 hours postpartum. It has been also known to complicate amniocentesis. The onset is sudden with collapse, hypoxia, cyanosis, and hypotension followed by cardiopulmonary arrest. It may be heralded by seizures.

If undelivered there may be tetanic uterine contraction with subsequent fetal distress. It was initially considered that the tetanic contractions precipitated the embolism of amniotic fluid into the uterine veins and maternal circulation. The tetanic contraction now appears to be a result of AFE with the insult causing the release of catecholamines as a normal human response to shock, causing uterine contraction as a direct effect of noradrenaline (also called norepinephrine) on uterine musculature. The previously held belief that AFE was precipitated by oxytocin-induced labour and overcontraction has not been borne out by recent studies.

Any one of the major manifestations may dominate the picture or not occur at all, which may confuse the initial picture. Death will result in 61–86% of cases, although this may be an overestimate as there may be milder presentations that currently remain undiagnosed. Of the survivors, only 15% remain neurologically intact as a result of the initial profound hypoxia.

The fetus fares badly as well. If it is *in utero* at the time of AFE, 80% survive but half have neurological sequelae, secondary to profound hypoxia. Survival, not surprisingly, is related to timing of delivery. If delivered within 15 minutes, intact survival occurs in 67%. Thereafter, death or neurological sequelae are the most likely outcome.

The diagnosis of AFE can be problematic. Histological findings of fetal squames or mucin in the pulmonary vessels or aspirates from pulmonary artery catheter lines are not sensitive or specific and the diagnosis of AFE is a clinical one.

Management

This is mainly supportive aiming to maintain the blood pressure > 90 mm Hg systolic, urine output > 25 mL/hour, and arterial oxygen tension > 8 kPa and to correct any clotting abnormality. Senior help should be summoned immediately and appropriate consultation made, e.g. with a haematologist, anaesthetist, and respiratory physician. Standard cardiopulmonary resuscitation (CPR) should be instituted immediately if indicated either because of cardiac arrest or dysrhythmia.

- High-concentration oxygen should be administered and the woman intubated if indicated.
- Left ventricular failure leading to hypotension is common but may be treated with volume expansion to increase preload, followed by dopamine if hypotension persists.
- Internal monitoring with pulmonary artery catheterization aids fluid replacement, which may be complicated.
- After the initial volume expansion, fluid should be restricted to prevent pulmonary oedema and respiratory distress, which may rapidly ensue.
- Clotting anomalies should be treated with fresh frozen plasma or fresh whole blood if available.
- High-dose steroids may be given, although there is no supporting evidence for their use.
- In the event of cardiopulmonary arrest maternal survival is very low. The resuscitation is more difficult in the presence of a gravid uterus. Therefore in the presence of arrest immediate Caesarean delivery for the sake of the fetus and for adequate resuscitation of the mother should be undertaken.
- Sufficient staff should be summoned to allow continued resuscitation of the mother.

Chapter 44

Venous thromboembolism (VTE) in pregnancy

407

Thromboembolic disease remains the leading cause of maternal death (48/268 deaths = 2.1/100 00 maternities in triennium 1997–99 in the UK). VTE risk rises sixfold in pregnancy (0.3–1.6% of UK pregnancies: 20–50% occur antenatally—in any trimester—but they become more common as pregnancy advances).

There is an increased risk with:
- Immobility.
- Increased body mass index (BMI).
- Increasing maternal age.
- Increasing parity.
- Smoking.
- Air travel.
- Surgery (Caesarean section).
- Family history of deep vein thrombosis (DVT)/VTE (50% of those with VTE have thrombophilia syndrome).
- Blood group other than O.
- Caucasian race.
- Sickle cell disease.
- Women with lupus anticoagulant with risk of arterial and venous thrombosis, which may occur in atypical veins such as in the arm on in the portal circulation.

Investigate any unexplained calf or chest symptoms on the same day. Often symptoms/signs are not clear-cut.

Previous or family history

In patients with a recurrent history of VTE or a family history strongly suggestive of VTE, perform a thrombophilia screen:
- APCR (activated protein C resistance, ↓ factor V breakdown by protein C—genetic mutation in factor V molecule (Leiden mutation)). The Leiden mutation is the most common abnormality with heterozygotes for this mutation having a 10-fold increased risk of DVT. Rare homozygotes have a 100-fold increased risk of DVT.
- Antithrombin III deficiency (70% risk of developing DVT).
- Proteins C and S deficiency.
- Homocystinuria.
- Lupus anticoagulant ± anticardiolipin antibodies (especially if there is a history of arterial VTE or a bad obstetric history, e.g. recurrent miscarriage, eclampsia, intrauterine growth restriction (IUGR), intrauterine fetal death (IUFD), placental abruption).

Liaise with haematologists should there be any doubt about the risk of DVT/pulmonary embolism (PE).

Deep vein thrombosis and pulmonary embolism

Deep vein thrombosis (DVT)

- *Incidence in pregnancy.* 0.5–1.4%.
- *Presentation.* Acutely painful swollen leg in the absence of trauma.
- *Signs.*
  —Calf and thigh commonly affected—turgid and tender.
  —Dorsiflexion of the calf may elicit pain (Homan's sign—poor clinical discriminator).
  —Of such patients 30% do not have a DVT when assessed by venography.
- *Risks.* PE and post-phlebitic syndrome (skin swelling, ulceration).
- *Investigations.*
  —Limited venography with shielding of the maternal abdomen in 2nd or 3rd trimesters may be undertaken if clinically indicated.
  —Ultrasound imaging + Doppler flow studies/colour Doppler (clot imaging, lack of vein compressibility, lack of vein dilatation during Valsalva manoeuvre) are good techniques for diagnosing proximal vein thromboses (iliac, etc.) but not distal vein thromboses (e.g. in calf veins).
  —Radio-nucleotide venography (do not use ^{125}I in pregnancy). *NB.* Calf vein thromboses seldom embolise.
  —Consider magnetic resonance imaging (MRI) for investigation of suspected pelvic vein thromboses.

Pulmonary embolism (PE)

- *Incidence in pregnancy.* 0.3–1.2%. Small emboli may cause unexplained pyrexia, syncope, cough, chest pain, and breathlessness.
- Pleurisy should be considered due to embolism unless there is high fever or purulent sputum (pleurisy is rare in pregnancy).
- Large emboli may present as collapse with chest pain, breathlessness, and cyanosis.
- *Signs* include: raised jugular venous pressure (JVP), third heart sound, and parasternal heave.
- *Risks.* Untreated PE carries a maternal mortality of 13%.
- *Investigations.*
  —Chest X-ray.
  —Electrocardiograph (ECG) may be normal (Classic pattern of 'S1, Q3, T3' may be normal in pregnancy).
  —Blood gases may show decreased p_aO_2 (partial arterial pressure of oxygen) and decreased or normal p_aCO_2 (due to hyperventilation as a consequence of chest pain and hypoxia).
  —Ventilation/perfusion scans are safe in pregnancy, but instigate treatment whilst awaiting test.
  —Consider MRI ± spiral computer tomography.

409

Counselling and prophylaxis

During pre-pregnancy counselling initiate a thrombophilia screen when indicated and explain the risks to the mother and fetus from VTE and its treatment.

Prophylaxis

- *Low-risk group*, e.g. single episode of thromboembolism + no additional risk factors. Antenatal prophylaxis should be considered and postpartum prophylaxis employed.
  —Start heparin 7500 IU SC (subcutaneous) bd (twice daily) or low-molecular-weight heparin (LMWH) when the mother presents at delivery. Continue for 1-week post-partum, then heparin, LMWH, or warfarin for 5 weeks.
- *High-risk group*, e.g. multiple thromboembolic episodes or single episode + risk factor (thrombophilia screen positive).
  —Start heparin 10 000 IU SC bd or LMWH (enoxaparin 40 mg od (once daily) or fragmin 5000 IU SC od) at 4–6 weeks in advance of the gestation at which the previous thromboembolism occurred (counsel regarding bone demineralization). Continue heparin 7500 IU SC bd or LMWH through labour and delivery. Continue for 1-week postpartum, then heparin, LMWH, or warfarin for 5 weeks.
- *Thrombophilia screen positive patients*, e.g. those women who are 'screen' positive but have not had a VTE themselves.
  —All women will require postpartum prophylaxis for a minimum of 6 weeks.
  —In addition, many will need antenatal prophylaxis, the timing of treatment instigation and its nature being dependent on the individuals' specific risk factors. Protein C- or S-deficient patients are likely to require 10 000 IU heparin (or equivalent) bd: fully anticoagulate only if antithrombin III deficient, or homozygous for factor V Leiden mutation. Otherwise, only anticoagulate if delivered by lower segment Caesarean section (short course for 5 days postpartum—see below).
- *Patients with prosthetic heart valves.*
  —Full anticoagulation is essential throughout pregnancy.
  —In such patients it may be necessary to continue warfarin, even in the 1st trimester, with frequent monitoring of the INR (international normalized ratio; aim for levels of 3–4.5), prior to conversion to heparin at 36 weeks.
  —Liaise with haematologists throughout the pregnancy.

411

Treatment

Acute phase
This is characterized by massive emboli that are usually fatal. Treatment consists of cardiac resuscitation with consideration of pulmonary embolectomy. Consider streptokinase or tissue plasminogen activator treatment in life-threatening emergencies if surgery is not available.

Give bolus intravenous (IV) injection of up to 10 000 IU heparin and then commence infusion aiming to achieve an activated partial thromboplastin time (APTT) value that is twice that of the control. This can usually be achieved with infusion rates of 1000–2000 IU/hour, but may require individual dose regimens (e.g. 30 000 IU made up to 48 mL with 0.9% saline solution to run over 24 hours).

Chronic phase

Antenatal treatment
Treat for 1 week on IV heparin, then consider long-term SC heparin (10 000–15 000 IU bd) or LMWH equivalent (enoxaparin 40 mg od with final dose dependent on patient's weight) or change to warfarin.
- Heparin use is associated with osteopenia (1:100 patients: reversible) and thrombocytopenia, which is very rare and unpredictable, but is reversible. May be mild and symptomless or may be due to the development of heparin-dependent antibodies associated with thromboses.
- In the event of osteopenia or thrombocytopenia stop heparin and convert to warfarin.
- Alopecia (very rare and unpredictable, but reversible) with long-term use.
- No known fetal risks from heparin, as it does not cross the placenta.
- Heparin is continued throughout labour (reduce dose to 7500 IU bd at the onset of labour).
- Epidural anaesthesia is contraindicated.
- There is no evidence of increased risk of postpartum haemorrhage (PPH). If there is significant bleeding at delivery consider protamine sulfate (reverses effect of heparin—dose calculated by neutralization test).

Warfarin
Fetal risks of warfarin prevent its use. It is teratogenic at any stage of pregnancy (chondrodysplasia punctata; asplenia; diaphragmatic hernia). It may be associated with bleeding problems in the fetus resulting in optic atrophy, microcephaly, and other central nervous system defects.

Postnatal treatment
Either commence warfarin within the first few days with e.g. 10 mg/10 mg/5 mg regimen checking INR thereafter for dose adjustment or continue LMWH for 6 weeks postpartum or post-thrombosis if the embolism occurs postnatally. Breastfeeding is safe with warfarin. Liaise with the haematology department for better control.

44 Venous thromboembolism (VTE)

Treatment failure despite adequate anticoagulation

- DVT. Consider delivery as symptoms are exacerbated by obstruction to venous flow by gravid uterus.
- PE. Placement of an inferior vena cava filter above bifurcation, but below renal vessels, should be considered. Use a local anaesthetic procedure via percutaneous puncture of unaffected femoral vein.
- Septic PE (rare). DVT source is often the pelvic veins. It is characterized by recurrent PEs + high fever and secondary bronchopneumonia. Treatment is by antibiotics in addition to anticoagulants.

Prophylaxis against VTE at Caesarean section

Delivery by lower segment Caesarean section (LSCS) increases the risk of VTE 2–10-fold. A risk assessment of all patients undergoing LSCS should be performed and prophylaxis instituted as appropriate. This is discussed in Chapter 34.

Recommended further reading

Drife, J. and Lewis, G. (eds.) (1998). *Why mothers die. Report on Confidential Enquires into maternal deaths in the UK, 1993–96.* The Stationery Office, London.

de Sweit, M. (1995). Thromboembolism. In *Medical disorders in obstetric practice*, 3rd edn (ed. M. de Sweit), pp. 116–142. Blackwell Scientific Publications, Oxford.

Royal College of Obstetricians and Gynaecologists (RCOG) (1995). *Report of the RCOG Working Party on prophylaxis against thromboembolism in gynaecology and obstetrics.* RCOG, London.

Chapter 45

Psychiatric disorders in pregnancy

415

Pregnancy evokes joy in the majority of women with planned pregnancies but still constitutes a very stressful event. Psychiatric illness in pregnancy may be an onset of a new disorder or an exacerbation of an old problem.

Up to two-thirds of pregnant women have some psychological symptoms in pregnancy. These include anxiety, labile mood, irritability, and depression. However, serious psychiatric disorders are probably less common in pregnancy than in non-pregnant women.

- 1–2% of pregnant women have a psychiatric disorder although not all will seek or need treatment.
- The incidence of psychiatric disorder in pregnancy is higher in the first and third trimesters than in the second.
- An unplanned pregnancy may be associated with anxiety and depression in the first trimester.
- General discomfort, poor sleep, and fears about the impending labour and delivery and normality of the baby may cause anxiety and depression in the third trimester.
- The stress of childbirth and the lifestyle changes that come with a newborn baby may precipitate psychiatric illness. This is more likely in the presence of domestic/marital problems, unplanned/unwanted pregnancy, or a personal/family history of mental illness.

The booking history should include history of mental illness and abuse of alcohol and psychoactive substances. The classification of psychiatric disorder is outlined in the American Psychiatric Association's *Diagnostic and statistical manual*, 4th edition (DSM-IV) of 1993.

Antenatal disorders

Major mood disorders include depression (unipolar affective disorder) and manic–depressive illness (bipolar affective disorder).

- Features of depression include fatigue, feelings of worthlessness, poor concentration, poor appetite, and suicidal thoughts.
- Severe depression in pregnancy is usually a pre-existing illness and the treatment needs to be continued.
- Schizophrenia has higher psychiatric morbidity than any other psychiatric disorder. Its main clinical features include delusions, hallucinations, incoherence, and inappropriate affect. It also has a significant genetic component—the offspring carries a 5–10% schizophrenia risk when one parent is affected. Women have a later age of onset compared to men, such that the illness may not manifest until well into the childbearing age.

45 Psychiatric disorders in pregnancy

Effects of medication on pregnancy

- *Risks to the pregnant woman.* A severe pre-existing psychiatric illness, if untreated, is a major threat to the life and well-being of a pregnant woman. It is necessary for her to continue with medication until medical advice can be sought regarding alteration or discontinuation. Cessation of medication carries the risks of relapse and self-harm, which may far outweigh possible risks to the fetus.

- *Substance abuse.* Psychiatric disorders may be associated with substance abuse, e.g. alcohol, tobacco, and narcotic drugs with the associated risks to mother and baby (see Chapter 17).

  Teratogenicity. Before prescribing medication the physician should ask a psychiatric patient if she is intending to become pregnant as it may be possible to avoid medication with established teratogenicity. Associations between psychotropic drugs and fetal malformation include the following.

  —Lithium carries a teratogenic effect on the fetal heart, associated with 1% risk of Ebstein's anomaly. There is also a risk of lithium toxicity in the newborn.

  —Phenytoin is associated with cleft lip and palate, cardiac malformations, microcephaly, and growth restriction.

  —Benzodiazepines have an unconfirmed link with cleft lip and palate but neonatal hypotonia and respiratory depression are established risks.

  —Antidepressants include tricyclic antidepressants, monoamine oxidase inhibitors (MAOIs), and selective serotonin uptake inhibitors (SSRIs). Although SSRIs are newer than the other two groups, antidepressants generally have not been shown to have a teratogenic effect.

  —Phenothiazines make up the largest group of antipsychotic medications. They are not associated with an increased risk of teratogenicity. Most patients on antipsychotics have a high risk of relapse if their medication is withheld.

- *Neonatal withdrawal symptoms.* As psychotropic drugs cross the placenta, a neonate may manifest signs of exposure to the drugs, e.g. floppiness, poor feeding, and respiratory depression from benzodiazepine therapy or neonatal goitre from lithium.

- *Breastfeeding.* Most psychotropic drugs are secreted into breast milk. Maternal therapeutic doses of benzodiazepines and lithium may result in breast milk levels sufficient to affect a neonate. Breastfeeding may have to be avoided in mothers on these medications. The amounts of antidepressant and anticonvulsant medication secreted into breast milk do not have a significant effect on babies.

Postpartum disorders

Mental illness predating a pregnancy has a high risk of recurrence in the puerperium.

Postpartum 'blues'

About 50% of postpartum women experience brief episodes of mood lability, tearfulness, poor sleep, and irritability, starting around the third postpartum day and reaching a peak lasting 1 to 2 days. This is most common in primiparous women and is not related to delivery complications. There is often a background of anxiety and depressive symptoms in the third trimester of pregnancy. The condition usually resolves spontaneously without treatment in a few days. Reassurance and support are the mainstays of management.

Postnatal depression

This is a non-psychotic depressive illness in the postnatal period, affecting about 10% of women in the postnatal period. Clinical features include poor sleep, poor concentration, irritability, poor appetite, and decreased libido. The recurrence rate in subsequent pregnancies may be up to 70%. Mild cases either need no treatment or can be treated by their general practitioner and rarely see a psychiatrist. Most cases resolve within 6 months of delivery. However, many mild cases are missed and may continue to suffer from depression, and up to 75% of sufferers may be inadequately treated. Lack of social and domestic support may precipitate or compound postnatal depression, the extra pressures of caring for a child being an unbearable additional burden. Postnatal depression may lead to a disturbed mother–infant relationship that progresses into a vicious cycle of worsening of the mother's condition and further poor relationship with the child.

Management should involve reassurance and support from the partner and other family members. Input from a social worker and attendance at support groups of women with similar problems is of value. Severe cases should be referred to a psychiatrist, and treatment options include anxiolytics, antidepressants, and electroconvulsive therapy (ECT). Antidepressant medication is indicated if the depression lasts for longer than a month.

Puerperal psychosis

Puerperal psychosis has an incidence of up to 1 in 200, resulting in 1 in 600 postpartum women being admitted into a psychiatric unit. Peak incidence is at about 2 weeks postpartum. Primiparous women are more susceptible, and up to 20% of these patients have a previous history of bipolar mood disorder. The recurrence risk in a future pregnancy is up to 25%. The condition may be depressive, manic, or schizophrenic. Onset is usually within 2 weeks of delivery. There is an associated suicide rate of up to 5% and an infanticide rate of up to 4%. The patient needs to be hospitalized for treatment as well as for the protection of the baby from neglect, mishandling, or infanticide. Despite the risk to the baby, it is inappropriate except in cases of severe psychotic disturbance to separate the baby from the mother. Admission into a 'mother and baby unit' is ideal. Mothers who keep their babies with them bond, recover better, and stay in hospital for shorter periods than those separated from their babies. The underlying psychosis is treated with appropriate antidepressant or antipsychotic medication or ECT.

Of cases of puerperal psychosis, 70% make a full recovery, but the risk of further psychosis is up to 50% overall and 20% in a future puerperium.

45 Psychiatric disorders in pregnancy

recommended further reading

Cunningham, F.G., MacDonald, P.C., Gant, N.F., Leveno, K.J., Gilstrap, L.C., Hankins, G.D.V., and Clark, S.L. (1997). Neurological and psychiatric disorders. In *William's obstetrics* (ed. F.G. Cunningham, P.C. MacDonald, N.F. Gant, K.J. Leveno, L.C. Gilstrap, G.D.V. Hankins, and S.L. Clark), pp. 1255–72. Appleton and Lange, Stamford, Connecticut.

Gelder, M., Gath, D., Mayou, R., and Cowen, P. (1996). Psychiatric aspects of obstetrics and gynaecology. In *Oxford textbook of psychiatry* (ed. M. Gelder, D. Gath, R. Mayou, and P. Cowen), pp. 394–9. Oxford University Press, Oxford.

Puri, B.K., Laking, P.J., and Treasaden, I.H. (1996). Psychiatry of menstruation and pregnancy. In *Textbook of psychiatry* (ed. B.K. Puri, P.J. Laking, and I.H. Treasaden), pp. 231–44. Churchill Livingstone, Edinburgh.

Chapter 46

Fibroids and ovarian cysts in pregnancy

421

Fibroids in pregnancy

Fibroids are benign smooth muscle tumours of the myometrium and may be present in as many as 1 in 5 women over the age of 35. They are more common in Black compared to Caucasian women.

Effects of fibroids on pregnancy

Fibroids tend to be responsive to oestrogen and therefore generally enlarge in size during pregnancy due to increased vascularity, oedema, hypertrophy, and hyperplasia of fibromuscular tissues.

- Occasionally fibroids may be mistaken for fetal parts.
- Fibroids may also undergo softening and flattening during pregnancy and this may make them indistinguishable from the normal uterus.
- The presence of fibroids often results in the uterus measuring large for dates.
- Implantation over a submucous fibroid may be associated with a risk of miscarriage.
- In early pregnancy, impaction of the fibroid may lead to urinary retention and the initial management is that of a retroverted gravid uterus.
- Later on in pregnancy, fibroids in the lower segment or cervical fibroids may prevent engagement of the head and result in persistent abnormalities of lie/presentation.
- Fibroids *per se* do not interfere with uterine action though it is believed that they may predispose to postpartum haemorrhage (PPH) as the fibroid in the lower segment may interfere with contraction and retraction of the uterus. It may therefore be worthwhile having intravenous (IV) access *in situ* with cross-matched blood if there are large or multiple fibroids especially in the lower segment.
- If Caesarean section is required the principle is to avoid interfering with the fibroids unless unavoidable. If the latter is the case, there may be a risk of uncontrollable bleeding and a need for Caesarean hysterectomy.
- In the puerperium uterine involution may appear to be slower than expected.
- Other potential problems in the puerperium due to the presence of fibroid may be infection in the fibroid and secondary PPH.

Two of the complications that fibroids may undergo are more common in pregnancy—infarction/red degeneration and torsion.

Red degeneration

Red degeneration is thought to be a result of the fibroid outgrowing its blood supply. It presents with acute abdominal pain requiring opiate analgesia and tenderness over the fibroid. Clinical signs may include localized peritonism and guarding. There may be associated constitutional symptoms such as vomiting and pyrexia and a leucocytosis. The management involves supportive treatment with bed rest, analgesia, and reassurance that it is often common for signs and symptoms to persist for 7–10 days. The differential diagnosis includes abruption, appendicitis, or urinary tract infection/pyelonephritis. The pattern of illness together with results of bacteriological investigations and observation of the clinical course will lead to the correct diagnosis.

Torsion

Torsion of a pedunculated fibroid may occur during pregnancy or soon after delivery in the puerperium where uterine involution and laxity of the previously tense abdomen predispose to increased mobility of the abdominal contents.

Presentation may be as an acute abdomen, the diagnosis being suspected in the presence of a known history of one or more pedunculated fibroids. The differential diagnosis includes ovarian cyst accident, volvulus, appendicitis, spontaneous rectus sheath haematoma, or renal colic/pyelonephritis.

Management is surgical removal of the fibroid.

Ovarian cysts in pregnancy

423

Ovarian cysts of varying sizes may occur. The majority are small (3–4 cm) and persistent follicular cysts. The other main groups of benign ovarian tumours in pregnancy are the cystadenomas and dermoid cysts, the latter being twice as common in pregnancy than in the non-pregnant state. Malignant disease of the ovary is rare in pregnancy.

Effects of ovarian cysts on pregnancy

Impaction of the ovarian cyst may lead to retention of urine. The sheer size of the ovarian cyst may be responsible for discomfort. Later in pregnancy a large ovarian cyst may predispose to failure of engagement of the fetal head and mal-presentation, whilst in labour there may be a risk of obstructed labour.

Ovarian cysts in pregnancy may undergo the same complications as in the non-pregnant state. Torsion of an ovarian pedicle is most likely to occur in early preg-nancy and in particular at the end of the first trimester or in the puerperium. Haemorrhage into the cyst may occur as a result of increased vascularity and this in turn may lead to rupture of the cyst. Cyst rupture may also follow impaction in labour. In the majority of cases, however, the cyst remains asymptomatic.

Management

Management depends on the nature, size, and problems posed by the cyst. In general, with cystadenomas and dermoids that are asymptomatic, treatment is deferred till after the delivery. If acute complications arise such as torsion, these need to be dealt with at any gestation. If elective surgery in pregnancy is con-templated this is best done at around 16 weeks where the risk of miscarriage and preterm labour are less and access to the pedicle is easy. Provided engagement of the head has occurred and labour is progressing satisfactorily, no special action needs to be taken in labour. If a Caesarean section is needed for obstetric indi-cations, the cyst should be dealt with at the same time. Otherwise, an elective admission should be organized for the postnatal period.

Chapter 47

Malignancy and pre-malignancy of the genital tract in pregnancy

Cervix

Cervical cancer complicates 0.02–0.4% of pregnancies. Up to 7% of cervical carcinomas are diagnosed at the time of pregnancy. Cervical carcinoma is the most common genital tract malignancy to present in pregnancy.[1]

Presentation

Between one- and two-thirds of women with invasive lesions are asymptomatic. Of these, roughly 50% are detected by cervical cytology. The most common presenting symptom is vaginal bleeding. Any woman with a history of recurrent painless bleeding in pregnancy not due to placenta praevia should be referred for colposcopy to exclude cervical neoplasia.

Management

- *Early invasive disease.* Diagnosis is usually made by a colposcopically directed biopsy or wedge biopsy of the cervix. Treatment is by cone biopsy. There is an increased risk of haemorrhage. Despite the increased risk of miscarriage following cone biopsy in pregnancy, 80% of pregnancies will deliver at term and the overall fetal survival rate is 90%. Further treatment can then be deferred until 6 weeks postpartum.

- *Stage 1B.* If the disease is diagnosed after 24 weeks, the pregnancy can be allowed to continue until viability. Treatment is then by radical hysterectomy and lymphadenectomy or radiotherapy. If delivery is by Caesarean section this can be combined with radical hysterectomy. The prognosis is the same whichever method of treatment is used. If disease is diagnosed before 24 weeks, a delay in treatment is not recommended. Termination of pregnancy can be combined with surgical treatment. If radiotherapy is used this will usually induce miscarriage although after 16 weeks termination of pregnancy may be required before proceeding to intracavity radiotherapy.

- *Advanced disease.* Stage 2b or more advanced disease should be treated by radiotherapy. If the pregnancy has reached viability this can be carried out after delivery of the fetus by Caesarean section.

Prognosis

Five-year survival depends mainly on the stage of disease at the time of diagnosis. It ranges from 74% for patients with stage 1B lesions to 16% for stage 3/ disease. The prognosis for stage 1 disease is the same as that for non-pregnant women, although the prognosis for advanced disease is poorer. The overall prognosis tends to be worse for women diagnosed in the later stages of pregnancy because a higher proportion of women have stage 2 or more disease. When analysed by stage there is no significant difference in survival between patients diagnosed in the first and third trimesters. Delaying treatment of early stage disease by up to 16 weeks to allow the fetus to reach viability does not appear to affect long-term prognosis.

Pre-invasive disease

Interpretation of cervical cytology can be difficult during pregnancy and, unless clinically indicated, routine cervical screening should be deferred until after pregnancy is completed. Women with evidence of dyskaryosis on cervical cytology should be referred for colposcopy to differentiate pre-malignant from invasive disease. The increased vascularity of the cervix accentuates the colour difference between normal and (aceto-white) neoplastic epithelium. If an area of atypical epithelium is identified, this should be biopsied, if clinically suspicious of high-grade cervical intraepithelial neoplasia (CIN) or invasive disease. There is some increased risk of bleeding following biopsy during pregnancy but the risk of miscarriage is low. Colposcopic assessment without biopsy may be acceptable if there is no suggestion of invasive disease on cytology and colposcopy and the assessment is carried out by an experienced colposcopist. If biopsy confirms CIN, a conservative approach to treatment is usually adopted. Repeat colposcopy is carried out between 24 and 34 weeks and again at 8–12 weeks postpartum. If this confirms the continued presence of CIN, treatment should be delayed until the third or fourth month postpartum because of the increased risk of bleeding prior to this. Pregnancy does not appear to affect the rate of progression from low- to high-grade CIN nor that from CIN to invasive disease.

427

Ovarian carcinoma

Between 1 in 80 and 1 in 300 pregnancies are complicated by the presence of ovarian cysts.[1] The majority of these will be benign, the most common being functional ovarian cysts (follicular cysts, corpus luteum). The most common solid, benign ovarian cysts found in pregnancy are mature cystic teratomas (dermoid cysts). Mucinous cystadenomas are the most common epithelial neoplasm. Between 2 and 5% of ovarian cysts in pregnancy will be malignant with an overall incidence of between 1 in 8000 and 1 in 20 000 pregnancies. Of malignant tumours in pregnancy 25% will be dysgerminomas.

Diagnosis

Most lesions are asymptomatic and diagnosed following palpation of a abdominal or pelvic mass or on routine ultrasound scanning for fetal viability or abnormality. Symptoms usually arise as a result of complications such as torsion or rupture of the cyst causing abdominal pain, nausea, vomiting, and local tenderness. Torsion (but not haemorrhage and rupture) is more common in pregnancy and in the puerperium than at other times (complicates 10–15% of tumours). Torsion most commonly occurs between 10 and 16 weeks. Ultrasound examination should be arranged to distinguish ovarian cysts from other types of pelvic mass. Definitive diagnosis can only be made by removal of the cyst at laparotomy.

Management

Asymptomatic cysts < 5 cm can be left and monitored by ultrasound. They will usually resolve without treatment after delivery. Those 5–10 cm in size with no abnormal features can be either managed conservatively as above or aspirated under ultrasound guidance and the fluid examined cytologically.[2] Laparotomy is indicated for cysts that are persistently more than 10 cm in diameter, are enlarging, or contain abnormal features on ultrasound scan (complex multilocular or solid areas). Unless indicated earlier because of an acute surgical complication of the cyst such as torsion, laparotomy is usually performed during the mid-trimester at 16 weeks (by which time the pregnancy is not dependent on the corpus luteum and miscarriage is less likely).

- Benign lesions are treated by unilateral cystectomy or salpingo-oophorectomy.
- Stage 1 ovarian carcinoma can be treated by unilateral salpingo-oophorectomy providing that there is no obvious invasion of the capsule or involvement of the contralateral ovary and no ascites.
- Patients with more advanced disease should be treated by total abdominal hysterectomy and bilateral salpingo-oophorectomy.
- Where the diagnosis is made in the second trimester, a decision will need to be made on a case by case basis as to whether to delay treatment to allow the pregnancy to reach viability.
- Where possible, patients with suspected ovarian cancer should be managed in a specialist cancer unit. This is especially important for patients with malignant germ-cell tumours where it may be possible to preserve reproductive function and even the pregnancy in which the tumour is diagnosed by appropriate chemotherapy.
- Although chemotherapeutic agents are teratogenic in the first trimester, malformation rates do not appear to be increased in women treated in the second or third trimesters.

Vulval malignancy

Vulval carcinoma is rare in pregnancy, the peak incidence of the disease being in the 60–70 year age group. Vulval intraepithelial neoplasia (VIN) is however seen in younger women.

Diagnosis

Pre-malignant disease is commonly asymptomatic. The most common presenting symptom is pruritus. Signs such as fissuring, ulceration, or raised areas indicate the possibility of invasive disease. Colposcopic assessment may be helpful in identifying the extent of disease but the diagnosis should be confirmed by biopsy.

Treatment

- *Pre-malignant disease*. Treatment of VIN can be deferred until after the pregnancy is completed.
- *Malignant lesions*. Management is essentially the same as for the non-pregnant woman. Early invasive disease, where the depth of penetration is no more than 1 mm, can be treated by wide, local excision. Where more invasive disease is diagnosed after 36 weeks, treatment is usually deferred until after delivery. At earlier gestations vulvectomy and node dissection can be performed without having to terminate the pregnancy. If the vulval wound has healed there is no contraindication to vaginal delivery.

429

References

1 Singer, A. (1989). Malignancy and premalignancy of the genital tract in pregnancy. In *Turnbull's obstetrics* (ed. G. Chamberlain), Chapter 43, p. 657. Churchill Livingstone, Edinburgh.

2 Buckley, C.H. (1989). Is needle aspiration of ovarian cysts adequate for diagnosis? *British Journal of Obstetrics and Gynaecology* **96**, 1021.

Chapter 48

Perinatal mortality

The perinatal mortality rate has been defined as the total number of all babies born dead from 24 weeks gestation (stillbirths) and of all live born babies that die in the first week of life regardless of gestational age at birth (neonatal deaths) per 1000 livebirths and stillbirths. A late neonatal death is one that occurs from 7 days to 27 completed days of life, whereas a postneonatal death includes deaths from 28 days onwards but under 1 year.

The perinatal mortality rate at present in the UK is around 8.7 per 1000. Direct comparison with other developed countries may be misleading due to slight variations in definition. Perinatal mortality rates are much higher in the developing world, up to 10-fold higher than in the developed world. Possible causes for this vast discrepancy are malnutrition and susceptibility to infection.

Over the last 60 years where data on perinatal mortality has been collected in the UK, there has been a steady improvement in perinatal mortality. Not surprisingly, the major contribution to the improvement has been through public health measures leading to a healthier population through better nutrition and health education. The role of the medical profession must not, however, be underestimated.

In an attempt to further reduce the risk of fetal and neonatal loss from 20 weeks of pregnancy through to the first year of life, the Confidential Enquiry into Stillbirths and Deaths in Infancy (CESDI) was set up. The aim of CESDI is to identify risks that are attributable to suboptimal care through review of a sample of anonymous casenotes by an expert panel.

Classification of perinatal deaths

The Wigglesworth classification of perinatal deaths uses a pathophysiological approach where causes of death are arranged in a hierarchical mutually exclusive order. This classification has been extended for use in the CESDI reports as follows:
- Congenital malformations (lethal or severe).
- Antepartum fetal deaths.
- Deaths due to intrapartum asphyxia, anoxia, or trauma.
- Neonatal deaths due to immaturity.
- Infection.
- Other specific causes.
- Accident or non-intrapartum trauma.
- Sudden infant death (cause unknown).
- Unclassifiable.

Causes of perinatal mortality

In the 1996 CESDI report the four most common causes of perinatal mortality were prematurity, congenital malformations, antepartum fetal death, and intrapartum asphyxia.

Prematurity

Although prematurity accounts for only 1 in 12 births, this group is overrepresented among the neonatal deaths with 1 in 2 neonatal deaths having been premature babies. There have been dramatic improvements in the survival of very premature infants through improvements in neonatal care as well as the beneficial antenatal intervention of corticosteroid administration to the mother at least 24 hours prior to delivery. The most common causes of morbidity and mortality in premature babies are respiratory distress syndrome, overwhelming sepsis, and neurological and gastrointestinal problems.

Congenital malformations

Malformations account for 1 in 6 of perinatal deaths in the UK. There has been a change in the pattern of congenital abnormalities over the last 2 decades with a reduction in open neural tube defects. This has been brought about by maternal serum alpha-fetoprotein (MSAFP) screening and subsequently by routine ultrasound scanning in pregnancy. Detection of the abnormality offers the woman the possibility of termination of the affected pregnancy. It is hoped that the recent advice regarding periconceptual folic acid will actually further reduce the incidence of neural tube defects (NTDs). With the reduction in NTDs, the predominant group of fetal abnormalities are those of the cardiovascular system where ultrasound diagnosis has not got the same sensitivity as that for NTD screening.

433

Antepartum deaths

Antepartum fetal death includes fetal loss due to a variety of causes (such as placental abruption) but also a significant proportion of unexplained fetal losses. In a special review of antepartum fetal death the fifth CESDI report concluded that almost one-third of cases were unexplained, while in a quarter of the cases there was evidence of intrauterine fetal growth restriction. The incidence of placental abruption and abnormal glucose tolerance in this group as a whole was almost 10%.

Intrapartum asphyxia

The risk of a baby dying in labour is less than 1 in 1000 but in the 1994 annual CESDI report almost 1300 normally formed babies greater than 1.5 kg in weight died intrapartum. In the 873 cases reviewed, care was criticized as suboptimal in 78%. The main criticisms focused on inadequate recognition of antenatal risk factors, poor interpretation of and failure to act on cardiotocograph (CTG) abnormalities, and poor resuscitation of the newborn. These recommendations highlighted the need for critical appraisal of the training, supervision, and practice of both obstetricians and midwives and has led to moves to develop guidelines and educational programmes to achieve and maintain the competence required for intrapartum care and fetal monitoring.

Conclusion

The perinatal mortality rate appears to have plateaued since the late 1980s. If further improvements are to be made it is important to reduce the avoidable causes of perinatal loss particularly suboptimal intrapartum care. There is also a need to direct research towards antepartum fetal loss and how this could be predicted and prevented.

Maternal mortality

435

There are in excess of half a million maternal deaths worldwide each year and there is a huge worldwide variation in maternal mortality rates. Based on the World Health Organization (WHO) figures from 1988, North America, Europe and what was then the USSR account for just 1.6% of that year's total number of maternal deaths worldwide. The high maternal mortality in the developing world can be attributed to the high fertility rate with poor access to contraception, unsafe abortion practices, absence of a primary health-care system, and often lack of access to any form of health-care professional or institution.

Maternal mortality—steps taken in the past

Obstetricians have taken the lead in clinical audit for many years by collection of information on maternal mortality rates since 1847. The most notable improvements in maternal mortality rates in the UK occurred in the period 1935 to 1985 due to:

- General improvement in public health.
- Better training of midwives and obstetricians, through the Midwives act of 1902 and 1936, and the establishment of the Royal College of Obstetricians and Gynaecologists (RCOG) in 1929.
- The use of antibiotics such as penicillin and sulfonamides dramatically cut down the deaths due to puerperal sepsis.
- Prevention and treatment of postpartum haemorrhage (PPH) by administration of ergometrine.
- Development of safe blood transfusion practice.
- The introduction of effective and simple family planning options such as the combined oral contraceptive pill (COCP) helped reduce parity and average family size.
- The 1967 'Abortion Act' and the legalization of abortion led to the elimination of illegal abortion and the associated complications.

Since 1985 there has been little change in the overall maternal mortality rate, but this does not mean that maternal deaths have reached an irreducible low.

Since 1951 there has been a thorough system of reviewing maternal deaths and the publication of triennial reports. The system initially covered England and Wales, with similar practices elsewhere in the UK, but the last four triennial reports have covered the whole of the UK. All maternal deaths during pregnancy and within the following year are collated, made anonymous, and the causes of death assessed by expert panels to determine whether there were aspects of substandard care. The triennial reports then highlight areas of substandard care and make recommendations as to how improvements can be made.

Classification of maternal deaths

The definitions used by the Confidential Enquiry into Maternal Deaths in the UK (CEMD) are as follows.

Maternal death. Death of a woman while pregnant or within 42 days of termination of pregnancy from any cause related to or aggravated by pregnancy or its management but excluding accidental or incidental causes.

Direct death. Death resulting from obstetric complications of the pregnant state; from interventions, omissions, or incorrect treatment; or a chain of events resulting from the above.

Indirect deaths. Deaths resulting from previous existing disease or disease that developed during pregnancy and that was not due to obstetric causes but that was aggravated by the physiological effects of pregnancy.

Late deaths. Deaths occurring between 42 days and 1 year after abortion, miscarriage, or delivery due to direct or indirect maternal causes.

Fortuitous deaths. Deaths from unrelated causes that happen to occur in pregnancy or the puerperium.

In the 1997–1999 triennium 2 123 614 maternities were recorded and there was a total of 378 maternal deaths reported to the CEMD. The leading causes of maternal mortality are given in the following sections.

Direct causes

Thrombosis and thromboembolism

These accounted for 35 deaths (rate of 16.5 deaths per million maternities). Deaths from thromboembolism were predominantly after pulmonary embolism (PE) and occurred at any stage of pregnancy (including the first trimester) and the puerperium (slightly more common compared to the antenatal period). The report highlighted the point that close attention is needed with symptoms such as chest and leg pains to exclude PE or deep vein thrombosis (DVT) by means of the appropriate investigations. Thrombosis and thromboembolism have always been among the leading causes of maternal mortality and guidelines were drawn up to identify patients at high risk for appropriate thromboprophylaxis. The last triennium has seen a decline in maternal deaths due to this cause.

Hypertensive disorders

These account for 15 deaths (rate of 7.1 deaths per million maternities). In this group cerebral (7 cases) and hepatic (2 cases) complications appear to be the main causes of maternal mortality. The recommendations of CEMD highlighted the need to formulate and update protocols for the management of pre-eclampsia and eclampsia, with a senior clinician having the overall responsibility of management of the patient especially with respect to fluid management. Severe life-threatening hypertension should be treated effectively. $MgSO_4$ is the anticonvulsant drug of choice in the treatment of eclampsia. Multiple pregnancies are increased risk of pre-eclampsia. The report also recommended antenatal education of all women to recognize the symptoms associated with pre-eclampsia and seek professional help urgently.

Amniotic fluid embolism

This accounted for 8 deaths showing a decrease from previous reports. For the last two reports, a clinical diagnosis was accepted without the absolute requirement of post-mortem histopathological confirmation. There appear to be no consistent common factors to identify risk. Thus a confidential amniotic fluid embolism register has been set up at Bradford Royal Infirmary. The entry criteria are cardiac arrest or acute hypotension, acute hypoxia (cyanosis, dyspnoea, or respiratory arrest), coagulopathy, or any combination of the above during labour, at Caesarean section, or within 30 minutes of delivery with no other clinical condition or potential explanation.

Early pregnancy deaths

These accounted for 17 cases, 13 of these were due to ectopic pregnancies, 2 following spontaneous miscarriage, and 2 following legal termination of pregnancy (TOP). The main criticism in association with deaths in the ectopic pregnancy group was delay in diagnosis and inappropriate management. It highlighted the need to constantly keep in mind the possibility of pregnancy which can easily be confirmed or refuted by serum β-hCG (beta-human chorionic gonadotrophin), and that an empty uterus in woman with a positive pregnancy test may potentially indicate an ectopic pregnancy. The CEMD also highlighted the importance of timely senior and often multidisciplinary involvement where there is unexpected decline in patient's condition after what is generally an uncomplicated process such as spontaneous miscarriage. Senior medical staff should attend to difficult surgical cases. The possibility of unusual presentation mimicking gastrointestinal disorders must be taught to medical and nursing students and emphasized in textbooks.

Sepsis

This accounted for 14 deaths and there is now clear evidence to support the use of prophylactic antibiotics at Caesarean section. Women with prolonged rupture of membranes who develop fever should be carefully assessed by senior staff. Where patients are systemically seriously ill, antibiotic treatment on the advice of a microbiologist should be instituted while awaiting bacteriological cultures.

Haemorrhage

This accounted for 7 maternal deaths. The points that emerged from the CEMD report were that anterior placenta praevia with a previous uterine scar may be associated with severe uncontrollable haemorrhage at the time of Caesarean section necessitating recourse to Caesarean hysterectomy. Hence, involvement of a very experienced operator from the onset is recommended. Other recommendations that emerged from the report highlighted the importance of regular 'fire drills' and agreed protocols for the management of emergencies such as obstetric haemorrhage that can become life-threatening very rapidly.

Genital tract trauma

This accounted for 2 maternal deaths in the 1997 to 1999 triennium. The report of the previous triennium (1994–96) had 5 deaths, one due to uterine and vaginal lacerations following instrumental delivery, with the remaining four due to uterine ruptures. The report reiterated the recommendations of the 5th CESDI report of maternal and fetal vigilance during induction of labour in the presence of a uterine scar and the importance of the involvement of an experienced obstetrician in the antenatal and intrapartum care planning of such patients.

Anaesthesia

There were only 3 cases directly due to anaesthesia and in these cases care was deemed substandard. The safety of obstetric anaesthesia is such that the risk of death is one per million maternities. This has been achieved through greater use of epidural and regional anaesthesia in place of general anaesthesia and ready access to intensive care facilities when required.

Indirect deaths

Cardiac deaths

There were 35 deaths due to cardiac disease. Heart disease was the commo cause of maternal death. Those who have pulmonary vascular disease have 30% risk of mortality. The CEMD emphasized the importance of joint obste ric and cardiological management of patients with severe or complex heart d ease with the individuals with pulmonary hypertension being especially at hi risk. The use of oxytocin may compromise a woman with severe cardiac disea Obscure febrile illness may suggest the possibility of endocarditis. Aortic disse tion in pregnancy should be kept in mind in women with severe chest pain pregnancy. Chest X-rays should not be withheld. Echocardiography is the inve tigation of choice for diagnosis of aortic root dissection.

Psychiatric deaths

There were 42 deaths in this group, of which 28 were due to suicide. The impo tance of screening for psychiatric disorders and substance abuse at booking well as the availability of a psychiatrist with an interest in managing the perin tal mental health service is recommended. Women who have serious mental ness should be counselled about possible recurrence following the pregnancy

Other indirect deaths

This group accounted for 75 deaths, the largest single group being women w diseases of the central nervous system: a total of 34 cases of which 11 were ca of subarachnoid haemorrhage and 9 were cases of epilepsy, and the rest we due to other causes. The recommendations that emerged highlighted the impo tance of multidisciplinary decision-making and management. As regar epilepsy, educating relatives about positioning patients in the recovery positi following a fit and also educating the pregnant women to avoid having a ba when alone and to use the shower instead to avoid the possibility of drownir following a fit.

Part 2

Gynaecology

History and physical examination of the gynaecological patient

It is best to have an outline on which the gynaecological history can be taken and presented. This avoids inadvertent omission of important details and allows for a systematic and concise presentation of the facts. Please be polite, introduce yourself (your name & designation) to the patient and the purpose of your discussion. A suggested outline is as follows:

Current history

- *Name, age and parity*
- *Detailed history of present complaint* - One should be able to establish the presenting complaints. A brief history relevant to the presenting complaints must be taken. There must be some organisational logic in history taking.

e.g. Abnormal menstrual loss – Distinguish between a regular or irregular pattern of bleeding. Attempt to quantify amount of loss by indicating the number of sanitary pads used in a day, presence of blood clots and the need to use two pads at one time ('flooding'). The social impact of the heavy periods such as absence from work during menses due to associated pain, weakness or flooding is important.

e.g. Pelvic pain – Establish the duration, site and nature of pain and possible relationship with the time in the menstrual cycle. Aggravating and relieving factors. Radiation of the pain and associated symptoms e.g. vomiting, fever, dysuria.

e.g. Vaginal discharge – Describe odour, colour, consistency, amount and presence of blood. Relationship to the period and associated itching or irritation is relevant.

Past medical, family, and social history

This is an inquiry into the reproductive history that includes past obstetric, gynaecological, menstrual, contraceptive and smear histories. This should be followed by past medical and surgical history. Family and social history should not be forgotten.

- *Menstrual history*
  Menarche (age when periods began)
  Cycle (interval between the first days of two consecutive periods)
  Duration of period
  State first day of the last menstrual period (L.M.P.)
- *Past Obstetric history* - Describe outcomes and details of previous pregnancies. If there were many pregnancies, it is appropriate to summarise, e.g. 5 previous full term spontaneous vaginal deliveries. Operative deliveries and any important issue such as miscarriage and fetal loss should be noted.
- *Past Gynaecological history* - Details of gynaecological history other than the presenting complaint should include details of previous cervical smears, previous gynaecological problems and any surgery (e.g. pelvic inflammatory disease or endometriosis).

History and physical examination

- *Contraceptive history* – The methods used, duration of use, acceptance, current method, side effects and plan for the future.
- *Past Medical and Surgical history* - Past medical and surgical history may have some bearing to the current problem or its management.
- *Drug allergies* - This is vital information and should be **prominently displayed** in the notes. Failure to do so may cause severe illness or death of the patient.
- *Social history* - This should include the impact of the present problem on the patient's life. Smoking, drinking, drug abuse and living conditions may be relevant to the current problem or to the management planned.

447

Physical examination

This should always start with the general examination of the patient followed by cardiovascular and respiratory systems.

The gynaecological examination encompasses both an abdominal as well as a vaginal pelvic examination that includes bimanual palpation. A bimanual examination should be preceded by inspection of the vulva, vagina and cervix using a speculum. In specific circumstances, a rectal examination may be indicated.

Abdominal examination

The fundamental steps in an abdominal examination should be followed, i.e. inspection, palpation and percussion. Auscultation may be relevant especially in cases of acute abdomen and post-operative examinations.

Inspection

Abdominal distension, if any, should be noted and if present look for visible evidence of masses. If surgical scars are present they should be correlated to the past history.

Palpation

Guarding, tenderness and rebound tenderness are important signs to elicit in any one presenting with an acute abdomen. After performing a routine light palpation of the whole abdomen with the right hand, it is important to switch to the left hand and feel for pelvic masses. This is an important difference between gynaecological and surgical examination that allows the clinician to detect any masses that may rise out of the pelvis.

Percussion/auscultation

Percussion is useful to distinguish between a solid mass (dull) and distended bowel (tympanic). In the presence of a vague mass on palpation in an obese individual or when one is tensing the abdominal wall percussion is useful to identify the possibility of the mass and also in defining the borders of a mass. It is useful to demonstrate ascites or collection of blood. Shifting dullness and fluid thrill need to be demonstrated appropriate to the situation.

The pelvic examination

The pelvic or vaginal examination is the most challenging part of the gynaecological physical examination. It is a potential source of embarrassment to the woman and should be conducted in a sensitive manner in privacy accompanied by a suitable chaperon. Exposure should be in a manner needed to carry out the examination. The abdomen should be covered up to and just below the knees. It should be performed gently, otherwise it can be uncomfortable. A well performed pelvic examination gives good information about the genital tract and pelvic organs. It is thus an indispensable part of the gynaecological assessment and is to the gynaecologist the equivalent of a rectal examination to the surgeon.

Position

The pelvic examination can be performed in the dorsal, lithotomy or Sim's position. Sim's position is a modification of the left lateral position and is ideal for examination of a woman with utero-vaginal prolapse or vesico-vaginal fistulae. The lithotomy position, in which both thighs are abducted and feet suspended from lithotomy poles is usually adopted when performing vaginal surgery. The dorsal position is most commonly used for routine outpatient gynaecological examinations such as when obtaining a cervical smear.

Technique

The steps in performing a pelvic examination are:

- inspection of the external genitalia
- speculum examination of the vagina and cervix
- bimanual examination of the uterus and adnexae.

Inspection

Inspect the vulva and external genitalia. It is useful to imagine a series of circles surrounding the vaginal introitus and then to describe your findings from the outermost to the innermost circle. For example, one could begin with describing the mons pubis and pubic hair distribution, the labia majora and minora, the clitoris, urethral meatus and vaginal introitus.

Speculum examination

Two vaginal speculae are commonly used – the Sim's (duck-billed) speculum and Cusco's or bivalve speculum. Sim's speculum is used in the Sim's position and is most useful for the examination of utero-vaginal prolapse. Cusco's speculum is most frequently used and is described below.

The labia minora are parted with the index and middle fingers of the left hand to obtain a good view of the introitus. A well-lubricated and warm bivalve speculum is held in the right hand with the main body of the speculum in the palm and the closed blades projecting between the index and middle fingers. This grasp is intended to keep the blades opposed and prevent inadvertent opening of the speculum while it is being inserted. In the lithotomy position, the speculum is usually inserted with the handle inferior while in the dorsal position, the handle should be superior. The speculum is advanced gently along with gentle pressure on the posterior wall of the vagina to open the potential space. Take note that the axis of the vagina is directed slightly towards the rectum. Open the speculum only when it can not be advanced further. The cervix may be visualised. If it cannot be seen, the speculum is either above or below the cervix as the blades are in the anterior or posterior fornix of the vagina. It will then be necessary to close the speculum, withdraw it slightly, change its direction and advance it before opening it again. The vaginal skin is rugose and that over the cervix is smooth, usually there is mucus close to the cervical os, there will be a convex anterior vaginal fornix or a concave posterior fornix – one or more of these features may come into view that may help to change the direction of the speculum.

Removal of the speculum requires as much care as insertion. It is essential that the blades are held open as the speculum is withdrawn until the ends of the blades are distal to the cervix. Otherwise, closing the blades on the cervix will cause pain. The speculum must be completely closed as the ends of the blades come out through the introitus.

Digital examination

The digital bimanual examination helps to identify the pelvic organs. The bladder should be emptied prior to this examination. The index and middle finger of the right hand are inserted into the vagina with the palmar aspect facing upwards. Feel the consistency of the cervix. The left hand is placed on the abdomen and bimanual palpation commenced. The purpose of bimanual palpation is to bring the abdominal wall close to the pelvic organs by pressing at the appropriate place on the abdominal wall and also by shifting the pelvic organs or masses towards that hand. One should feel these organs or masses between the vaginal and abdominal hands. First, the uterus is felt with the vaginal fingers placed on the cervix and the hand on the lower midline above the uterine fundus. Then, the adnexae can be palpated between the vaginal fingers placed in the lateral fornices and the abdominal hand over the respective iliac fossa. An anteverted uterus is easily palpated bimanually but a retroverted one may not be. Retroverted uteri can be assessed by feeling the body of the uterus with the vaginal fingers via the vaginal wall of the posterior fornix. If a pelvic mass is discovered, its size, consistency and mobility are determined. Uterine masses may be felt to move with the cervix when the uterus is shifted upward while adnexal masses will not. If adnexal masses are suspected there should be a line of separation between the uterus and the mass and the mass should be felt distinctly from the uterus. However, pedunculated masses from the uterus may give the impression of an adnexal mass and an adnexal mass adherent to the uterus may give the impression of a uterine mass. The consistency of the mass may be of help to distinguish the origin in some cases. An ultrasound examination may be necessary to define it better.

Summary of the clinical problem

At the end of history taking and examination the clinical problem should be summarised in a manner that would provide the important differential diagnosis or some pointers towards the investigations needed to derive at the diagnosis. The summary should include salient points from the past medical, surgical, obstetric and gynaecological history that may influence the treatment.

This summary should be explained to the patient and the information provided should be understood by her in order for her to decide whether to proceed with the investigations and/or to accept the treatment. This should also form the basis for a reply to her Family practitioner.

451

Gynaecological anatomy

The anatomy of the female genital tract comprises the pelvic wall, the pelvic cavity and its contents, and the perineum.

The pelvic walls

These consist of the bony pelvis and pelvic floor muscles.

- *Anterior wall*. Pubic bone and its rami, symphysis pubis, and urogenital membrane.
- *Posterior wall*. Sacrum, coccyx, piriformis muscle, and sacrotuberous and sacrospinous ligaments.
- *Lateral wall*. Part of the pubic bone below the pelvic inlet, obturator membrane, sacrotuberous and sacrospinous ligaments, and obturator internus muscle with its covering fascia.
- *Inferior wall* (*pelvic floor*). Levator ani and coccygeus muscles and their covering fascia. It is incomplete anteriorly to allow the passage of the urethra and vagina.

The pelvic cavity

This contains the rectum, sigmoid colon, terminal coils of ileum, ureters, bladder, female genital organs, visceral pelvic fascia, and peritoneum.

Ovaries

Each ovary is oval-shaped, measuring 4 × 2 cm, and is attached to the broad ligament by the mesovarium. The ovarian ligament supports the ovary and connects it to the lateral margin of the uterus. Before puberty, the ovaries are smooth, but they get progressively scarred with age. Postmenopausal ovaries are shrunken and have a surface pitted with scars.

Tubes (Fallopian tubes)

Each tube is about 10 cm long; lies in the upper border of broad ligament, and runs laterally from the uterine cornu to the ovary. A tube is divided into four parts: funnel-shaped infundibulum and its fimbriae; wide ampulla; narrow isthmus; and the intramural part that pierces the uterine wall.

The Fallopian tubes, ovaries, and associated connective tissue (parametria) are collectively called the *adnexae*. They are palpated bimanually in the lateral fornices and, if normal, cannot be felt except in a very relaxed and slim woman.

- On pelvic examination look for masses and tenderness.

Uterus

This is a hollow, pear-shaped organ with thick muscular walls that measures about 8 cm (length) × 5 cm (breadth) × 2.5 cm (anteroposterior (AP)) in a young nulliparous adult. It is divided into fundus, body, and cervix. The mucin-secreting glands on the surface of the cervix lubricate the vagina. The opening or the os of the cervical canal is circular in nulliparous women and slit-like in the parous. The peritoneum is draped over the uterus, forming an anterior uterovesical fold, a posterior recto-uterine fold, and, laterally, the broad ligament.

Relations of the uterus

Anterior: uterovesical pouch, superior surface of the bladder, anterior fornix of the vagina.

Posterior: recto-uterine pouch (of Douglas), coils of ileum or sigmoid colon.

Lateral: contents of the broad ligament (Fallopian tubes, round ligament, ovarian ligament, uterine and ovarian vessels, vestigial mesonephric remnants), ureter, lateral vaginal fornix.

Positions

In most women, it lies in an anteverted and somewhat anteflexed position.

Anteverted. The long axis of uterus is bent forward on the long axis of the vagina, almost at right angles.

Anteflexion. The long axis of the body of the uterus is bent forward at the level of the internal os with the long axis of the cervix.

Retroversion. The fundus and body are bent backward and therefore lie in the pouch of Douglas.

Retroflexed. The body of the uterus is bent backward on the cervix.

Among normal women, 20% have a retroverted uterus. A full bladder will push the uterus backward and mimic retroversion.

Supports

The supports of the uterus are the levator ani and perineal body, transverse cervical ligaments (also called cardinal ligament or Mackenrodt ligament), uterosacral ligaments, and pubocervical ligament.

Look for: uterine position, size, mobility, and tenderness; cervical ectopy; cervicitis; discharge; polyps and pain on moving the cervix (cervical excitation tenderness).

455

Vagina

The vagina is an empty, distensible, muscular tube, extending upwards and backwards from the vulva to the uterus. It is about 8 cm long, with its upper half above the pelvic floor and the lower half within the perineum. It is attached circumferentially at its upper end to the cervix, which divides the vaginal lumen into an anterior, a posterior, and two lateral fornices.

Relations:

—Anteriorly: bladder and urethra.

—Posteriorly: pouch of Douglas, ampulla of the rectum, and perineal body.

—Laterally: ureter, levator ani, urogenital diaphragm, and bulb of the vestibule.

Look for: Inflammation, discharge, prolapse.

Perineum

This is the part of the pelvic inlet that lies inferior to the pelvic diaphragm. When seen from below with the thighs abducted, it is diamond-shaped and bounded anteriorly by the symphysis pubis, posteriorly by the tip of the coccyx and laterally by the ischial tuberosity. The perineum is artificially divided into an anterior urogenital and a posterior anal triangle.

- *Contents of urogenital triangle*: vulva and urethral and vaginal orifices.
- *Contents of anal triangle*: anus and ischiorectal fossa with the pudendal canal of Alcock in its extreme lateral position.

Vulva

This is the name applied to the external female genitalia (Fig. 50.1). It consists of the mons pubis, labia minora, labia majora, the vestibule (with the clitoris, ducts of paraurethral glands, ducts of the Bartholins glands, hymen, and vaginal and urethral orifices), and the perineum. The hymen when broken (by tampons or intercourse) leaves tags at the entrance to the vagina.

- *Look for*: rashes, atrophy, ulcers, lumps, and deficient perineum.

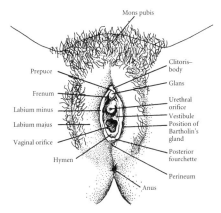

Fig. 50.1 External genitalia. (Taken from *The Oxford handbook of clinical specialities*, 6th edn (ed. J. Collier, M. Longmore, and P. Scally), p. 9, © 2003 by permission of the publisher Oxford University Press.)

457

Malformations of the female genital tract

The incidence is difficult to ascertain but it is estimated that 1% of phenotypic females have some abnormality of the genital tract. Of these, 40–50% are associated with renal tract abnormalities and 15% with an absent kidney. Vulval and gonadal anomalies are dealt with in Chapter 52.

Malformations of the uterus

The incidence is difficult to define. Malformations include absent uterus (Müllerian agenesis or hypoplasia), fusion anomalies of the uterus, and cervical atresia.

Absence of the uterus

The uterus may be absent or so rudimentary as to be incapable of functioning. This is usually associated with absence of vagina and primary amenorrhoea. It may be associated with a blindly ending lower vagina, suggesting androgen insensitivity (XY with testes) or XX chromosome complement with ovaries.

Treatment

There is no corrective treatment available. Give psychological support. If there is androgen insensitivity, remove any testicular tissue to avoid risk of malignancy and provide oestrogen replacement therapy.

Fusion anomalies

These are more common and result in a variety of well-recognized uterine shapes such as bicornuate uterus and subseptate uterus.

- Diethylstilboestrol exposure is associated with a T-shaped uterus.
- Unilateral atresia of one mesonephric duct results in a unicornuate uterus with a single Fallopian tube, usually associated with unilateral absence of a kidney.
- Unilateral partial atresia of the mesonephric duct results in the presence of a rudimentary horn, which may communicate with the well-developed side.
- In a didelphic uterus, there are two completely separate uterine cavities, two cervices (which often unite externally), the vagina may be septate, and there may be associated ipsilateral absence of the kidney. It could be asymptomatic or present with cryptomenorrhoea and haematoma.

Presentation

Fusion anomalies may be asymptomatic and only diagnosed on investigation of recurrent pregnancy loss, primary infertility, urological abnormalities, or menstrual disorders. In pregnancy, they may be associated with miscarriage, poor intrauterine fetal growth, malpresentation, and adherent placenta.

Investigations

Hysterosalpingogram: if a double cervix, contrast should be injected into both cervical canals. Cervical atresia is a rare but serious malformation, which is due to the failure to develop of the cervical portion of the fused Müllerian ducts. The uterus may be normal or didelphic. If attempts to create a cervical opening are not effective, tubo-ovarian masses and peritonitis could develop, requiring hysterectomy.

Malformations of the vagina

These occur in 1:4000 to 1:10 000 female births. They are the second commonest cause of primary amenorrhoea. 50% are associated with renal anomalies and 12% with anomalies of the bony skeleton.

Absence
- If there is a rudimentary or no uterus due to congenital absence of the Müllerian duct (Mayer–Rokitansky–Kuster–Hauser syndrome), it presents at about age 16 years with primary amenorrhoea. Sexual characteristics are normal because the ovaries are normal.
- If secondary sexual characteristics are not well developed, consider androgen insensitivity syndrome (XY female).
- 15% have major renal defects.
- If the uterus is present and the majority of the vagina is absent, the presentation is with amenorrhoea, cyclical abdominal pain, and haematometra with a palpable mass. Sexual characteristics are normal.

Disorders of vertical fusion
There could be a high (46%), middle (35%), or low (19%) transverse vaginal septum or intact hymen. The usual presentation is as a teenager with cryptomenorrhoea, cyclical abdominal pain, and haematocolpos. She may also have pressure symptoms of urinary frequency or retention.

Lateral fusion defects
There may be a complete or partial septum, lying in the midline in the sagittal plane. These defects may be associated with a double uterus and cervix or with a single uterus. They are usually an incidental finding or they may present with dyspareunia. When associated with unilateral vaginal obstruction, they present with abdominal pain, haematometra, and haematocolpos. Careful examination is needed. Otherwise, it will be missed, as it is associated with menstrual flow from other side.

Diagnosis
- There should be a careful examination of the vulval appearance and sexual characteristics, and evidence of retained blood in vagina or upper or lower part of genital tract should be sought.
- There should be an ultrasound scan of the pelvis investigating the uterus, ovaries, haematometra, haematocolpos, and the level of defect.
- Intravenous urogram (IVU).
- Chromosomal analysis is needed if vagina is absent. May require gonadectomy if XY.

Management
- *Absence.*
  —Psychological counselling.
  —If non-functioning uterus: vaginal dilators; vaginoplasty.
  —If coexisting functional uterus: release of retained menstrual blood; creation of neo-vagina.
- *Vertical fusion defect.*
  —Obstructed hymen: cruciate incision through hymen.
  —Low/middle septum: transvaginal removal of septum and re-anastomosis of vaginal segments.
  —High septum: abdomino-perineal surgery.
- *Lateral fusion defect.* Resection of septum.

Wolffian duct anomalies

Remnants of lower part may present as vaginal cysts and those of upper part as para-ovarian cysts (epoophoron and paroophoron). Small vaginal cysts do not necessarily need removal. If causing symptoms (usually dyspareunia) it should be removed surgically. Large or painful para-ovarian cysts require surgical exploration.

Chapter 52

Intersex

Basic concepts in sex differentiation

Understanding intersex requires an insight into factors that are prerequisite in sexual development. The gonads, genital ducts, and external genitalia (Table 52.1) are normally interlinked in their development, but they can develop independently in aberrant conditions.

- *The gonads*. The SRY (sex-related Y) gene is the only gene required from the Y chromosome in testis determination. We do not know whether SRY is an activator of genes involved in testis determination, a suppressor of genes involved in ovarian differentiation, or both. More genes upstream and downstream to SRY have been identified in the cascade leading to gonadal differentiation.[1]
- *The genital ducts*. Males and females have both the Wolffian (male) and the Müllerian (female) genital ducts. The neutral state is the female genital ducts. Its suppression requires a Müllerian inhibitory factor released from the testes.
- *External genitalia*. These develop under hormonal influence. The genital tubercle forms the phallus or the clitoris. The urethral fold forms the shaft of penis or labia minora. The genital swelling forms the scrotum or labia majora.

Basic principles in management

- The fundamental step at the birth of an intersex neonate is to rule out a life-threatening process.
  —Immediate threat to life. Congenital adrenal hyperplasia (CAH).
  —Late threat to life. Gonadal tumour formation particularly in neonates with 45X/46XY or neonates with 46XY and gonadal dysgenesis. Tumour formation in women with androgen insensitivity syndrome (previously known as testicular feminization syndrome) increases after the age of 15.
- Decision-making on the gender. Expert advice may be required to determine the sex of rearing, with the aim of providing close to natural secondary sexual organs and preserving fertility. The suitability of external genitalia for sexual life should be the most important determinant in one or the other gender role. The determination of the sex of rearing and any simple corrective feminizing surgery may be performed before discharge. True hermaphrodites probably should be raised as females. The decision on sex of rearing should be reinforced by continued support and counselling to parents, relatives, and the child as he or she continues to develop.
- Preservation of fertility. CAH patients can be fertile if treated early and true hermaphrodites are potentially fertile if an ipsilateral ovary is present.

Some conditions of intersex are described in Table 52.2.

Table 52.1 Basic concepts in sex differentiation

	Differentiation of ducts		
	Wolffian duct	**Müllerian duct**	**Mesonephros**
In the male	Epididymis, ductus deferens, seminal vesicles	Remnant forms appendix testis	Regress, may form ductuli efferentes joining rete testis
In the female	Remnant may form Gartner's cyst at side of uterus or vagina	Tubes, uterus, upper 4/5 of vagina	Regress, may form epoophoron or paroophoron in the broad ligament

Table 52.2 Conditions of intersex

Congenital adrenal hyperplasia (CAH)

Autosomal recessive, enzymatic defect in cortisol synthesis (most common is 21-hydroxylase). Lack of negative feedback leads to excess ACTH that overstimulates the mineralocorticoid and the androgen pathways. Severity depends on degree of enzyme defect:
- Severe neonatal CAH virilization of female fetus and salt losing; vomiting, diarrhoea, weight loss, dehydration. Diagnosis may be delayed in males as no physical finding at birth.
- Non-salt-losing CAH: mild virilization; may present in childhood with genital overgrowth and increase in weight.
- Late-onset CAH: presents at puberty; early & excess sexual hair; clitoromegaly; delayed menarche; lack of puberty progression.

Diagnosis: family history; clinical findings; excess metabolites proximal to 21-hydroxylase particularly 17-hydroxyprogesterone. Electrolyte levels will indicate the mineralocorticoid status; genetic studies confirm the diagnosis.

Treatment. Cortisol replacement; salt supplementation to neonates; correction surgery of female genitalia if necessary; psychological support to parents and child.

The XY female
- Failure of androgen production due to anatomical testicular failure (pure gonadal dysgenesis or mosaicism). There is a uterus and an upper vagina.
- Failure of androgen production due to enzymatic testicular failure. There is no uterus or upper vagina.
- End-organ insensitivity: 5-alpha reductase deficiency resulting in no conversion of testosterone to dihydrotestosterone (DHT). There is no uterus or upper vagina. Inactive androgen receptors (absent gene on X).

The XX male

Normal external genitalia, but underdeveloped with hypospadias. Positive H-Y antigen. Unlikely to present to gynaecologist.

True hermaphrodites

Both ovary and testis are present. Male or female may dominate. Most are 46XX, but also can be 46XX/XY, 46XY, 46XY/47XXY.

Androgens from: luteoma, polycystic ovary, Krukenberg tumour. Gestogens derived from testosterone

Variable masculinization but no metabolic defect.

467

Management of intersex

Even mild deviations from normal anatomy at birth or in childhood may represent potential intersex disorders. This should encourage specific questioning about drug use during pregnancy, the family history of women without periods and queries about family members who had ambiguous external genitalia. A full examination for other endocrine and other physical anomalies should be undertaken.

Examination

It is imperative that an experienced clinician performs the examination. This should include evaluating the size of the genital tubercle (clitoris/phallus), palpating the labioscrotal pouches and inguinal canals for any masses, identifying the urethra, and identifying the vagina and cervix if necessary by using a paediatric cystoscope. Rectal examination may at times be helpful in palpating the uterus. Table 52.3 lists anomalies that may be found and their possible causes.

Conditions confused with intersex

- Labial adhesion (confused with vaginal agenesis) is rare at birth. It can be acquired as early as 6 weeks of age and occurs more frequently before 12 months. The aetiology remains unclear and infection does not necessarily result in fusion. However, *Candida* and *Herpes simplex* infection can cause labial adhesions.[2, 3]
- The presence of notches and bumps on the hymen's rim are common findings at birth. The decrease in oestrogen levels after birth and ageing to pre-puberty results in a decrease in the number of these findings.[4]
- Hymenal septa, hymenal clefts, and imperforated hymen are abnormal findings but not intersex.
- In pre-pubertal girls, a vaginal opening more than 4 mm is distinctly rare in the absence of a history of sexual abuse.[5]
- Virilizing adrenal tumours may produce sufficient masculinization of the external genitalia to simulate sexual ambiguity.

Investigation

- Ultrasonography with Doppler may be useful for hydrocele or inguinal masses.
- Cord blood (risk of contamination) and peripheral blood samples should be sent for karyotyping, testosterone, and 17-hydroxyprogesterone.
- Fluorescent *in situ* hybridization (FISH) and polymerase chain reaction (PCR) are particularly valuable for Y DNA.
- 17-hydroxyprogesterone, electrolytes, and renin will indicate the mineralocorticoid status and are diagnostic for CAH.
- The HLA complex in families can be studied as necessary to determine whether they are normal, heterozygotes, or affected.

Treatment

Physiological replacement of cortisol in CAH patients, plus mineralocorticoid if needed, will suppress adrenocorticotrophic hormone (ACTH) secretion and remove the stimulation of excessive androgen synthesis. Increased dosages are needed during periods of stress, but excessive therapy may suppress growth. A subsequent pregnancy in couples with a CAH child has a 1:4 chance of being affected. Steroids can be given. However, to be effective this should begin before the diagnosis can be made by chorionic villus sampling (CVS). This will involve treating 7–8 pregnancies (males or unaffected females) for each female diagnosed. The safety of long-term steroid treatment is yet unknown.

The decision on the sex of rearing should be made on the basis of the suitability of external genitalia for sexual life in one or other gender role. The female role is often chosen in the XY female. Inappropriate gonads for the chosen gender role should be removed and hormone replacement therapy (HRT) is given at puberty.

In true hermaphrodites, menstruation and/or breast development may occur and, if brought up as male, then total abdominal hysterectomy (TAH) and bilateral salpingo-oophorectomy (BSO) and mastectomy should be performed. Traditionally, surgical construction of female genitalia has been done. Further studies are needed to assess a possible psychosocial impact of central nervous system (CNS) exposure to high androgens in the female and the presence of ambiguous genitalia.

Follow-up during childhood is essential to monitor for tumour formation, remove contradictory pelvic gonads, perform reconstruction surgery, and measure levels of follicle-stimulating hormone (FSH), luteinizing hormone (LH), and testosterone. Support groups and continued counselling of the child and parents are essential as the child continues to develop. New possible therapies are antiandrogens and aromatease inhibitors.[6]

Table 52.3

469

Anomaly	Possible causes
Clitoral enlargement	CAH; asymmetrical gonadal dysgenesis; hermaphroditism
Cryptorchidism	Undescended testes, but also 46XX, 45X/47XYY.
Inguinal or labioscrotal masses	Androgen insensitivity syndrome; Rokitansky syndrome
Large testicles with hypospadias	Fragile-X syndrome
Sex ambiguity	CAH; XY female; XX male; true hermaphrodite; excess androgens

References

1 Birk, O.S. et al. (2000). The LIM homeobox gene Lhx9 is essential for mouse gonad formation. Nature 403, 900–13.

2 McCann, J., et al. (1990). Genital findings in prepubertal girls selected for non-abuse: a descriptive study. Pediatrics 86, 428–39.

3 DeMarco, B.J. (1987). Labial agglutination secondary to herpes simplex II infection. American Journal of Obstetrics and Gynecology 157 (2), 296–7.

4 Berenson, A.B. (1993). Appearance of the hymen at birth and one year of age: a longitudinal study. Pediatrics 91 (4), 820–5.

5 Goff, C.W., et al. (1989). Vaginal opening measurement. American Journal of Diseases in Children 143, 166–8.

6 Merke, D.P. and Cutler, G.B., Jr (1997). New approaches to the treatment of congenital adrenal hyperplasia. Journal of the American Medical Association 277, 1073–6.

Chapter 53

Physiology of normal menstruation and the ovarian cycle

Menstruation is the shedding of the functional upper two-thirds (layer) of the endometrium after sex steroid withdrawal. The role of the functional layer is to prepare the uterus for implantation. The basal endometrial layer (lower one third) provides tissue for regeneration during the following cycle. This shedding process, which consists of three phases (menstrual, proliferative, and secretory) is repeated approximately 300–400 times during a woman's reproductive life. It also occurs in primates and bats. Menstruation indicates that conception has not occurred.

Phases of the endometrial cycle (Fig. 53.1)

The proliferative phase

This phase is associated with increasing ovarian follicular growth and therefore increasing levels of ovarian oestrogen, which leads to repair and growth of the glandular, stromal, and vascular components of the endometrium. Endometrial glands towards the end of the proliferative or follicular phase are short, straight, and narrow, measuring up to 5 mm in height.

The secretory phase

After ovulation, progesterone becomes the dominant steroid, and its early effect is to inhibit and stop epithelial proliferation, which occurs 2–3 days after ovulation. During this secretory or luteal phase, initial glandular and vessel growth within a progesterone-dominated endometrium leads to increasing tortuosity of glands and coiling of spiral vessels. The *lumina* of the endometrial glands gradually fill with glycogen-rich secretion. This phase lasts around 14 days, and is ended by the demise of the corpus luteum, and therefore progesterone production, unless implantation occurs.

Implantation, on days 21–22 of a 28-day menstrual cycle, is followed by further dramatic morphological changes. Otherwise, the gradual fall of progestogen and oestrogen from the mid-secretory phase onwards causes other changes that finally lead to menstruation.

The menstrual phase

Gradual withdrawal of ovarian sex steroids causes slight shrinking of the endometrium, and therefore the blood flow of spiral vessels is reduced. This together with spiral arteriolar spasms, leads to distal endometrial ischaemia and stasis. Extravasation of blood and endometrial tissue breakdown lead to the onset of menstration.

Of the menstrual loss, 50% is thought to occur during the first 24 hours, and the rest thereafter. An estimated volume of approximately 80 mL is expelled.[1] A loss of over 80 mL is considered to be heavy—menorrhagia—although the volume lost is poorly related to patient perception of loss.[2] Various mechanisms are thought to have an important role to play in the control of menstrual loss.

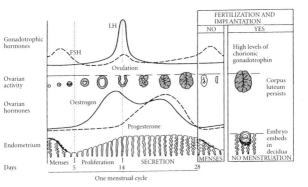

Fig. 53.1 Pituitary, ovarian, and endometrial cycles. (Taken from *The Oxford handbook of clinical specialities*, 6th edn (ed. J. Collier, M. Longmore, and P. Scally), p. 9, © 2003 by permission of the publisher Oxford University Press.)

Endometrial haemostasis

In parallel with the endometrial ischaemic changes already described, progesterone also destabilizes lysosome membranes, leading to the release of active enzymes and prostaglandins. These active enzymes cause further local tissue necrosis, including vascular damage. The functional endometrium is therefore shed in tandem with local bleeding.

On shedding the functional endometrium and ending a sequence of changes designed to nourish an implanting embryo, various complex mechanisms come into play to control and limit bleeding, balanced with active fibrinolysis to avoid clot formation. Absence of fibrinolysis would subsequently lead to the formation of intrauterine adhesions and reduced fertility.

Prostaglandins

Endometrial prostaglandin (PG) concentrations are now known to be low during the proliferative phase of the menstrual cycle, and increase during the latter part of the secretory phase. The two main endometrial PGs have antagonistic effects on the spiral arteriolar system. PGE_2 is a vasodilator and $PGF_{2\alpha}$ a vasoconstrictor.[3] Women with menorrhagia are thought to have a higher local concentration of the vasodilator PGE_2, which can respond to therapeutic doses of prostaglandin synthetase inhibitors.

- Prostacycline (predominantly from the myometrium) is also a vasodilator and also reduces platelet aggregation.
- Prostaglandins are known to play a key role in the onset of human parturition and myometrial contractility and also promote endometrial haemostasis by inducing uterine contractions.

Other agents

*Platelet activation factor*s likely to make a direct contribution to endometrial haemostasis have also been shown to stimulate the release of vasoconstricting PGE but not $PGF_{2\alpha}$. Other potent vasoconstrictors of small vessels in the human uterus have now been identified—a group of peptides termed *endothelins*.[4]

Endometrial regeneration

At the end of menstruation, the basal endometrium—glandular, stromal, and vascular—grows and develops to form the subsequent functional endometrial component. This process begins soon after the onset of menstruation. The aim of certain surgical approaches for women with menorrhagia is the complete or near complete destruction of the basal endometrium, leading to amenorrhoea.

The cellular and molecular processes of endometrial repair are poorly understood, but several agents are thought to play a role in endometrial regeneration.[5]
- Interleukins.
- Interferons.
- Epidermal growth factors.
- Insulin-like growth factors.

The proliferative effect of oestradiol on the endometrium is probably mediated by basal endometrial tissue release of the above factors, and many others not yet clearly implicated.

The ovarian cycle

The uterus is a target organ, and menstruation is an active response to changes in the ovarian steroid signals. Therefore, no account of normal menstruation would be complete without a brief review of the ovarian cycle and its physiology.

Follicular growth

Each ovary contains approximately 250 follicles at birth, and in every cycle a small cohort of follicles develop, and some become sensitive to the pituitary gonadotrophin FSH (follicle-stimulating hormone). What induces initial follicular growth and renders a few follicles responsive to FSH remains speculative, but increased sensitivity is paramount to antral follicular development. Follicular oestrogen synthesis is essential for uterine priming, but is also part of the positive feedback that induces the pituitary LH (luteinizing hormone) surge and subsequent ovulation. The growth of the follicle and oocyte over such a short period of time is dramatic. A pre-ovular human follicle can grow up to 25 mm, and an oocyte enlarge from 15 μm to over 100 μm. Inhibin is also thought to be produced by the dominant pre-ovulatory follicle, and its role probably is to suppress FSH levels, and therefore cause other follicles to become atretic.

Corpus luteum

Progesterone production by the corpus luteum is regulated by LH, and subsequently hCG (human chorionic gonadotrophin) if pregnancy occurs. The continuation or cessation of secretion of progesterone in the corpus luteum then controls the onset of menstruation. If pregnancy fails to occur, luteal regression as a probably age-related phenomenon, leads to reduced responsiveness to LH and subsequent luteolysis. With implantation of a blastocyst and hCG secretion the endometrium is sustained and menstruation delayed.

Implantation is a process that includes an embryo reaching the inner uterine wall and penetrating the epithelium and the underlying circulation of the receptive endometrium. This process starts 2–3 days after the fertilized egg enters the uterus. Soon after trophoblastic invasion of the myometrium, hCG is produced by the conceptus. This luteal support with sustained progesterone production is crucial during the first weeks of pregnancy to avert endometrial regression.

The pituitary cycle

Follicular development and ovarian steroidogenesis are regulated by gonadotrophins FSH and LH released from the anterior pituitary. Pulsatile release of gonadotrophin-releasing hormone (GnRH) from the hypothalamus at the start of the cycle stimulates the release of FSH and follicular development in the ovary. Fourteen days before menstruation in a 28-day cycle, the rising level of oestrogen leads to a surge of LH and ovulation.

53 Physiology of normal menstruation

References

1 Hallberg, L., Hogdahl, A.M., Nilsson, L., *et al.* (1966). Menstrual blood loss—a population study. *Acta Obstetrica et Gynaecologica Scandinavica* **45**, 320–51.

2 Chimbira, T.H., Anderson, A.B., and Turnbull, A. (1980). Relation between measured blood loss and patient's subjective assessment of loss, duration of bleeding, number of sanitary towels used, uterine weight and endometrial surface area. *British Journal of Obstetrics and Gynaecology* **87**, 603–9.

3 Baird, D.T., *et al.* (1996). Prostaglandins and menstruation. *European Journal of Obstetrics and Gynaecology and Reproductive Biology* **70**, 15–17.

4 Campbell, S. and Cameron, I.T. (1998). The origins and physiology of menstruation. In *Clinical disorders of the endometrium and menstrual cycle* (ed. I.T. Cameron, I.S. Fraser, and S.K. Smith), pp. 13–30. Oxford University Press, Oxford.

5 Critchley, H.O.D., Kelly, R.W., and Kooy, J. (1994). Perivascular expression of chemokine interleukin-8 in human decidua. *Human Reproduction* **9**, 1406–9.

Chapter 54

Paediatric and adolescent gynaecology

Common childhood conditions

Vaginal discharge

Neonates
Circulating maternal oestrogens exert a physiological effect on the female fetus and it is normal to see a clear, odourless discharge in the early neonatal period. In around 10% of cases it will be bloodstained as a result of endometrial stimulation by the maternal oestrogens. The discharge settles as the levels of maternal hormone in the newborn decline after birth.

Older children (ages 2–7yrs most commonly)
Vulvovaginitis (infection of the vaginal introitus): often presents with recurrent green/yellow discharge, pruritis, or inflammation. Swabs should be taken from introitus below the hymen. The infection is almost exclusively bacterial in origin (*Haemophilus influenzae*, *Staphylococcus*, *Streptococcus*, coliform bacteria and rarely is it due to *Candida* in this age group. Growth of *Gonococcus*, *Trichomonas*, or *Gardnerella* suggests sexual abuse. Treatment consists of appropriate antibiotics, hygiene and clothing advice, and avoidance of constipation.

Pruritis vulvae
This is a collective term for vulval irritation due to a variety of causes in the absence of discharge.
- Threadworms (*Enterobius vermicularis*). Common, diagnose using the sellotape test.
- Non-specific vulvitis. This may be due to a number of dermatological conditions, e.g. eczema, psoriasis, contact dermatitis. They are rarely confined to the vulva.
- Lichen sclerosus. Usually a self-limiting condition in childhood without malignant predisposition. Relapses are not uncommon.
- Warts. Usually due to auto-inoculation from hand lesions or transmitted from the hands of carers. Usually self-limiting, but may require more definitive treatment.

Labial adhesions
These are the most commonly seen condition in toddlers. They develop secondary to chronic inflammation and are usually asymptomatic but may obscure the urethral opening and give rise to urinary symptoms. Treatment consists of reassurance and topical oestrogen cream in 2 weekly cycles until the adhesions separate. Surgery is rarely needed.

Bleeding from the vagina/blood-stained discharge
This should always be investigated. Around 90% will be due to the presence of a foreign body causing an offensive bloody discharge. This requires examination under anaesthetic (EUA) to remove the foreign body.
- Trauma (e.g. straddle injuries) is a common cause of genital bleeding. Tears involving the posterior fourchette or hymen are *not* caused by this mechanism and are suspicious of sexual abuse.
- If no obvious cause is found, rarer causes must be considered, e.g. vaginal tumours/Munchausen's by proxy.

Puberty

Puberty is a recognized continuum of changes that begins around the age of 9 years in girls. Marshall and Tanner[1] described and staged the changes occurring in puberty in terms of breast development or thelarche (stages 1–5), pubic hair development or adrenarche (stages 1–5), and an end growth spurt, with the onset of menstruation or menarche occurring on the downward slope of the growth velocity curve (current average age of menarche is 12.8 years).

Precocious puberty

Pubertal changes before the age of 8 years are considered to be precocious and are divided into two categories.

- True or central precocious puberty: premature activation of the hypothalamo-pituitary-ovarian axis (HPO axis)
  —*Causes*. Largely idiopathic. Can be secondary to brain abnormalities, e.g. hamartomas, hydrocephalus.
  —*Treatment* depends on the cause. Gonadotrophin-releasing hormone (GnRH) analogues are used to postpone puberty until a more appropriate age and to optimize adult height potential.
- Pseudo-precocious puberty. A process independent of the HPO axis. It is much rarer than true precocious puberty.
  —*Causes*. In girls it is often due to an oestrogen-secreting tumour, McCune–Albright syndrome.

When hirsutism/virilization occurs with precocious puberty, late-onset adrenal hyperplasia and adrenal tumours must be excluded.[2]

Delayed puberty

This presents with primary amenorrhoea with or without the presence of secondary sexual characteristics.

Girls with absence of both menses and secondary sexual characteristics by age 14

Possible causes are as follows.

- *Constitutional delay* is by far the most common cause often with a positive family history.
  —Treatment consists of ruling out other causes and reassurance. The induction of puberty can be considered if there are psychological problems.
- *Chronic systemic disease*, e.g. endocrine disorders, cystic fibrosis, chronic renal failure, coeliac disease, emotional or physical neglect.
  —Treating the underlying cause usually triggers puberty.
- *Absence of ovarian function*, e.g. due to premature ovarian failure or due to abnormal gonadal development or gonadal dysgenesis. The majority will have Turner's syndrome.
  —Treatment relies on good psychological support especially regarding fertility issues, induction of puberty, and long-term maintenance of oestrogen levels. Gonadectomy may be necessary if any Y chromosome is present due to increased malignant potential.
- *Hypothalamo-pituitary dysfunction* due to tumours, genetic conditions, or idiopathic.
  —The underlying cause should be treated if possible and, if due to a non-reversible cause, puberty should be induced.

54 Paediatric and adolescent gynaecology

Girls with normal secondary sexual characteristics but absent menses by age 16

Possible causes are the following.

Constitutional delay is again the most common cause, usually with a family history.

Absent uterus/endometrium due to:

—Complete androgen insensitivity syndrome (46 XY female). Treatment is with oestrogen replacement and gonadectomy because of malignant potential. Vaginal reconstruction surgery may be needed and psychological support is vital.

—Rokitansky–Kutser–Hauser syndrome (46XX, absent uterus and upper vagina, associated renal and vertebral anomalies). Treatment might involve vaginal reconstructive surgery. Psychological support is essential especially regarding fertility issues (assisted conception).

Absent vagina/imperforate hymen presents with cyclical abdominal pain, pelvic mass, and absent menses. Treatment is to incise hymen, excise septum, or fashion lower vaginal opening to allow menstrual flow to pass.

Induction of puberty

This aims to mimic the gradual increase in ovarian function at puberty. Treatment is with an incremental ethinyl oestradiol regime in 6 monthly increments. When breakthrough bleeding occurs or when the 20–30 mg dose is reached, progesterone is added for endometrial protection. This is usually the combined pill but hormone replacement therapy (HRT) preparations are also used.

References

Marshall, W.A. and Tanner, J.M. (1969). Variations in the pattern of pubertal changes in girls. *Archives of Disease in Childhood* **44**, 944–54.

Garden, A.S. (1998). *Paediatric and adolescent gynaecology*. Arnold, London.

Chapter 55

Menstrual problems—amenorrhoea, oligomenorrhoea, and dysmenorrhoea

Secondary amenorrhoea is defined as complete cessation of menstrual cycles for a minimum of 6 months. Failure to start menstruating by the age of 16 (14 associated with absent breast development) is described as *primary amenorrhoea*. The aetiology and management of these symptoms are often similar apart from a few specific causes of primary amenorrhoea. The causes of amenorrhoea and their frequencies are given in Table 55.1.

Oligomenorrhoea is defined as menstrual bleeding at intervals of between 35 days and 6 months. This occurs frequently in practice but only needs investigating if it is persistent or associated with other problems.

The aims of investigations for these conditions should include the following.
- To reach a diagnosis, and to address patients' concerns.
- To detect serious causes requiring specific treatment:
  —Anorexia nervosa.
  —Tumours: hypothalamic, pituitary, ovarian
- To detect incidental or secondary conditions that affect general health and require further unrelated treatment.
  —Oestrogen deficiency.
  —Unopposed oestrogen.
- To manage ongoing subfertility: assess the need for ovulation induction and inform woman of prognosis.
- To give sound contraceptive advice on the basis of formal diagnosis.

Genital tract causes

- *Congenital Müllerian duct disorders* cause primary amenorrhoea with abnormalities of varying severity. With functioning ovaries, cyclical symptoms are often present and so is secondary sex hair growth—not so in testicular feminization. Similarly, a haematocolpos—most commonly caused by an imperforate hymen—leads to cyclical abdominal pain.
- *Asherman's syndrome* or endometrial fibrosis[1] is now often induced surgically to achieve amenorrhoea or light periods in women with menorrhagia. It is rarely seen following surgical trauma or pelvic tuberculosis infection.
- *Cervical stenosis* is also very rare and in most cases caused by surgical trauma after repeat surgery for cervical intraepithelial neoplasm (CIN). Laser endocervicectomy is the treatment of choice.

Hypothalamic disorders

The arcuate nucleus of the hypothalamus secretes pulses of GnRH (gonadotrophin-releasing hormone). This is transported in the capillary plexus down the pituitary stalk to the anterior part of pituitary, where GnRH stimulates the synthesis of luteinizing hormone (LH) and follicle-stimulating hormone (FSH).

Primary hypothalamic failure
This occurs in various conditions and presents with clinical evidence of GnRH deficiency. Any central nervous system tumours, e.g. gliomas, can be associated with amenorrhoea, but the latter is of little consequence and often occurs with

her anterior pituitary hormone deficiencies. More important from the ndocrine viewpoint is congenital GnRH deficiency, which results in poorly eveloped females with absence of menarche (isolated gonadotrophin defi- ency). This can occur in association with anosmia due to a coexisting congen- al abnormality of the olfactory bulb and is thought to be X-linked (Kallman's yndrome).

ypothalamic functional disorders

hese are the most common causes of secondary amenorrhoea. The majority of uses are related to emotional/psychological stress, weight loss, or excessive hysical exercise.[2] They are most common in teenagers.

ith loss of body mass the onset of amenorrhoea is often abrupt and cycles do ot return immediately after the weight is regained.[3] Severe gonadotrophin eficiency is seen in anorexia nervosa. Oestrogen hormone replacement therapy ust be considered in the management of such patients.

able 55.1 Causes of amenorrhoea with frequency

Cause	Frequency (%)
Polycystic ovarian disease	33
Hypothalamic disorders	35
Hyperprolactinaemia (prolactinoma in 50%)	20
Primary ovarian failure	12
Thyroid disease	1
Adrenal causes	< 1
Anatomical causes	< 1

487

Pituitary dysfunction

- *Primary failure*. Sheehan's syndrome, which is due to postpartum hypotension with subsequent anterior pituitary gland necrosis, is now rare. Tumours causing compression of the pituitary stalk or lesions causing damage to the pituitary gland—empty sella syndrome—lead to amenorrhoea either by destruction of the gonadotrophes and gonadotrophin deficiency or by causing hyperprolactinaemia by interfering with the negative feedback effect of dopamine secretion and transport along the pituitary stalk.
- *Pituitary functional disorders*. Hyperprolactinaemia is by far the most common pituitary disorder causing amenorrhoea. Prolactin secretion from the pituitary lactotrophes is inhibited by dopamine transported down the pituitary stalk from the hypothalamus.

Causes of hyperprolactinaemia
Physiological causes
Pregnancy and *lactation* are by far the most common causes of hyperprolactinaemia, followed by *stress* and *exercise*. Some women find initial hospital visits very stressful. Therefore estimation of prolactin levels needs to be repeated after subsequent visits.

Nipple stimulation at times of sexual foreplay can cause both increased prolactin levels and subsequent galactorrhoea. A detailed and cautious history is essential.

Pharmacological causes
Any drug that antagonizes dopamine receptors or acts as a neurotransmitter can cause hyperprolactinaemia. Phenothiazines and other drugs used to treat psychiatric conditions have been implicated, together with methyldopa, opiates and oestrogens. If uncertainty exists regarding a certain drug, further information must be obtained from a Drugs Information Unit.

Pathological causes
- Moderate hyperprolactinaemia (less than 1750 mU/L) occurs in patients with hypothyroidism and similarly in association with polycystic ovarian syndrome, possibly caused by increased unopposed oestrogen in the latter.
- A *primary* pituitary neoplasm may produce excessive prolactin.
  —*Macro-prolactinomas* (diameter greater than 10 mm) are associated with very high levels of prolactin (8000 mU/L or more).
  —*Micro-prolactinomas* usually have lower levels of prolactin (less than 3000 mU/L) and do not always require ongoing treatment with dopamine agonists.

Diagnosis and management
For diagnosis repeat serum prolactin estimates and thyroid function tests must be performed. Pituitary imaging by computerized tomography (CT) or magnetic resonance imaging (MRI) and formal visual field evaluation are essential to reach a diagnosis, but also as part of ongoing surveillance of primary hyperprolactinaemia.

Treatment is for subfertility or symptomatic galactorrhoea or oestrogen replacement to avert long-term complications of hypogonadism.

- *Bromocriptine* is effective in over 90% of patients with a prolactinoma. Galactorrhoea also decreases in the vast majority of patients. Side-effects include nausea, dizziness, and postural hypotension. These can be reduced by incremental and split dosage regimes starting with a 1.25 mg dose taken before bedtime with the aim of increasing to a target dose of 7.5 mg.
- *Carbegoline*, a potent and long-acting dopamine agonist, offers new therapeutic options.[4] The recommended initial dose is 0.25 mg twice weekly aiming for a maximum of 1 mg twice weekly. Carbegoline is better tolerated than bromocriptine.
- *Transphenoidal surgery* as part of the management of prolactinomas is now mostly limited to patients with dopamine agonist resistance or marked intolerance.

Hyperprolactinaemia and fertility

There is no benefit in performing serum prolactin levels with ongoing subfertility in women who have regular menstrual cycles. Confusion can instead arise in the rare event of finding high levels of non-bioactive macro (big) prolactin levels. Not much is known about this condition which does not affect fertility.

Unless there is a coexisting problem, regular menstrual cycles return and so does fertility in the majority of women with prolactinomas once the prolactin levels are normalized with dopamine agonists.

Treatment during pregnancy

During pregnancy, the normal pituitary gland is known to enlarge.
- The risk of a treated microprolactinoma enlarging significantly during pregnancy is extremely low. Therefore treatment can be stopped once pregnancy is diagnosed.[5]
- A macroprolactinoma must be treated and tumour shrinkage to within the sella and normal fields confirmed prior to considering a pregnancy. Treatment can be stopped once pregnancy is diagnosed. There is controversy about the need for surveillance during pregnancy.
  —Visual fields during the second and third trimester are often performed, although sudden and unpredictable acute suprasellar extension rarely occurs. If suspected, therapy with a dopamine agonist is resumed after confirmation by MRI.

489

Gonadal failures

The primary ovarian disorders include the following.
- Premature ovarian failure.
- Autoimmune disease.
- Destruction.
- Sex chromosomal abnormalities.

Premature ovarian failure

The menopause occurs before the age of 40 in 1% of women, and in more than two-thirds the aetiology remains unknown. This is termed *premature ovarian failure* and accounts for approximately 10% of amenorrhoeic women. This can occur at any age, and may present with absence of menarche—primary amenorrhoea. The main candidate gene for premature ovarian failure—hypergonadotrophic hypogonadism—is possibly the FSH receptor gene.

Autoimmunity

Based on the presence of auto-antibodies (thyroid and, less frequently, ovarian antibodies) autoimmunity has been estimated to be the cause of ovarian damage in 20–30% of women with primary ovarian failure. Treatment with glucocorticosteroids has been reported to restore fertility in this subgroup. Spontaneous resumption of ovulation may occur.

The resistant ovary syndrome

Another small subgroup of women with clear hypergonadotrophic amenorrhoea of unknown cause does, after a period of time, resume spontaneous menstrual cycles and even conceive—the *resistant ovary syndrome*. The place for exogenous gonadotrophin therapy in this subgroup remains unclear.

Destruction

Radiotherapy and *chemotherapy* for neoplastic conditions are increasing causes of premature ovarian failure, e.g. treatment of lymphomas. Freezing of ovarian tissue is now offered to women prior to therapy, but future use has not as yet been clearly defined.

In the older age group *surgery* is a common cause of premature menopause, requiring hormone replacement therapy.

Sex chromosomal abnormalities

Turner's syndrome (XO ovarian dysgenesis) is the most commonst chromosome abnormality. It presents with primary amenorrhoea, short stature, and sexual infantilism. Patients with Turner's mosaics very occasionally develop secondary sexual features and menstruate. Other forms of abnormalities including 46XY gonadal dysgenesis and testicular feminization are discussed in Chapter 52.

The treatment of Turner's syndrome includes growth hormone and oestrogens, both causing a growth spurt. The oestrogen should be started from about the age of 10–11 to stimulate normal secondary sex characteristic development (first year 5 μg/day, second year 10 μg/day, and third year 20 μg/day). A withdrawal bleed is likely to occur any time after 10 μg/day and, when it occurs, a combined oestrogen/progestogen prepration should be introduced.

Investigations of amenorrhoea/oligomenorrhoea

- *Serum FSH.* Raised in primary ovarian failure. Normal size ovaries by scan and autoantibodies suggest autoimmune ovarian failure.
- *Serum LH.* Raised in polycystic ovary (PCO), but normal level is of no diagnostic value.
- *Serum prolactin.* Raised level is diagnostic of hyperprolactinaemia.
- *Serum testosterone.* Requested only if there is associated hirsutism. Significantly raised levels (over 7 nmol/L) are suspicious of tumour.
- *Thyroid function test.*
- *Progestogen challenge test.* A negative test is suggestive of oestrogen deficiency due to primary or secondary (hypothalamic/pituitary) ovarian failure. A positive test suggests oestrogenized endometrium as in PCO.
- *Chromosome analysis.* Important in certain patients with primary amenorrhoea.
- *Diagnostic imaging.* Lateral X-ray, CT, or MRI of pituitary fossa in all women with suspected secondary amenorrhoea of hypothalamic/pituitary origin.
- *Pelvic ultrasound* is useful to investigate the structure of ovaries and the size of the uterus including endometrial thickness.

Dysmenorrhoea

Crampy lower abdominal pain radiating to the back and legs associated with menstruation is a common symptom in women of reproductive age. Primary dysmenorrhoea in adolescents usually occurs in the absence of pelvic pathology. Secondary dysmenorrhoea is pain that develops later in reproductive life and is more likely to be associated with pelvic pathology.

Primary dysmenorrhoea

This starts soon after menarche with the onset of ovular cycles. It is suprapubic, tends to be worst on the first day of menstruation, and improves thereafter. Patients with primary dysmenorrhoea have been shown to have increased frequency and amplitude of myometrial contractions mediated by prostaglandins.

- *Investigations* of primary dysmenorrhoea are predominantly to exclude any pelvic pathology and are similar to those for secondary dysmenorrhoea (see below).
- *Treatment.* Over 80% of women with this condition respond to therapy with *nonsteroidal anti-inflammatory* drugs (NSAIDs) started 24–48 hours before the onset of pain. Mefenamic acid 500 mg or ibuprofen 400 mg three times a day are often prescribed. Side-effects are mostly gastrointestinal.[6]
  - —The use of combined oral *oestrogen/progestogen* contraceptives leading to anovulatory cycles is a useful second line of management that should be continued for 9–12 months if symptom improves. Otherwise, investigations are stepped up as per secondary dysmenorrhoea.

Secondary dysmenorrhoea

This exhibits various patterns depending on the underlying pathology.

- The presence of dyspareunia is significant, and the associated pelvic/lower abdominal pain occurs either intra/postmenstrually, starts premenstrually, or only occurs on days 1 and 2 of the menstrual cycle. This is discussed in detail in Chapters 65–7.
- The pattern of secondary dysmenorrhoea caused by an endometrial polyp is similar to that seen with submucous fibroids and usually occurs at the beginning of menstruation.

Investigations planned are determined by the history and clinical examination findings. Investigations may include basic haematological investigations and erythrocyte sedimentation rate (ESR) or C-reactive protein with or without microbiological swabs from the genital tract followed by ultrasound, laparoscopy, and/or hysteroscopy.

The *treatment* of secondary dysmenorrhoea is that of the underlying condition discussed in the relevant chapters.

493

References

1 Schenker, J.G. and Margalioth, E.J. (1982). Intrauterine adhesions: an updated appraisal. *Fertility and Sterility* **37**, 593–610.

2 Boydon, T.W., Pamenter, R.W., Grosso, D., Stanforth, P., Rotkis, T., and Wilmore, J.H. (1982). Prolactin responses, menstrual cycles, and body composition of women runners. *Journal Clinical Endocrinology & Metabolism.* **54**, 711–714.

3 Warren, M.P. and Vande Wiele, R. L. (1973). Clinical and metabolic features of anorexia nervosa. *American Journal of Obstetrics and Gynaecology* **117**, 435–49.

4 Bevan, J.S. and Davis, J.R. (1994). Cabergoline: an advance in dopaminergic therapy. *Clinical Endocrinology (Oxf.)* **41**, 709–12.

5 Soule, S.G. and Jacobs, H.G. (1995). Prolactinomas: present day management. *British Journal of Obstetrics & Gynaecology* **102**, 178–81.

6 Anderson, A.B. (1981). The role of prostaglandin synthetase inhibitors in gynaecology. *Practitioner* **225**, 1460–70.

Chapter 56

Dysfunctional uterine bleeding

Dysfunctional uterine bleeding (DUB) is defined as excessively heavy (> 80 ml per month) or prolonged uterine bleeding in the absence of systemic or genital tract pathology. It is a diagnosis of exclusion. It affects 10% of women[1] and is the most common cause of iron deficiency anaemia and gynaecological referrals. Although up to 30% of women report symptoms of heavy or prolonged menstrual bleeding (menorrhagia), this is confirmed on objective measurement in fewer than a third of cases. Dysfunctional uterine bleeding is divided into ovulatory, which is associated with regular painful periods, and anovulatory, which is more common in the postmenarcheal and perimenopausal age groups.

Diagnosis

History
Ask about age, parity, fertility, current contraception, and previous treatment for abnormal uterine bleeding. To assess the heaviness of bleeding ask about the duration of the periods, amount, sanitary protection used, and whether the women passes clots during menstruation. The presence of bleeding between the periods or a recent onset of pain at the time of menstruation are suggestive of pelvic pathology.

Examination
A general examination may reveal signs of thyroid disease, anaemia, or clotting disorders. An abdominal examination should precede a pelvic examination. All women with abnormal genital tract bleeding must have a speculum examination to visualize the cervix and vagina to exclude any local cause. A cervical smear is taken if not recently performed. On pelvic examination check for uterine enlargement (fibroids) or the tender, fixed uterus typical of pelvic inflammatory disease or endometriosis.

Investigations
Abnormal bleeding can occur in early pregnancy. If there is any possibility of pregnancy this should be excluded by a pregnancy test. A full blood count (FBC) to exclude anaemia should be carried out for all women complaining of abnormal uterine bleeding. Thyroid function tests and a hormone profile are not usually required unless otherwise clinically indicated. Pipelle endometrial sampling, hysteroscopy (as an out-patient or day case surgery under general anaesthesia), and transvaginal ultrasound scan should be carried out to exclude endometrial pathology for patients above 40 years. Below the age of 40 the risk of endometrial cancer is very low, and endometrial sampling is not normally required for regular heavy periods. Irregular bleeding warrants hysteroscopy and sampling to rule out endometrial pathology.

Medical management

The treatment of DUB should be with the simplest regimen with the fewest side-effects that is effective. First-line therapy is medical and will depend on the patient's need for contraception and on whether irregularity of the cycle is a problem. Regardless of which therapy is chosen treatment should be reviewed after 3 months and, if there is no response, the patient should be referred for further investigation.

Patients with a regular cycle who do not require contraception

- *Tranexamic acid* (antifibrinolytic). This is the most effective first-line drug.[2] It acts by inhibiting tissue plasminogen activator (a fibrinolytic enzyme that has raised levels in women with DUB) and reduces menstrual blood loss (MBL) by around 50%. The dose of tranexamic acid is 1 g three to four times a day during menstruation. The side-effects are mainly gastrointestinal symptoms. It is contraindicated where there is a history of thromboembolic disease.
- *Nonsteroidal anti-inflammatory drugs* (NSAIDS) such as mefenamic acid are effective, well tested, and tolerated. They act by inhibiting cyclo-oxygenase and this blocks myometrial prostaglandin PGE_2 receptors. NSAIDs reduce MBL by 25% and are also analgesic drugs, so they are often used as a first-line treatment in the presence of dysmenorrhoea. Mefenamic acid is commonly used at a dose of 500 mg three times a day for 5 days during menses. The main side-effect is gastrointestinal irritation.

Patients with an irregular cycle or who need contraception

- The *combined oral contraceptive pill* (COCP) is commonly used especially in the younger age group. It reduces MBL by 20%, helps to regulate periods, and provides contraception. The mode of action is by inhibition of ovulation, production of inactive endometrium, and possibly by reduction in endometrial prostaglandin synthesis and altered fibrinolysis. See Chapter 75 for further details on side-effects and contraindications.
- In the perimenopausal age group sequential combined *hormone replacement therapy* (HRT) can be used in a similar way to regulate the cycle and reduce mean blood loss.
- *Progestogens.* Synthetic progestogens (e.g. norethisterone 5 mg 8-hourly from day 12–26 or day 5–26) are the most popular drugs prescribed in general practice in the UK for the treatment of menorrhagia even though they have minimal or no effect on MBL. Progestogen therapy can be of value in regulating an irregular cycle. The main side-effects are weight gain, bloating, and androgenic symptoms such as acne.
- *Levonorgestrel-releasing intrauterine contraceptive device (Mirena)* releases 20 µg of levonogestrel per 24 hours over 5 years. The modes of action of levonogestrel are a reduction in endometrial prostaglandin synthesis, the production of inactive endometrium, and a reduction in endometrial fibrinolytic activity. It reduces MBL by 86% after 3 months.[3]
- If a copper intrauterine contraceptive device is already *in situ*, either treat with tranexamic acid/NSAIDS or change to levonogestrel intrauterine device. Patients should be warned that irregular bleeding is common during the first 3 months after insertion.
- Depo-provera used for contraception is also associated with reduced MBL and amenorrhoea in some women.

econd-line medical treatment

Danazol (100 mg 6–24 hourly) is a synthetic steroid that acts in a number of ways. It inhibits steroid synthesis, blocks the androgen and progesterone receptors, and inhibits pituitary gonadotrophins.[4] These actions combine to inhibit endometrial growth. Its use is limited by the androgenic side-effects (acne, hirsutism, breast atrophy, and weight gain) and high cost.

Gonadotrophin-releasing hormone analogues (GnRH-a) downregulate the pituitary and inhibit follicle-stimulating hormone (FSH) and luteinizing hormone (LH) production. They are highly effective in producing amenorrhoea in DUB but treatment is limited to 6 months because of the risk of osteoporosis.

Ethamsylate, which acts by preventing the breakdown of capillaries, is ineffective in reducing menstrual blood loss.

Surgical management

For patients who have completed their family and have failed medical management, surgical management can be considered.

Endometrial ablation or resection (hysteroscopic procedures)

These are useful alternatives to hysterectomy in cases of DUB. Approximately 75% of women obtain a satisfactory improvement in their symptoms and the recovery time is significantly less than that for hysterectomy. About 40–50% of patients become amenorrhoeic after endometrial ablation, with a further 20–30% reporting reduced menstrual bleeding. 20–30% of patients have no improvement, and up to 10% require further treatment such as hysterectomy. The procedure can be performed using laser photovaporization, electrosurgical resection or ablation by resectoscope, or intrauterine thermal coagulation (balloon procedures). These procedures are less effective in women under 35 or where pain is a significant associated symptom or when the uterus is enlarged. They are contraindicated if future fertility is desired. GnRH-analogues for 8 weeks prior to surgery are often used to thin the endometrium. These procedures can be carried out as day-case surgery, offer quick recovery, and are highly effective with significant reduction in menstrual blood loss. There is a small risk of serious complications such as uterine perforation, haemorrhage, or fluid overload.

Hysterectomy

Hysterectomy is one of the most common major operations in the UK. It is the definitive treatment for patients with DUB, with a higher rate of patient satisfaction than in hysteroscopic endometrial ablation at 6 months. By the age of 60 20% of all women in the UK have had a hysterectomy. More than 40% of hysterectomies are for DUB.[6] Hysterectomy can be performed abdominally, vaginally or laparoscopically. Abdominal hysterectomy carries a higher risk of morbidity than vaginal hysterectomy, so vaginal hysterectomy is the route of choice unless contraindicated. Selecting one approach over another depends on various factors, such as age, parity, history of pelvic surgery, desire for ovarian preservation, and the presence of pelvic disease (such as endometriosis or adhesions). Abdominal hysterectomy should be reserved only for a small group of patients who cannot be offered the less invasive approaches (vaginal or laparoscopic hysterectomy).[7] Complications of hysterectomy include:

- *Intraoperative*: bleeding, damage to pelvic organs, and anaesthetic.
- *Postoperative*: bleeding, wound infection and dehiscence, thromboembolism, ureteric or vesical fistula, chest and urinary tract infection.
- *Long-term complications* are prolapse and early ovarian failure.

References

Irvine, G.A. and Cameron, I.T. (1999). Medical management of dysfunctional uterine bleeding. *Baillière's Clinical Obstetrics and Gynaecology* **13** (2), 189–202.

Prentice, A. (1999). Medical management of menorrhagia [fortnightly review]. *British Medical Journal* **319**, 1343–5.

Barrington, J.W. and Bowen-Simpkins, P. (1997). The levonorgestrel intrauterine system in the management of menorrhagia. *British Journal of Obstetrics and Gynaecology* **104**, 614–16.

Weeks, A.D. and Duffy, S.R.G. (1996). Abnormal uterine bleeding: diagnosis and medical management. *Progress in Obstetrics and Gynaecology* **12**, 309–26.

Overton, C., Hargreaves, J., and Maresh, M.A. (1997). A national survey of the complications of endometrial destruction for menstrual disorders: the MISTLETOE study. *British Journal of Obstetrics and Gynaecology* **104**, 1351–9.

Royal College of Obstetricians and Gynaecologists (RCOG) (1998). *Evidence-based clinical guidelines—the initial management of menorrhagia.* RCOG, London.

Reich, H., Ribeiro, S.C., and Vidali, A. (1999). Hysterectomy as treatment for dysfunctional uterine bleeding. *Baillière's Clinical Obstetrics and Gynaecology* **13** (2), 251–69.

Chapter 57

Termination of pregnancy (TOP)

Termination of pregnancy (TOP) is defined as the removal of pregnancy from the uterus in a manner that does not anticipate subsequent survival of the fetus. The laws governing TOP vary from country to country.

Over 150 000 TOP procedures are performed each year in England and Wales with 55% carried out by the National Health Service (NHS) and the rest in private clinics (e.g. British Pregnancy Advisory Service, Marie Stopes) operating on a charitable basis.

Termination of pregnancy in the UK

TOPs in the UK are performed under the legal umbrella of the 1967 Abortion Act (amended as the *Human Fertilisation and Embryology Act*, 1990). Two doctors need to decide in good faith that one or more of five conditions apply and complete Form HSA 1. The five conditions are:

(a) The continuance of the pregnancy would involve risk to the life of the pregnant woman greater than if the pregnancy were terminated.

(b) The termination is necessary to prevent grave permanent injury to the physical or mental health of the pregnant woman.

(c) The pregnancy has not exceeded its 24th week and the continuance of the pregnancy would involve risk, greater than if the pregnancy were terminated, of injury to the physical or mental health of the pregnant woman.

(d) The pregnancy has not exceeded its 24th week and the continuance of the pregnancy would involve risk, greater than if the pregnancy were terminated, of injury to the physical or mental health of any existing child(ren) of the family of the pregnant woman.

(e) There is substantial risk that if the child were born it would suffer from such physical or mental abnormalities as to be seriously handicapped.

Of TOPs 98% are done under clauses (a)–(d).

- No practitioners are under any duty to participate in abortion procedures they have a conscientious objection provided that this does not involve risk of grave permanent injury or death to their patient.
- Dedicated clinics and operating lists may achieve better counselling and lower operative complication rates.
- It is advisable to care for TOP patients separate from other gynaecological cases especially those with infertility/miscarriage.
- Confidentiality is essential in the management of women seeking termination and it may be necessary to make it clear to patients that it is always maintained, especially so for teenagers seeking TOP without parental awareness.

Management prior to termination of pregnancy

- A full clinical check should be carried out, especially menstrual history and gestational age.
- Arrange an ultrasound scan if there is any doubt about gestational age.
- Check Hb and blood group. (Cross-match is not routinely indicated: may need anti-D if mother is rhesus-negative).
- Genital tract swabs should be taken for chlamydia, gonorrhea, and bacterial vaginosis and any infection should be treated preoperatively. If swab results are not available, antibiotic prophylaxis should be used.
- Take a cervical smear if due, especially if patient had been defaulting recall.
- Counsel on the procedure and complications. Providing written information is advisable as this can be read and better understood at the patient's leisure.
- Discuss and arrange future contraception but avoid sterilization at TOP. The unplanned pregnancy is often a result of inadequate or total lack of contraception and the consultation provides a valuable opportunity to address this.

Consent

Valid consent is necessary, after full counselling. The use of written information is becoming more widespread. Although parental involvement is ideal, girls under 16 may sign consent for TOP if they decline parental involvement and doctors feel they are 'mature' enough (Gilick competent) to comprehend their circumstances.

Methods

First trimester

- *Vacuum aspiration*. This is usually a day-case procedure under general anaesthesia but may be performed under paracervical block. Vacuum aspiration is the conventional method used from 7 to 12 weeks gestation. The cervix is primed with vaginal prostaglandin preoperatively and dilated to 8–12 mm at surgery. A plastic aspiration cannula is used with a vacuum device to empty the uterus and an oxytocic is administered to reduce blood loss and risk of perforation.
- *Medical TOP*. Up to 9 weeks gestation, oral mifepristone (RU 486) 600 mg followed 48 hours later by vaginal prostaglandin e.g. misoprostol 600 µg or gemeprost 1 mg PV (per vagina) will produce complete abortion in 95%, incomplete abortion in 4%, and failure in under 1%.
- Surgical procedure is avoided in 95% of cases.

Second trimester

- *Dilatation and evacuation* (D&E). This is a similar procedure to first-trimester vacuum aspiration but needs further cervical dilatation and removal of fetal parts with forceps. It also needs considerable skill to minimize complications.
  —The risk of cervical incompetence is increased as a result of the degree of dilatation necessary and there is a higher risk of major complications, e.g. uterine perforation and visceral damage.
  —It is not suitable for cases of fetal abnormality when post-mortem examination is recommended.
- *Hysterotomy*. This is now rarely used for TOP. It may rarely be appropriate in cases of conjoint twins in mid-trimester when vaginal expulsion may not be feasible.
- *Medical TOP*
  —*Medication by oral route*. Oral mifepristone 600 mg followed 36 to 48 hours later by 1 mg of gemeprost vaginally. Administration of gemeprost 1 mg, 3-hourly, to a maximum of 5 pessaries is licensed for mid-trimester TOP. Other published, but unlicensed regimes include 200 mg oral mifepristone followed by vaginal misoprostol 400 µg and 200 mg oral mifepristone followed by 6 hourly gemeprost 1 mg.
  —*Medication by vaginal route*. Vaginal gemeprost 1 mg 3-hourly (maximum 5 in 24 hrs) or misoprostol (200–600 µg) 4- to 6-hourly results in abortion within 24 hours in 85% of cases. The fetus, although non-viable, may be born alive, causing undue distress to staff and patients. The advantage of this method is that surgery is avoided and the fetus delivered intact for post-mortem examination in cases of fetal anomaly.
  —*Medication by extra-amniotic route*. A self-retaining catheter is passed through the cervix into the extra-amniotic space and a continuous infusion of PGE_2 is given until the cervix is sufficiently dilated to allow catheter balloon to be expelled, followed by an oxytocic infusion.

—*Medication by intra-amniotic route.* This is currently the recommended method after 20 weeks gestation. Amniocentesis is performed, 100–200 mL of liquor removed, and replaced with 80–120 g of 20% urea and up to 5 µg of PGE_2. This usually produces fetal death before expulsion, reducing the distress to patients and staff. Continuous ultrasound scanning is essential for the procedure, to prevent intravascular injection, leading to coagulopathy and cardiogenic collapse.

etal demise can also be achieved by intracardiac KCl injection or air emboliza-
on under ultrasound guidance.

Complications

The majority (over 95%) of TOPs are undertaken on otherwise healthy young women for personal and social reasons. Complaints and litigation are not that uncommon when complications occur. Complication rates depend on stage of gestation, method of termination, skill of operator, and coexisting conditions e.g. uterine abnormalities.

Haemorrhage

The incidence is 1.5/1000 under 13 weeks gestation and 8.5/1000 over 20 weeks gestation. Significant haemorrhage (needing blood transfusion) at the time of TOP or soon after is rare in the first trimester. It is more likely with a retained placenta in the second trimester. Secondary haemorrhage, usually from infection, if not promptly treated can result in significant blood loss.

Infection

In the presence of chlamydia, gonorrhea, and bacterial vaginosis, there is a high risk of postoperative pelvic inflammatory disease (PID), which may result in infertility. This risk is minimized by taking swabs preoperatively and by using prophylactic antibiotics at the time of TOP. Preoperative metronidazole 1 g rectally and erythromycin 1 g orally, or postoperative doxycycline 100 mg twice daily for 7 days will provide sufficient cover. A single dose of azithromycin is also effective. Uncomplicated TOP does not impair fertility but if other problems occur it may result in subfertility and the patient is likely to reflect adversely on the TOP.

Major complications leading to hysterectomy, although rare, imply loss of fertility. These aspects should be discussed during counselling.

Retained products of conception (RPOC)

This has an incidence of 1–2%. It may sometimes necessitate repeat uterine evacuation. Antibiotic cover should be given if repeat evacuation is being considered. The risks of infection and perforation are higher than at the first procedure.

Ultrasound is sometimes useful in diagnosis but blood clots are commonly seen making diagnosis difficult. Clinical features must therefore be foremost in the diagnostic process.

Uterine perforation

The incidence is 1–4/1000. This may go unnoticed at time of TOP and present later as abdominal pain and tenderness or shock. When suspected at TOP a laparoscopy is indicated to confirm. If bleeding from the perforation is significant, laparotomy and suturing is indicated. Otherwise, it may be possible to treat conservatively, including antibiotic cover. It is still necessary to complete the TOP and this should be done under laparoscopic control or at the laparotomy.

During mid-trimester D&E, bony fetal parts may lacerate/perforate the uterus. When a suction cannula has been inserted into a perforated uterus, visceral damage should be thoroughly sought and if found it should be repaired, usually by laparotomy. A bowel surgeon or other appropriate surgeon should be involved. If perforation has occurred into the broad ligament, the damage to blood vessels may be such that hysterectomy may be required to control haemorrhage.

Failure to abort

The incidence is 2.3/1000 for surgical TOP and 6/1000 for medical TOP.

Failure to abort is more likely at early gestations. The Royal College of Obstetricians and Gynaecologists recommends that suction TOP be avoided under 7 weeks. Skilled operators can usually recognize that less tissue has been obtained by suction than expected.

Unknown multiple pregnancy or bicornuate uterus may lead to failure to abort as one fetus may be completely spared or the suction cannula introduced only into the empty horn.

Ectopic pregnancy may also be missed, especially when coexisting with intrauterine pregnancy (heterotopic pregnancy). If ectopic pregnancy is suspected during a TOP procedure, a diagnostic laparoscopy is indicated.

Products of conception are not routinely sent for histological examination after TOP performed for 'social' indications. Unlike medical TOP, follow-up is not usually arranged for surgical TOP and thus there may be a delay in diagnosing failure to abort. The risk may be reduced by giving verbal and written instructions on what to expect after TOP, e.g. rapid cessation of pregnancy symptoms and return of menstruation in about 4 weeks. If in doubt, follow-up with ultrasound scan and serum beta human chorionic gonadotrophin (β-hCG) is prudent.

Cervical trauma

Incidence is < 1%. Cervical trauma is usually minor in form, e.g. lacerations from forceps used in holding the cervix and creation of a false passage. If a false passage is created, it is extremely difficult to find the cervical canal. Postponement with cervical priming at a later date may be necessary.

- Damage to the circular fibres of the cervix may result in cervical incompetence.
- Dilatation beyond 10 mm is usually necessary for D&E and this is more likely to cause cervical incompetence. Cervical priming with misoprostol 400 µg or gemeprost 1 mg reduces the risk of trauma to the cervix.

Rhesus isoimmunization

Anti-D globulin should be given in appropriate dosage to prevent Rh isoimmunization of Rh-negative women.

Hysterectomy

Rarely, haemorrhage is uncontrollable and hysterectomy unavoidable. Every effort should be made to contact the patient's family to discuss the problem while the patient is under anaesthetic. A full explanation should be given to patient/and family as soon as possible after the procedure.

Complications (*continued*)

Psychological sequelae

Because TOP is often sought because of personal and social difficulties, feeling of guilt are common after the procedure. Preoperative counselling shoul ensure that patients have given careful thought to their options. Further post operative counselling should be arranged when indicated. This may includ social services input if appropriate. If a patient has doubts about undergoing th procedure preoperatively, it is best to allow some time for her to reach a definit decision before committing to TOP. A small number of women may appea unable to decide for themselves. It is advisable that a medical practitioner doe not decide what is best for them.

Recommended further reading

Office for National Statistics (1997). *Abortion statistics 1995* (*England and Wales*), Series AB no. 22. HMSO, London.

Department of Health and Social Security (DHSS) (1986). *Family planning services for young people*, Health Circular HC (FP0(86)1). DHSS, London.

Argent, V.P. (2000). Induced abortion. *The Obstetrician and Gynaecologist* 2 (2), 31–6.

Royal College of Obstetricians and Gynaecologists (RCOG) (2000). *The care of women requesting induced abortion*, Evidence-based guideline no. 7. RCOG, London.

MacKenzie, I.Z. (1992). Pregnancy termination. In *Prenatal diagnosis and screening* (ed. D.J.H. Brock, C.H. Rodeck, and M. Ferguson-Smith), pp. 675–87. Churchill Livingstone, New York.

Ectopic pregnancy

Ectopic pregnancy is implantation occurring outside of the uterine cavity. affects 11.5 per 1000 pregnancies in the UK. The number of cases has doubl over the last 10 years, although this may be in part due to better methods diagnosis. It is the major cause of maternal mortality in the first trimester pregnancy (4% of maternal deaths, 4 deaths/10 000 ectopic pregnancies).

Aetiology

Tubal transit of the fertilized ovum takes approximately 3–4 days and depen on the patency of the Fallopian tube, the action of the ciliated epithelium lini of the tube, tubal peristalsis, and relaxation of the tubal isthmus. If tubal tran is delayed, implantation occurs on the papillary fronds, eventually leading obliteration of the tubal epithelium, invasion of the muscularis layer of the tul and perforation into the retroperitoneal space. If rupture does not occur, t blood and embryo are either expelled from the tube (tubal abortion) or rea sorbed. A minority of pregnancies re-implant in the peritoneal cavity and su vive into the third trimester.

- Factors associated with an increased risk of ectopic implantation include previous tubal surgery and ectopic pregnancy, failed sterilization or intrauterine contraceptive device (IUCD), pelvic inflammatory disease (PID), and assisted reproductive techniques.

Presentation

Of ectopic pregnancies, 97% occur in the Fallopian tubes, the most common si being in the ampullary region. 25% of cases occur in the narrower tubal isthm where rupture and early presentation are more likely and 3% implant on tl cervix, ovary, or peritoneum. Simultaneous intrauterine and tubal ectopic pre nancies (hetero-ectopics) occur in 1 in 3000 to 1 in 30 000 pregnancies.

- 15% of cases present acutely with abdominal pain, amenorrhoea, and haemodynamic compromise.
- Patients may complain of shoulder tip discomfort because of referred pair as a result of irritation of the diaphragm from intraperitoneal haemorrhage.
- There may be a history of syncope or feeling faint.
- Irritation of the pelvic peritoneum causes pain on defecation and diarrhoe or pain on micturition.
- In most cases the history will be more chronic.
- Typically, ectopics present after 6–8 weeks of amenorrhoea but they can present at any stage of pregnancy (or when there is no history of a missed period).
- There may be associated vaginal bleeding. This is due to shedding of the decidual lining of the uterus rather than bleeding from the ectopic itself and is usually lighter than that seen with miscarriage. Classically, it occurs after the onset of symptoms of abdominal pain, whereas that from miscarriage tends to precede abdominal pain. The abdominal pain tends to be more unilateral than that seen with miscarriage.
- Ectopic pregnancies may also be identified when an early pregnancy ultrasound scan is performed or suspected following a uterine evacuation for suspected miscarriage when the histology report fails to show any evidence of chorionic villi but a decidual reaction (Arias–Stella reaction).

514

Diagnosis

Clinical

Ectopic pregnancy should be excluded in any woman with pain or irregular bleeding in early pregnancy. There may be a history of risk factors. On examination look for signs of intraperitoneal haemorrhage including abdominal tenderness (95%), peritonism, abdominal distension, or pain on movement of the cervix (cervical excitation, 50%). If there is pelvic tenderness it will tend to be localized more to one adnexa and there may be an adnexal mass (63%). The cervical os will be closed.

Ultrasound

The presence of an intrauterine gestation sac will usually exclude ectopic pregnancy but can be mimicked by the decidual reaction (decidual ring) associated with ectopic pregnancy (look for a yolk sac or fetal pole). An intrauterine gestation sac should be identified in an ongoing viable intrauterine pregnancy by 5 weeks or where the serum β–hCG (beta human chorionic gonadotrophin) level is greater than 1000 IU/L (by transvaginal scan; 6000 IU/L on abdominal ultrasound).

The presence of free fluid within the peritoneal cavity or of an adnexal mass in the absence of an intrauterine pregnancy is highly suggestive of an ectopic pregnancy. Rarely, it may be possible to identify an extrauterine fetal heartbeat.

hCG measurement

Following conception, hCG can be detected in the maternal serum within 7 days and in maternal urine by the time the first period would have been due had conception not occurred.

A negative urinary pregnancy test will exclude all but 3% of pregnancies and a negative serum hCG effectively excludes the possibility of ectopic pregnancy.

Quantitative serum hCG measurement is also of value in determining whether an intrauterine pregnancy should be seen on ultrasound (see above).

At lower levels of hCG, serial measurements 48 hours apart will show an increase of more than 66% in 85% of normal pregnancies and a suboptimal rise in more than 80% of ectopic pregnancies.

Laparoscopy

This remains the definitive method of diagnosis but is associated with a 1 in 500 risk of injury to the bowel or abdominal blood vessels. False-negative results occur in 4–5% of cases.

515

Management

Patients with suspected ectopic pregnancy should be referred for urgent hospital assessment.

- Pelvic examination should be delayed until facilities for resuscitation and surgical treatment are available.
- Intravenous access should be secured and blood sent for group and cross-matching, full blood count, and serum saved for possible hCG measurement.
- If the patient is shocked, site two 14G cannulae and give colloid as fast as possible pending immediate transfer to theatre.
- In the acutely compromised patient, surgery should not be delayed to allow full preoperative transfusion.
- Rhesus-negative women should be given anti-D.

Surgical treatment

If there is evidence of acute intraperitoneal haemorrhage with haemodynamic compromise, arrangements should be made for immediate laparotomy and ligation of the bleeding point. This will usually involve removal of the tube containing the ectopic pregnancy. On no account should patients be transferred between hospitals in this condition. If no gynaecological team is available at the referring hospital, the help of a general surgical team should be sought. When the patient is haemodynamically stable, surgical treatment can usually deferred until normal working hours and time allowed for the results of ultrasound and hCG evaluation.

- Surgical treatment may be carried out laparoscopically or through a mini-laparotomy incision.
- Laparoscopic treatment is associated with lower postoperative morbidity and quicker recovery but requires the availability of suitably trained staff and appropriate theatre equipment.
- In either case treatment may be by removal of the Fallopian tube (salpingectomy) or by aspiration of the ectopic through an incision in the wall of the Fallopian tube (salpingotomy).
- If the contralateral tube is healthy, both procedures are associated with similar intrauterine pregnancy rates in subsequent pregnancies but conservative surgery is associated with a higher risk of recurrence of ectopic pregnancy.
- Of cases treated by conservative surgery, 5–10% will be complicated by the presence of persistent trophoblastic tissue requiring further surgical or medical treatment. Follow-up with serial hCG measurements is therefore required.

Medical treatment

Suitable patients are those who are haemodynamically stable, have a serum hCG of less than 10 000 IU/L, have no evidence of extrauterine fetal heart activity on ultrasound, and are able to comply with the need for protracted follow-up.

- Systemic methotrexate at a dose of 50 mg/m^2 is given as an intramuscular (IM) injection and the patient followed with serial hCG measurements until these become negative.
- An initial rise in hCG levels following treatment and some abdominal discomfort are common.
- Tubal rupture may still occur and a falling hCG level does not exclude this possibility.
- Surgery will be required in 5–10% of cases.
- Patients must avoid alcohol and excessive exposure to sunlight following treatment and should be advised to avoid becoming pregnant again for at least 6 months.

rognosis

llowing a single ectopic pregnancy, 60–70% of women wishing to have further
egnancies will have an intrauterine pregnancy. Of subsequent pregnancies,
–15% will be ectopic. The likelihood of recurrence is determined principally
the condition of the remaining Fallopian tube and the rest of the pelvis at the
ne of treatment, although recurrence is slightly more common following con-
vative surgery. Patients should be advised about the need to seek medical
vice and to have an early ultrasound scan in subsequent pregnancies even if
ey are asymptomatic to confirm an intrauterine pregnancy.

Trophoblastic disease

This is a group of disorders characterized by abnormal placental development. The chorionic villi are hydropic with vacuolation of the placenta and destruction of the normal stroma. Trophoblastic disorders affect 1.5 per 1000 pregnancies in the UK. There is considerable geographical variation in incidence, the highest incidence being in countries of the Far East.

Aetiology

Trophoblastic disease is thought to arise by fertilization of the oocyte by diploid spermatozoon or by two haploid sperm. If this occurs in the absence any female nuclear material, the resulting conceptus is diploid (46XX) and is *complete mole*. If associated with female nuclear material, the conceptus will triploid and a *partial mole* (69XXX or 69XXY). Risk factors are maternal age previous history of trophoblastic disease, and blood group A.

Pathology

- *Benign trophoblastic disease* is usually either a complete hydatidiform mole where there is no evidence of an embryo or a partial hydatidiform mole, which may be associated with an embryo (usually abnormal). Other types of trophoblastic disease include invasive moles, placental site reaction, trophoblastic tumour, and hydropic change.
- *Malignant trophoblastic disease* (choriocarcinoma) complicates approximately 3% of complete moles, although in 50% of cases of choriocarcinoma there is no history of immediately preceding trophoblast disease. It may also occur following normal pregnancy.

Presentation

Trophoblastic disease typically (50% of cases) presents at about 14 weeks (range 8–24 weeks) with symptoms of vaginal bleeding and is usually diagnosed initially as a threatened miscarriage.
- The uterus is large for dates in 50% of cases.
- Enlarged ovarian theca-lutein cysts (see below) may cause abdominal pain if they rupture or undergo torsion.
- Products of conception containing small vesicles may be passed and there may be exaggerated pregnancy symptoms such as vomiting and early-onset pre-eclampsia (20%).
- The high circulating levels of human chorionic gonadotrophin (hCG) have a thyroid-stimulating hormone (TSH)-like action and can cause clinical thyrotoxicosis.
- Choriocarcinomas may present with the symptoms of distant metastases (cerebral, pulmonary).

Diagnosis

- Ultrasound.
  - —A 'snowstorm' appearance with multiple highly reflective echoes and areas of vacuolation within the uterine cavity suggests molar disease.
  - —In a partial mole a gestation sac with a fetus may also be present.
  - —Large ovarian theca-lutein cysts may be present on the ovaries as a result of the high hCG levels and take up to 4 months to resolve after treatment.
- Other imaging such as chest X-rays, computerized tomography (CT), or magnetic resonance imaging (MRI) may be indicated to exclude pulmonary or cerebral metastases if choriocarcinoma is suspected.
- The diagnosis of molar disease is usually confirmed by histological examination of products of conception removed at the time of uterine evacuation.
- Histological confirmation of metastatic deposits of choriocarcinoma is not usually required and may be dangerous.
- The diagnosis of metastatic disease is made by a combination of high levels of hCG in the absence of a pregnancy and the characteristic findings of secondaries (cannonball appearance) on imaging.

Management

Surgery

Evacuation of the uterus is carried out under general anaesthetic by an experienced surgeon. Preoperatively, blood should be taken for serum hCG levels, full blood count (FBC), cross-matching, and urea and electrolytes (U&Es). The anaesthetist should be warned about the possibility of thyrotoxicosis (risk of thyroid storm). There is an increased risk of uterine perforation and haemorrhage and the uterus may be enlarged due to collection of blood. Performing the procedure with an oxytocin infusion running may reduce the risk of haemorrhage but carries a theoretical risk of dissemination of trophoblastic material into the bloodstream.

If there is persistent bleeding after the initial evacuation, or evidence of persistent trophoblast within the uterus on imaging or hCG measurement, repeat evacuation may be performed after 10–14 days. If more than one repeat evacuation is required, the patient should be referred to a specialist centre for possible medical treatment.

Follow-up

The aim of follow-up is to detect persistent trophoblastic disease and choriocarcinoma.

- In the UK all patients are registered at one of three centres.
- Because all trophoblastic tumours produce hCG, patients can be monitored by measurement of urinary or serum hCG levels.
- These are checked fortnightly until the serum level is less than 2 IU/L and then monthly for 6 months following this if the hCG is negative within 6 weeks of treatment, or for 12 months and then 3-monthly for a further year if the hCG takes longer than 6 weeks to become negative.
- Patients should be advised to avoid another pregnancy until at least 6 months after the hCG level is less than 2 IU/L and to avoid using the combined oral contraceptive pill for at least 4 months.

Chemotherapy

All patients requiring chemotherapy are referred to specialist centres. Indications for treatment are a rising hCG level in the absence of a new pregnancy, an hCG persistently more than 20 000 IU/L by 4 weeks after treatment, persistent symptoms, or evidence of metastatic disease. Methotrexate is the mainstay of treatment (with folinic acid rescue).

Prognosis

- Overall 5-year survival is more than 99%.
- There is a 0.8–2.9% risk of recurrence in subsequent pregnancies after one mole and 15–28% after two moles.
- Patients are more likely to require chemotherapy if the initial hCG level is more than 100 000 IU/L, they are aged over 40, there are associated ovarian cysts, or when early use of the oral contraceptive pill or early pregnancy follows previous trophoblastic disease.
- Subsequent fertility does not appear to be impaired by chemotherapy and there does not seem to be an increased incidence of other chromosomal abnormalities.

Premenstrual syndrome

Premenstrual syndrome (PMS) is also known as premenstrual tension (PMT). It is a very common disorder affecting up to 95% of women. Rarely is it life-threatening but PMS has been cited as a factor in poor work performance, criminal acts, suicide, and even murder.

Aetiology and incidence

The aetiology is unknown but it is likely to be a consequence of the hormone changes over a normal menstrual cycle.
- It has been suggested that PMS symptoms are caused by various excesses or deficiencies of oestrogen or progesterone, but no consistent abnormality has been found.
- Side-effects caused by the progestogen component of cyclical hormone replacement therapy (HRT) are very similar to those with PMS, and the temporal relationship of symptoms to progesterone production in pre-menopausal women is strong.
- Serotonin and beta-endorphins have also been implicated.
- It is likely that PMS is an exaggerated endorgan response to the normal cyclical changes in ovarian hormones.

Estimates for the incidence vary from 5% to 95% of women being affected at some point. About 20% of women will seek help from their GPs for PMS symptoms. Typically, PMS is said to occur most frequently in the 30s and 40s, often after childbirth. However, it may be that this group of women simply reports it most frequently.

Symptoms and diagnosis

Symptoms fall into three main groups—physical, emotional, and behavioural (Table 60.1). Most women will experience at least one symptom but tolerate these without interference with their normal functioning.

Most women will self-diagnose PMS, but they may be mistaken in their interpretation of their symptoms. There is no objective method of measuring PMS but, for practical purposes, the diagnosis is made through the history, structured questionnaires, and the exclusion of competing diagnoses.
- Symptoms must be of sufficient severity to produce social, family, or occupational disruption and must occur in most menstrual cycles. They occur in the premenstrual phase, resolving or markedly improving at menstruation. Ideally, the symptoms should be monitored prospectively for 2 months with a menstrual diary.
- Various quality of life questionnaires have been used to attempt to quantify the amount of distress (e.g. Moo's menstrual distress questionnaire).
- Blood tests are unhelpful, except to exclude other causes of symptoms. Measurements of haemoglobin and thyroid function can be useful in this respect, whilst follicle-stimulating hormone (FSH) may be checked to exclude climacteric symptoms. Premenstrual symptoms may merge into climacteric symptoms in the 40s.

Table 60.1 Symptoms of PMS

Physical	Emotional	Behavioural
Backache	Anxiety	Violence
Headache	Irritability	Aggression
Breast tenderness/swelling	Fatigue	Clumsiness
Bloating/fluid retention	Depression	Loss of concentration
	Food craving	
	Anorexia	
	Mood swings	

Treatment

As there is no accepted aetiology for PMS, treatment remains empirical. In research studies looking at the effectiveness of treatments there is a large placebo response. This makes it difficult to show a true effect of treatment but treatment can be beneficial in clinical practice.

Active treatment can be chosen on the basis of treating the most severe symptoms first.

Non-hormonal therapy

- *Support and reassurance*. In milder cases, listening to the patient and acknowledging the problems can be helpful. Many women simply need the reassurance that the problem is being addressed by a sympathetic practitioner. Education and explanation of the physiological basis for the condition will ease frustration and anxiety. However, for the majority of women who approach a doctor, more help may be needed.
- *Stress management and relaxation techniques*. Various techniques have been tried and are of benefit to certain women. These include:
  —Yoga.
  —Hypnosis.
  —Music therapy.
  —Homeopathy.
  —Acupuncture.
  —Self-help groups, etc.
  If any of these appeal to the patient, then they can be encouraged. Side-effects are rare and avoidance of reliance on pharmacotherapy is seen as a benefit by many.
- *Exercise*. Aerobic physical exercise in the latter part of the menstrual cycle can be useful. The exercise causes an increase in endorphin production and this seems to have a 'mood-elevating' effect. Improvements may also come because the exercise usually takes the woman away from the stressful home environment for a while. Many women relish this form of treatment as it is seen as 'self-help'.
- *Vitamin B_6*. This is a co-factor in the synthesis of various neurotransmitters including serotonin and dopamine. This treatment may be useful for emotional and behavioural symptoms, but studies have shown only small advantages over placebo. There is some concern that overdosage may cause peripheral neuropathy.
- *Evening primrose oil*. Prostaglandin precursors such as linoleic and gammalinoleic acid are contained in the oil of the evening primrose flower. It is postulated that a deficiency of E series prostaglandins allows an increased response to circulating ovarian hormones. Some benefits are seen over placebo treatments (clumsiness, depression, headache, bloatedness). Like vitamin B_6, this treatment is available 'over the counter'.
- *Diuretics*. Only a few women truly experience premenstrual fluid retention and weight gain, although many think they have this problem because of perceived bloatedness. For women where there is a measurable weight gain, spironolactone is effective in the premenstrual phase.
- *Selective serotonin reuptake inhibitors* (SSRIs). It may be that women with serotonin deficiency are more sensitive to cyclical ovarian hormone changes and certainly there can be dramatic relief of PMS with SSRI drugs. They are usually taken throughout the cycle at a standard dose. They are most useful for psychological symptoms. Side-effects can limit the usefulness of long-term treatment.

60 Premenstrual syndrome

Hormone therapy

- *Progesterone supplements.* Many studies have looked at progesterone supplementation because of the belief that PMS is caused by progesterone deficiency. It has been given by various routes (suppositories, pessaries, injections, oral micronized). Although there is a wealth of anecdotal evidence suggesting benefits, placebo-controlled studies have shown disappointing results. It may be that progesterone has an anxiolytic effect in higher doses.
- *Progestogens.* Dydrogesterone has been used premenstrually but studies have shown disappointing results.
- *Combined oral contraceptive pill* (COCP). The response to treatment with the COCP is unpredictable—some women will gain benefit whereas others may get worse. However, it may be worth a trial for 3 months.
- *Bromocriptine.* Prolactin was at one time considered to be a potential causative agent for PMS. Treatment with bromocriptine is useful for cyclical breast symptoms but not for other symptoms.
- *Danazol.* Low doses of danazol (100 mg daily) have been shown to be beneficial in treating breast symptoms, without causing cycle suppression or severe side-effects. However, other PMS symptoms are not improved.
- *Oestradiol.* 17 beta-oestradiol implants (50–100 mg pellet 6-monthly) or transdermal oestradiol patch therapy (100–200 µg patch, used continuously) act by causing cycle supression. They can be very effective but in non-hysterectomized women a progestogen has to be given cyclically. This can reproduce PMS-like symptoms, which limits the usefulness of this regimen. However, by using the Mirena intrauterine system (IUS) as the progestogen component of treatment, systemic absorption is minimized and the acceptability of the treatment increased. Symptoms tend to return when treatment is discontinued and cyclical ovarian hormone production restarts.
- *Gonadotrophin-releasing hormone* (GnRH) analogues. PMS is usually eliminated when cycles are suppressed with GnRH analogues. In severe cases this treatment can bring prompt and welcome relief from symptoms. However, the ensuing oestrogen deficiency symptoms can be equally troublesome. These can be minimized by giving add-back therapy with livial or a continuous combined HRT. GnRH analogues are expensive for long-term treatment. If the patient has shown a good response, surgery may be the logical next step.

529

Surgery

For surgery to be effective, it is best to remove the ovaries and uterus, followed up with oestrogen-only HRT. If the uterus is left then treatment will need to include progestogens, which may give rise to the same symptoms again. Surgery is a big step to take and only justified in severe cases. It is usually best to give a trial of a GnRH analogue first to ensure that PMS will resolve when the ovaries are removed.

Chapter 61

Hirsutism/virilization

- *Hirsutism* in females is the growth of pigmented terminal hair in a typical male distribution pattern—face, chest, abdomen, and limbs. It is often associated with acne and seborrhoea.
- *Virilization* is the extreme of the spectrum. It includes baldness, voice changes, and clitoromegaly. This is a rare condition, but indicates a serious cause.
- Conversely, hirsutism not associated with menstrual disturbance is unlikely to be the result of serious underlying pathology.
- Excessive hair growth in women is difficult to define precisely—the amount that causes problems varies in different ethnic cultures.
- It is generally a subjective diagnosis, with facial hair being the most unacceptable.

The pilosebaceous unit

The process that regulates the growth and differentiation of hair follicles and sebaceous glands is not fully understood. At birth the skin is covered with short, fine, and unpigmented vellus hair. Scalp hair and eyebrows/eyelashes are non-sexual and grow continuously thereafter.
- At puberty, androgen production results in sex-hormone-dependent hair growth in the axillae and lower pubic triangle in both sexes.
- In the female, excessive androgen exposure at any time after puberty causes hirsutism, except on the scalp, where hair loss can occur in a male pattern.
- Hair follicles within the pilosebaceous unit go through successive phases of actively producing hair and resting hair—this is termed the *hair growth cycle* and can last up to 3 years.
- Human terminal hair growth is affected by several factors, with androgens being the most obvious regulator.

Androgen action in the hair follicle
Circulating unbound androgens diffuse into dermal papilla cells at the base of the hair bulb. Intracellularly, testosterone is converted by the enzyme 5α-reductase to 5α-dihydrotestosterone (DHT). This and other less bioactive androgens then bind to specific nuclear receptor proteins, eventually leading to slow protein synthesis.

The follicle increases in size, and is transformed from a small vellus follicle into a terminal hair-producing follicle. Men with 5α reductive deficiency have a female hair growth pattern.

Circulating androgens
The major androgens, produced by ovaries (25%), adrenals (25%), and peripheral conversion (50%), are testosterone, DHT, dehydroepiandrosterone sulfate (DHEAS), and androstenedione.

- Androgens have different potencies and binding affinities. These therefore determine the onset, severity, and progression of symptoms.
- Luteinizing hormone (LH) and insulin control ovarian androgen production via LH and insulin receptors found in the theca interstitial ovarian cells. Adrenocorticotrophic hormone (ACTH) controls adrenal androgen production.
- In women circulating testosterone is highly bound to sex-hormone-binding globulin (SHBG). Free testosterone is biologically active and small changes in SHBG can have marked effect on the biologically active free fraction available. *Hyperandrogenism* and *obesity* lower SHBG levels,[2] leading to higher levels of free active testosterone with 'normal' total testosterone levels. Androstenedione and DHEAS are not bound to SHBG.

Clinical evaluation

History

A detailed history, including age of onset and speed of progression of hirsutism and details of menstrual cycles may reveal the more common causes of hirsutism.

- Regular menstrual cycles and excessive hair on limbs and around lips only usually indicate *familial idiopathic hirsutism.*[3]
- Polycystic ovary syndrome (PCOS) is the most common cause of oligomenorrhoeic anovular hirsutism, starting in the late teenage years.
- Fast-progressing hirsutism of sudden onset leading to virilization is more likely to be associated with serious disease.

Examination

During examination the severity of the hirsutism can be graded using general descriptive terms or, more precisely, using the Ferriman and Galloway score (Table 61.1). Other signs of androgen production must be looked for—these will indicate the severity of androgen production. Hirsutism tends to be followed[1] in order by acne, oily skin, male hair pattern, breast atrophy, and clitoromegaly with deepening of the voice.

Acanthosis nigricans, indicating insulin resistance with PCOS, as velvety pigmented changes, can be seen around the neck and armpits.

Table 61.1 The Ferriman and Galloway scoring system. A score of 0 indicates absence of terminal hair

Score	Criteria
Upper lip	
1	A few hairs at outer margin
2	A small moustache at outer margin
3	A moustache extending from outer margin
4	A moustache extending to midline
Chin	
1	A few scattered hairs
2	Scattered hairs with small concentrations
3 & 4	Complete cover, light and heavy
Chest	
1	Circumareolar hairs
2	With midline hair in addition
3	Fusion of these areas, with three-quarter cover
4	Complete cover
Upper back	
1	A few scattered hairs
2	Rather more, still scattered
3 & 4	Complete cover, light and heavy
Lower back	
1	A sacral tuft of hair
2	With some lateral extension
3	Three-quarter cover
4	Complete cover
Upper abdomen	
1	A few midline hairs
2	Rather more, still midline
3 & 4	Half and full cover
Lower abdomen	
1	A few midline hairs
2	A midline streak of hair
3	A midline band of hair
4	An inverted V-shaped growth
Arm	
1	Sparse growth affecting not more than a quarter of the limb surface
2	More than this: cover still incomplete
3 & 4	Complete cover, light and heavy
Forearm, *thigh*, and *leg* are scored as for the arm	

535

Causes of hirsutism

- Idiopathic (familial) hirsuitism (IH).
- Ovarian:
  —PCOS.
  —Neoplasms.
  —Arrhenoblastoma.
  —Gonadoblastoma.
  —Hilus cell tumours.
  —Pregnancy luteoma.
- Adrenal:
  —Congenital adrenal hyperplasia (CAH).
  —Cushing's syndrome.
  —Neoplasms.
- Iatrogenic/drugs:
  —Anabolic steroids.
  —Danazol.
  —Phenytoin.
  —Androgenic progestogens—high doses.

Idiopathic (familial) hirsutism

This usually presents with excessive hair on the limbs and around the lips of mild to moderate severity. Androgen levels are normal, and menstrual cycles are regular. It affects between 5 and 15% of women, and is defined by some as the presence of hirsutism in the absence of ovulatory dysfunction, as determined by luteal progesterone if required.

Up to 30% of women with IH are satisfied to learn that they are healthy and are happy to continue with mechanical hair removal. The rest need medical therapy.

Ovarian causes of hirsutism

The clinical and hormone profile of PCOS, the most common cause of oligomenorrhaeic anovular hirsutism, is described in Chapter 62.[3] There is now a clear link between genetic insulin resistance and ovarian hyperandrogenism. At the extreme end of the PCOS spectrum, acanthosis nigracans (a manifestation of insulin resistance) and marked hyperandrogenism with virilization occur.[4] These usually coexist with abdominal obesity, which itself correlates with the presence of significant insulin resistance. Insulin also reduces production of SHBG in the liver, thus magnifying the effects of androgens.

- *Ovarian neoplasms* producing androgens are extremely rare. Serum testosterone levels are extremely high and often within the male biochemical distribution. Hirsutism rapidly progresses to frank virilization.
- Luteoma of pregnancy are benign hCG-driven tumours that can cause significant androgenic symptoms. Luteoma regress spontaneously after pregnancy.
- Occasional ovarian stromal hyperplasia seen in parallel with serous cystadenoma, teratomas, and other neoplasms can produce high levels of androstenedione causing androgenic symptoms.

Adrenal causes of hirsutism

- In CAH a partial block—enzyme defect—of cortisol synthesis results in increased levels of ACTH with subsequent increased androgen secretion. There are three such enzyme defects that lead to hyperandrogenism, the most common being 21-hydroxylase deficiency. Premature puberty is discussed elsewhere.

- A milder form of 21-hydroxylase deficiency can become apparent in early adult life causing amenorrhoea, hirsutism, and virilization—hence the term late-onset or incomplete CAH.[5] PCOS can occur in association with this form of CAH.

- Adrenal tumours resulting in hyperandrogenism without evidence of glucocorticosteroid excess are extremely rare—DHEAS levels are extremely high.

- Similarly, in Cushing's syndrome the well-described features are predominantly caused by excess glucocorticoid, and only extremely rarely present to a gynaecologist.

Investigations

Laboratory evaluation

The serum hormone evaluations of excessive androgen production are testosterone (total), androstenedione, DHEAS, 17α-hydroxyprogesterone, LH/FSH, SHBG with or without prolactin, and thyroid function tests. In women with menstrual cycles, the levels are best performed in the morning in the early follicular phase. Tests showing high levels should be repeated. High testosterone levels (above 5 nmol/L), although sometimes seen in PCOS, warrant further ovarian imaging investigations, as a very high DHEAS level necessitates exclusion of an adrenal neoplasm.

Adult-onset CAH is *not* always associated with a raised random 17α-hydroxyprogesterone level. If suspicious or when the level is mildly elevated, measurement should be repeated after an ACTH stimulation test.

Further investigations

- A 9 a.m. serum and 24-hour urinary cortisol should be estimated if Cushing's syndrome is suspected, and followed by a dexamethasone suppression test.
- Ultrasound and MRI/CT are the imaging investigations used if ovarian and adrenal neoplasms are suspected.

Treatment

Non-medical

- *Weight loss* remains an integral part of management,[6] and enhances other treatment modalities.
- *Destructive methods* can be used alone or in parallel with medical therapy. These methods either disguise or remove terminal hair—waxing, bleaching, shaving, electrolysis, or laser therapy.

Medical

- *Combined oral contraceptive pills* (COCPs) are most widely used and must be a combination that does not contain androgenic progestogen. COCPs will stimulate SHBG production, thereby reducing free testosterone levels; gonadotrophins will also be suppressed with a further reduction of adrenal androgen production. With combined preparations, as with other medical treatments, improvement in hirsutism is slow and no benefit will be seen for at least 6 months. Treatment must be continued for 18 months.
- The *anti-androgen* cyproterone acetate (CPA) is now often effectively used.[7] This compound binds to the androgen receptor and also has progestogenic activity. CPA further reduces serum androgen levels by hepatic enzyme induction, and therefore increased metabolic clearance of androgens.
- CPA is prescribed in a combination with ethinyloestradiol (EE) (Table 61.2). Both regimes in Table 61.2 provide good cycle control and contraception, but the reverse sequential one is best reserved for severe hirsutism because of side-effects. These are more frequently seen with higher doses and include loss of libido, weight gain, and, less frequently, headache and mood changes. If taken in early pregnancy, feminization of a male fetus is a risk.

- *Flutamide* is another anti-androgen, but is less commonly used.
- *Spironolactone*, an aldosterone antagonist, has a similar mode of action to that of CPA.[8] Doses of spironolactone range from 50 to 200 mg daily, but it should not be used long term for hirsutism in the UK.

CAH is treated with glucocorticoids, and surgery may be needed for other rare causes of androgen excess when specifically indicated.

Table 61.2 Combined regimen of cyproterone acetate (CPA) and ethinyloestradiol (EE)

	EE (μg)	CPA (mg)
Dianette	35	2
Reverse sequential regime	5–26 (30 days)	5–15 (100 days)

References

1 Hamada, K. *et al.* (1996). The metabolism of testosterone by dermal papilla cells cultured from human pubic and axillary hair follicles concurs with hair growth in 5-alpha-reductase deficiency. *Journal of Investigative Dermatology* **106**, 1017–22.

2 Plymate, S.R., Fariss, B.L., Bassett, M.L., and Matej, L. (1981). *Journal of Clinical Endocrinology and Metabolism* **52**, 1246–8.

3 Bernasconi, D., *et al.* (1996). The impact of obesity on hormonal parameters in hirsute and non-hirsute women. *Metabolism* **45**, 72–5.

4 Kahn, C.R., Flier, J.S., Ber, R.S., Archer, J.A., Gordon, P., Martin, M.M., and Roth, J. (1976). *New England Journal of Medicine* **294**, 739–45.

5 Azzis, R., Dewailly, D., and Owerback, D. (1994). *Journal of Clinical Endocrinology and Metabolism* **78**, 810–15.

6 Pasquali, R., Antenucci, D., Casimirri, F., Venturoli, S., Paradisi, R., Fabbri, R., *et al.* (1989). *Journal of Clinical Endocrinology and Metabolism* 173–9.

7 Barth, J.H., Cherry, C.A., Wojnorowstea, F., and Dawber, R.P. (1991). *Clinical Endocrinology* **35**, 5–10.

8 O'Brien, R.C., Cooper, M.E., Murray, R.M., Seeman, E., Thomas, A.K., and Jerums, G. (1991). *Journal of Clinical Endocrinology and Metabolism* **72**, 1008–13.

Chapter 62

Polycystic ovarian syndrome

Polycystic ovarian syndrome (PCOS) is one of the most common endocrine disorders, although its aetiology remains unknown. It was originally described as a clinical diagnosis based on the presence of oligomenorrhoea, hirsutism, and obesity—the classical Stein–Leventhal syndrome. This is now thought to be the extreme end of a spectrum. PCOS in modern practice applies to women who have classical ultrasound evidence of polycystic ovarian changes (enlarged ovaries with multiple cysts, 2–8 mm in diameter scattered around an echodense thickened central stroma)[1] and symptoms of oligomenorrhoea, obesity, and hyperandrogenism—all of varying degrees. Biochemical abnormalities—elevated luteinizing hormone (LH) to follicle-stimulating hormone (FSH) ratio, raised androgens, and reduced sex hormone-binding globulin (SHBG)—are also often seen, but ovarian morphology remains the most sensitive marker for PCOS.[1] A universally accepted definition, because of the heterogeneous nature of this condition, remains elusive.

PCOS is, however, not only an ovarian disease. Adrenal hyperactivity, abnormal pituitary hormone secretion, and changes in hepatic and adipose tissue functions are increasingly described in women with PCOS.

Features and prevalence of PCOS

PCOS is easy to recognize in its classical form, but only one or two of the three main components—anovulation, obesity, and hyperandrogenic features—are expressed in many women with PCOS. For example, hyperandrogenic women with PCOS can ovulate spontaneously and, conversely, anovulation in PCOS can occur in the absence of clinical or biochemical features of hyperandrogenic activity.

In the absence of a gold standard for diagnosis, the prevalence of PCOS in the general population cannot be precisely determined. An estimate of over 5% (documented range varies from 3 to 22%) makes PCOS the most common endocrine disorder depending on the criteria used. The symptoms of obesity, hyperandrogenism, and menstrual cycle disturbance are reported to occur in 38, 70, and 66%, respectively, of patients with an ultrasound diagnosis of PCOS.

Ultrasound and endocrine measurements

Laparoscopy with ovarian biopsy is too invasive, and does not form part of the diagnosis of PCOS. Transvaginal ultrasound is used instead.
- *Ultrasound criteria*:
  —Increased ovarian area/volume.
  —10 to 15 microcysts (< 10 mm diameter) organized in a peripheral rosary pattern.
  —Increased echogenicity of ovarian stroma.

Endocrine measurements
LH stimulates androgen secretion from theca cells of the ovary, while FSH regulates the function of the granulosa cells that convert androgens to oestrogens through the aromatase system—this being the pivot of mammalian female reproduction.

In PCOS *LH hypersecretion*,[2] which is particularly associated with menstrual disturbance and subfertility, occurs as measured by mean LH levels, peak frequency, and amplitude of LH pulses. In the early follicular phase the LH to FSH ratio is normally 1. In PCOS the persistently raised LH concentration (> 10 IU/L) leads to an increased LH to FSH ratio (in severe cases > 3:1). This endocrine feature appears to cause reduced fertility and increased rates of pregnancy losses.

Disturbed intraovarian regulation of ovarian androgen in PCOS leads to increased *testosterone* and *androstenedione* with subsequent reduction of SHBG.

Moderate *hyperprolactinaemia* is sometimes seen with PCOS[3]—this requires careful consideration and exclusion of other causes of hyperprolactinaemia.

In women who present predominantly with hirsutism, acne, and alopecia, adrenal androgens must be evaluated and congenital adrenal hyperplasia excluded. In PCOS, *17-alpha hydroxyprogesterone* is normal and *dehydroepiandrosterone sulfate* (DHEAS) levels are variable, but only moderately raised.

Obesity

Obesity, especially of the abdominal–visceral phenotype, is a common problem in PCOS. Of women with PCOS, 38% have a body mass index (BMI) above 25 kg/m². The BMI correlates with an increase in hirsutism, cycle disturbance, and subfertility.[4]

Weight gain starts in adolescence, when there is a normal degree of insulin resistance occurring. Probably inherited insulin resistance in PCOS, with a tendency to obesity, leads to further weight gain. This provokes further resistance and hypersecretion of insulin and a vicious cycle is established. Of women with PCOS, 11% have impaired glucose tolerance. Insulin also stimulates ovarian secretion of androgens worsening the hyperandrogenic status. Weight reduction in obese women with PCOS (BMI > 30 kg/m²) is an essential part of the management of this condition, which appears to have a strong genetic component. This is most likely to be dominant as suggested by family studies.

Management of PCOS

The therapeutic approach to individual women with PCOS is determined by the presenting problem caused by the underlying endocrinopathy. The need to lose weight in women with obesity and PCO is common to all management strategies.

Weight loss

Even moderate obesity (BMI > 27 kg/m^2) is known to be associated with a lower chance of ovulation, and women with central body fat distribution have more severe hirsutism and cycle disturbance.

In women with a BMI over 30 kg/m^2, weight loss is known to have a significant beneficial effect on endocrine function and ovulation, with improved fertility. With weight reduction, serum androgen and fasting insulin concentrations fall thus eventually improving hyperandrogenic symptoms, leading to spontaneous ovulation and increased fertility, with or without therapy. Ovulation induction (often involving expensive and potentially dangerous drugs) is known to be less effective when the BMI is over 30 kg/m^2. Pregnancy also carries greater risks in the obese.

Therapeutic strategies

Hirsutism affects over 70% of women with PCOS. Various drugs are available but the long-term outcome remains disappointing without weight reduction. This is further discussed in Chapter 61.

Cycle disturbance in women when fertility is not an issue can be treated with progestogens alone, or with combined preparations of oestrogens/progestogen. This will induce menstrual cycles and minimize the adverse effects of unopposed oestrogens, thus reducing the risk of endometrial hyperplasia, which may lead to atypical changes and, eventually, to endometrial adenocarcinoma. Thickened endometrium over 10 mm on ultrasound in association with PCO, amenorrhoea requires further management such as:

- Oligo/amenorrhoea:
  —Progestogens.
  —Combined oral progestogens and oestrogens.
- Dysfunctional uterine bleeding:
  —Progestogens.
  —Combined oral progestogens and oestrogens.

The combined preparations used should not contain 17 nortestosterone progestogens, which will further lower SHBG and increase free testosterone. Medroxyprogesterone acetate (MPA) is the ideal single progestogen to use—it also suppresses LH and ovarian androgen secretion.

Subfertility therapies

In women with regular cycles, anovulation must first be confirmed. In the majority with cycle disturbance it is helpful to assess oestrogen production prior to ovulation induction. A *progestogen challenge test* (MPA 30 mg daily for 1 week) performed after a negative pregnancy test is a simple way of investigating endogenous oestrogen, but it also facilitates onset of ovulation induction treatment.

62 Polycystic ovarian syndrome

Clomiphene citrate ovulation induction therapy

Clomiphene citrate and other forms of ovulation induction (unless the patient has longstanding amenorrhoea) should only be used after thorough subfertility investigations, including hysterosalpingogram or laparoscopy, confirming tubal patency. This change of practice has occurred following the recent evidence suggesting a likely link between ovulation induction and long-term risk of ovarian cancer.

In well oestrogenized PCOS patients (with normal FSH and prolactin levels) the first treatment of choice for induction of ovulation is the use of clomiphene—an anti-oestrogen. This is an oral therapy using 50 mg per day for 5 days starting on day 2 of a spontaneous or progestogen-induced bleed. Anti-oestrogens block the negative feedback of oestradiol on the hypothalamus and pituitary—this increases endogenous FSH levels, which promote follicular growth, leading to ovulation. Clomiphene also has a direct effect on the ovary's FSH-induced aromatase activity.

Clomiphene is an effective treatment for anovulation in appropriately selected women—obesity being the major correctable adverse factor. Although clomiphene is reported to induce ovulation in over 70% of patients, only 40% conceive. Up to 10 cycles of treatment can be considered after full discussion and counselling of the patients about the possible link between continued ovulation induction and ovarian cancer. This is mandatory if more than 6 cycles are to be used (this is because clomiphene is licensed for only 6 cycles in the UK). A subsequent pregnancy is reported to annul this risk.

Ovulation induction with clomiphene should only be performed in circumstances that allow access to ovarian ultrasound and endocrine monitoring. If ovulation does not occur using 50 mg daily, the dose should be increased to 100 mg daily. There is probably no benefit in increasing the dose of clomiphene if ovulation is shown to occur. A further increase, in 50-mg increments up to 200 mg, is advocated by some, but a daily dose of more than 100 mg rarely confers any benefit. When a dose of over 50 mg is used, the anti-oestrogenic possible adverse effect of clomiphene on the mid-cycle cervical mucus changes must be investigated by a mid-cycle postcoital test.

Gonadotrophin ovulation induction therapy

An injection of 5000 IU of human chorionic gonadotrophin (hCG), timed by the use of ultrasound to assess follicular growth, can be used to trigger ovulation. Ovulation occurs 24–36 hours later, and intercourse can be precisely timed.

Gonadotrophin ovulation induction therapy is indicated for clomiphene-resistant women with PCOS. Women who ovulate with clomiphene, but fail to conceive, are probably best served by moving to assisted conception, as opposed to an alternative method of ovulation induction.

Two regimens of gonadotrophins are widely used—daily or alternate day injections of gonadotrophins increasing the dose every 5–7 days, based on closely monitored follicular response. The usual starting dose is 75 units of gonadotrophin. There is no advantage in using gonadotrophin-releasing hormone (GnRH)

Management of PCOS (*continued*)

analogues in conjunction with gonadotrophins for ovulation induction in women with clomiphene-resistant PCOS, as there is no increase in the pregnancy rate.

The aim of monitoring by using ultrasound and serum oestradiol levels is to allow timing of the hCG injection to induce ovulation, without causing hazardous ovarian hyperstimulation.

Ovarian hyperstimulation syndrome (OHSS)

Some patients undergoing gonadotrophin stimulation show a marked response to the drugs, with multiple follicular development believed to result from an overproduction of oestrogen. To minimize the occurrence and severity of OHSS, gonadotrophin cycles are closely monitored. When this is suspected, further stimulation is withdrawn, hCG withheld and the treatment cycle is postponed. The pathophysiology of OHSS is still not completely understood so it is difficult to prevent and to treat. Although OHSS may occur after a spontaneous LH peak, this risk is much less than after the long-acting hCG preparations.

Hyperstimulation still provokes much fear because of morbidity needing intense treatment. Hyperstimulation is generally classified as mild, moderate, or severe (and, in all cases, there is excessive oestrogen secretion, with symptoms usually appearing 3–6 days after hCG administration/spontaneous ovulation).

- *Mild hyperstimulation* is defined as ovarian enlargement up to 5 cm diameter, accompanied by some mild abdominal swelling and pain. There is little cause for concern, and therapy should consist of rest at home, careful observation, and analgesia.

- *Moderate hyperstimulation* is defined as ovarian enlargement up to 12 cm diameter, accompanied by more pronounced symptoms, including abdominal distension and pain, nausea, vomiting, and occasional diarrhoea. Therapy includes bed rest and close observation to detect any progression to severe hyperstimulation in cases where conception has occurred. Hospital admission is sometimes required. Pelvic examination of the enlarged ovaries should be gentle, in order to avoid rupture of the cysts. In the majority of cases, symptoms should subside spontaneously within 2–3 weeks.

- *Severe hyperstimulation* is a rare but serious complication characterized by ovarian enlargement in excess of 12 cm in diameter. Symptoms include pronounced abdominal distension and pain, ascites, pleural effusion, haemoconcentration (packed cell volume (PCV) greater than 45%), reduced urine output, electrolyte imbalance, and, sometimes, shock. *Hospital admission is mandatory.* Treatment should concentrate on restoring fluid balance by giving intravenous (IV) fluids (colloids, rather than crystalloids) and heparin to prevent thromboembolism. In view of the recent concerns about its use, IV albumin is best avoided altogether. Patients should also be given oral intake of high protein fluids. A strict fluid balance chart should be kept as well as daily measurements of electrolytes, renal function, PCV, clotting screen, and serum albumin. Paracentesis may be indicated and performed under ultrasound guidance, if the abdominal discomfort is severe. The acute symptoms subside over several days. Symptoms may, however, be prolonged if conception occurs.

Results of gonadotrophin therapy

Range of reported pregnancy rate per cycle, 20–30%.

Range of reported multiple pregnancy, 10–35%.

Laparoscopic ovarian diathermy surgery

This has now replaced open ovarian wedge resection.[5] It is slowly replacing gonadotrophin therapy as the second-line therapy for clomiphene resistance in women with PCOS, and is thought to be equally effective. The risk of ovarian hyperstimulation and multiple pregnancy with gonadotrophin is replaced by the risk of peri-ovarian adhesions. The potential risk of ovarian destruction causing subsequent ovarian failure still remains an unanswered possibility.

Insulin-lowering medications

These are new adjuncts to the management of PCOS. Lowering insulin concentrations with metformin[6] or other similar agents improves hyperandrogenism by reducing ovarian enzyme activity that results in androgen production.

Although side-effects with these medications are rare, further evidence is awaited before widespread introduction into clinical practice.

References

Adams, J., Franks, S., Polson, D.W., Mason, H.D., Abdulwahid, N., Tucker, M., et al. (1985). Multifocal ovaries: clinical and endocrine features and response to pulsatile gonadotrophin releasing hormone. Lancet ii, 1375–8.

Singh (1981). Menstrual disorders in College students. American Journal of Obstetrics and Gynecology 140, 229.

Nahum, R., Thong, K.J., and Hillier, S.G. (1995). Metabolic regulation of androgen production by human cells in vitro. Human Reproduction 10, 75–81.

Stein, F.I. and Leventhal, M.L. (1935). Amenorrhoea associated with bilateral polycystic ovaries. American Journal of Obstetrics and Gynecology 29, 181–91.

Armar, N.A. and Lachelin, G.C.L. (1993). Laparoscopic ovarian diathermy: an effective treatment for anti-oestrogen resistant anovulatory infertility in women with the polycystic ovary syndrome. British Journal of Obstetrics and Gynaecology 100, 161–4.

Velasquez, E.M., et al. (1994). Metformin therapy in women with polycystic ovary syndrome reduces hyperinsulinaemia, insulin resistance, hyperandrogenaemia, and systolic blood pressure while facilitating menstrual regularity and pregnancy. Metabolism 43, 647–55.

Chapter 63

Vaginal discharge

Vaginal discharge may be physiological or pathological. It is likely to be physio logical if associated with menstruation, mid-cycle ovulation, and sexual excite ment. It is often pathological when associated with blood, pruritus, foul odou vulvulitis, ulcers, and soreness.

Causes

Physiological causes
The discharge is mucoid or white (leucorrhoea). Quantity and quality var throughout the menstrual cycle.
- Discharge is maximal at mid-cycle (ovulation), premenstrually, and with the use of intrauterine contraceptive devices or during sexual excitement.
- Coitus produces an increase in cervical and vaginal discharge together with semen.
- In pregnancy oestrogen causes mucus-secreting columnar epithelium to evert into the ectocervix causing an increase in vaginal discharge.
- Maternal oestrogen may cause a self-limiting vaginal discharge in neonates

Pathological causes
These vary in the premenarcheal, reproductive, and peri-/postmenopausal year with some degree of overlap. Premenarcheal causes include poor hygiene, for eign bodies (organic or inorganic), threadworms, sexual interference, and sar coma botryoides (rare and usually associated with a blood-stained discharge Vaginal discharge during the reproductive years may be due to the following.
- *Infections.* Candida albicans, Chlamydia trachomatis, Neisseria gonorrhoeae, Trichomonas vaginalis, Gardnerella vaginalis, Herpes genitalis, syphilitic chancre, or non-specific agents, e.g. Streptococci.
- *Neoplasms.* Benign or malignant and usually blood-stained.
- *Trauma or iatrogenic.* Sensitivity/allergy to contraceptive rubber, spermicidal creams, douching chemicals, retained products such as tampons, postabortum, or puerperal.
- *Local causes.* Examples include cervical ectropion or polyp, fistulae (urinary or faecal), A normal discharge but one conceived of as excessive and idiopathic. Peri-/postmenopausal vaginal discharge is often due to a low oestrogen state resulting in atrophic vaginitis. The discharge is quite often blood-stained.

It is important to exclude the above infective causes as well as any unreveale genital tract malignancy.

Diagnosis

Take a good history to include:
- Features of the discharge:
  —Nature (mucoid, serous, purulent, bloody).
  —Colour (clear, white, yellow-green, blood-stained).
  —Consistency (watery, viscid, curd-like).
  —Duration (continuous, intermittent).
  —Amount (the need for added protection such as pads).
- Associated symptoms—irritation, itching, burning.
- Frequency of attacks.

Relationship to menstrual cycle, sexual intercourse, pregnancy.
Hygiene practices—douching, use of tampons.
Risk factors and likelihood of sexually transmitted diseases.
Associated urinary tract infection.
Associated medical conditions, e.g. diabetes mellitus.
History of allergy to rubber/spermicides.
Drug history, especially antibiotics.
Last cervical smear.

Physical examination includes general and abdominal as well as pelvic examination.
The objective here is to establish the diagnosis (usually infective), determine the
extent of morbidity (any associated vulvitis or pelvic inflammatory disease), and
exclude a malignancy.

Investigations include cervical cytology, vaginal pH, saline wet mount, wet
mount on 10% potassium hydroxide solution (10% KOH), Gram stain of vaginal discharge, specimen for culture (high vaginal and endocervical swabs), and
colposcopy if indicated.

Diagnostic features of some common conditions

Candidiasis. Whitish to yellowish discharge with plaques at times. pH
slightly more acidic than normal (4.5–4.8), hyphae/pseudohyphae on
saline/10% KOH wet mount, Gram stain, culture (Nickerson's medium),
especially in recurrent cases (for *Candida glabrata*).

Trichomoniasis. Watery, grey-green frothy discharge. pH usually 5.0–6.0,
motile trichomonads visible on saline mount, culture (Stuart's medium).

Gardnerella vaginalis vaginitis. Watery grey offensive discharge. pH 5.0–5.5,
saline wet smear—demonstration of 'clue cells'. Application of 10% KOH
produces a fishy odour ('whiff test').

Mucopurulent cervicitis (Chlamydia trachomatis). Endocervical scrapings
should be taken. A direct immunofluorescent test using tagged monoclonal
antibodies against chlamydial surface antigens is a quick diagnostic test.
Culture in McCoy cell lines is possible.

Mucopurulent cervicitis (Neisseria gonorrhoeae). Demonstration of
intracellular Gram-negative diplococci; culture on Thayer–Martin medium.

Syphilis. Primary syphilis presents with painless, indurated ulcers.
Demonstration of treponeme by dark-field microscopy of a slide with
exudate from ulcer. Serologic tests: non-specific reagin type antibody tests
(rapid plasma reagin (RPR), the Venereal Disease Research Laboratory
(VDRL) test for syphilis) and specific antitreponemal antibody tests
(*Treponema pallidum* immobilization (TPI), fluorescent treponemal
antibody absorption (FTA-ABS), *Treponema pallidum* haemagglutination
(TPHA)).

Herpes genitalis. Tzank test to demonstrate multinucleate giant cells,
cultures of vesicular fluid.

Other diagnoses are unusual but they must be kept in mind. Make use of clinical examination, colposcopy, and biopsy if indicated.

Treatment of the common conditions

- *Candidiasis.*
  - —Polynes. Pessaries containing nystatin.
  - —Imidazoles: clotrimazole, miconaxole.
  - —Triazoles: fluconaxole, itraconazole.
  - —In recurrent infections, predisposing factors must be sought and treated
  - —The concomitant use of oral agents such as the triazoles helps eradicate gastrointestinal and subepithelial reservoirs, but liver function tests mus be monitored.
- *Trichomoniasis.* Metronidazole 200 mg tds (three times daily) for 5–7 days. Metronidazole 2 g single dose. Treatment should be undertaken concurrently by both partners.
- *Gardnerella vaginalis vaginitis.* Oral or topical metronidazole or topical clindamycin.
- *Mucopurulent cervicitis*
  - —*Chlamydia trachomatis.* Doxycycline 100 mg bd (twice daily) for 10 to 14 days. Erythromycin 500 mg qid (4 times a day) for 10 to 14 days.
  - —*Neisseria gonorrhoeae.* Treatment should aim at the penicillinase-producing strain. Ceftriaxone 250 mg given intramuscularly as a single dose.
- *Syphilis.* 2.4 million units benzathine penicillin. Erythromycin 500 mg qid for 15 days.
- *Herpes genitalis.* Local symptomatic relief with lignocaine jelly. Systemic therapy with oral acyclovir.
- *Atrophic vaginitis.* A diagnosis of exclusion after other infective and possibl neoplastic causes have been excluded. Topical oestrogen creams cause a reversal of symptoms within a week. Maintenance therapy with local application one to three times a week helps maintain a healthy vaginal epithelium. Hormone replacement therapy should be considered.
- *Other conditions.* Treatment will depend on the cause identified.

Principles to remember
- Neoplasia, though not common, must be looked for.
- If one sexually transmitted disease (STD) is identified, other STDs must be looked for and contact tracing and treatment of partner should be carried out.
- Refractory cases may need frequent intermittent therapy and are best dealt with by a specialist.
- Predisposing factors must be identified.

aginal discharge in obstetrics

inciples of management

An understanding of the management of vaginal discharge outside of pregnancy in the reproductive years.

Remember that vaginal discharge may be physiological in pregnancy.

A history of associated pruritus, blood-staining, purulent nature, vulvitis, ulceration, soreness, or foul odour would indicate a pathological cause.

Identification of the organism.

Modification or delay of treatment for fetal reasons.

Exclusion of leaking liquor in later pregnancy.

eatment for infective causes

Candidiasis.

—Nystatin pessaries: 1 tablet (100 000 IU) bd for 10 to 14 days.

—Clotrimazole: 500 mg (Canestin 1, Bayer) single pessary.

—Local antifungal cream (Canesten/Gyno-Travogen, Daktarin).

Trichomoniasis.

—Topical povidone–iodine.

—Metronidazole is contraindicated in the first trimester. In cases that need treatment in later gestation, use metronidazole 200 mg tds for 7 days (consider treating couple simultaneously).

Gardnerella vaginalis vaginitis.

—Oral amplicillin 500 mg 6-hourly for 1 week.

—For this infection, oral metronidazole may best be avoided in pregnancy because the risks might outweigh the benefits. Local metronidazole is effective.

Chlamydia trachomatis cervicitis.

—Erythromycin 500 mg qid for 14 days.

Neisseria gonorrhoea cervicitis

—Ceftriaxone 250 mg intramuscularly as a single dose.

Syphilis

—2.4 million units benzathine penicillin.

—Erythromycin 500 mg qid for 15 days.

Herpes genitalis

—The risk to the fetus must be kept in mind and third trimester management must be tailored to expose the fetus to minimum risk

—Topical acyclovir and lignocaine jelly for relief of symptoms.

Chapter 64

Lower genital tract infections

Most women experience lower genital tract infections at some time. Not all a[re] sexually transmitted. Vaginal discharge may also be physiological or due to [a] retained foreign body. If one sexually transmitted disease (STD) is diagnos[ed] there is an increased likelihood of others being present. Therefore patie[nts] should be treated in a genitourinary clinic where full bacteriological and se[ro]logical screening can be carried out. Treatment of women with STDs should [be] done in conjunction with screening and treatment of partners and follow-[up] tests of cure where possible.

Risk factors for STDs include multiple partners, pregnancies before the age of 2[?] being in the age group 15–34, previous termination of pregnancy (TOP), other previous STD, abnormal cervical cytology, local authority care, and prostituti[on].

A *sexual history* should include:
- Time since last intercourse.
- Type of intercourse (oral, vaginal, or anal).
- Contraception used.
- Number of previous partners.
- Menstrual history.
- Previous pregnancies.
- Previous treatment for STD in patient or her partner.
- History of travel abroad.
- History of intravenous (IV) drug use by patient or her partners.

Bacterial vaginosis

This is due to an overgrowth of anaerobic organisms such as *Gardnerella va[gi]nalis*, *Bacteriodes*, *Mycoplasma hominis*, and *Mobiluncus sp.* that are norma[lly] present in the vagina. It may occur in women who are not sexually active. It [is] more common in women undergoing termination of pregnancy and those wi[th] an intrauterine contraceptive device (IUCD) *in situ* or with pelvic inflammato[ry] disease (PID). It is associated with an increased risk of second trimester misca[r]riage, pre-term delivery, and pelvic infection after surgery.
- *Presentation* may be asymptomatic. The symptom is usually a white or pal[e] yellow vaginal discharge with an offensive fishy odour.
- *Diagnosis.* Characteristic vaginal discharge on examination. An increase in vaginal pH (use pH strips) to > 5.5. If a few drops of 10% potassium hydroxide are added to the discharge it produces a characteristic fishy sme[ll]. Microscopic examination may show 'clue cells' (squamous epithelial cells with small bacteria adherent to the wall). There will be large numbers of cocci and relatively few Gram-positive bacilli (Lactobacilli). The presence of the above anaerobes on culture from high vaginal swab is not diagnost[ic] by itself, as these can be isolated from normal vaginal flora.
- *Management.* Bacterial vaginosis may resolve spontaneously. Treatment is indicated if symptomatic, prior to termination of pregnancy, and in wome[n] with a previous history of second trimester miscarriage or unexplained pr[e] term delivery. Metronidazole 400 mg (200 mg if pregnant) twice daily for 5 days or 2 g as a single dose. Clindamycin 2% cream (1 applicator full at night vaginally for 7 days) is a suitable topical alternative. Recurrence afte[r] treatment is common.

Candida (Thrush)

There are several species of this yeast the most common being *Candida albicans*. It affects 75% of women at some time and an estimated 20% are carriers (in the gut). Predisposing factors include:

- Conditions or drugs that impair immunity.
- Antibiotics.
- Pregnancy or high-dose combined oral contraceptive pill (COCP).
- Diabetes or thyroid, parathyroid, or adrenal disease.

Presentation

Symptoms include vulval itching and soreness (worse at night), curdy white discharge (may also be thin and watery), dysuria, and dyspareunia. On examination look for an erythematous vulva with fissuring and white plaques in the vagina that are adherent.

Diagnosis

Diagnosis can be confirmed by culture or by the presence of Gram-positive spores and long pseudohyphae on wet preparation microscopic examination. The vaginal pH is usually normal. In recurrent infections look for anaemia, thyroid disease, and diabetes and consider acquired immunodeficiency.

Treatment

Asymptomatic women do not require treatment.

- Topical preparations such as clotrimazole 500 mg either as a single-dose pessary or as a cream for 14 days are usually effective.
- Recurrent or persistent infection can be treated by systemic antifungal agents such as fluconazole 150 mg (avoid in pregnancy; only effective against *C. albicans* strains).
- Treatment of the partner is usually recommended although re-infection may occur from the gut.
- Acetic acid jelly, e.g Aci-jel©, may prevent or relieve mild attacks.
- Advice about simple hygiene measure such as wiping the vulva from front to back, avoiding chemical irritants on the vulva such as bathsalts, and the use of cotton underwear may help.

Chlamydia

Chlamydia trachomatis, an obligate intracellular bacterium, is the most common cause of salpingitis and is present in up to 50% of genital infections the UK.

- *Presentation* is as vaginal discharge (cervicitis), urethritis, pelvic inflammatory disease, perihepatitis (Fitz–Hugh–Curtis syndrome), or Reiter's syndrome (arthropathy, rash, and conjunctivitis). It is commonly asymptomatic (80% of women) so patients undergoing procedures such as termination of pregnancy should be screened for infection.

- *Diagnosis.* *Chlamydia* can be cultured but requires special medium. The diagnosis is usually made by ELISA (enzyme-linked immunosorbent assay detection of antigen obtained by swabbing the endocervix. Polymerase chain reaction (PCR) or ligase chain reaction tests to detect bacterial DNA are more sensitive and can be performed on urine samples and vaginal swabs but are more expensive. Perihepatic adhesions may be seen at laparoscopy.

- *Treatment.* If untreated there is a significant risk of tubal damage and subsequent infertility.
  —Doxycylcine 100 mg twice daily for 10 days (avoid during pregnancy and lactation; use erythromycin 500 mg four times daily for 10 days).
  —Azithromycin 1 g is effective as a single-dose treatment.
  —Contact tracing of partners and treatment is essential to prevent re-infection.
  —Confirmation of cure should be obtained after treatment by repeat swabs.

Gonorrhoea

Neisseria gonorrhoeae is an intracellular Gram-negative diplococcus that grows columnar epithelium (incubation period 2–5 days).

Presentation. 50% of women are asymptomatic but 15% present as acute-onset PID with abdominal pain that may be associated with pronounced vaginal bleeding. May also cause bartholinitis/skeinitis, vaginal discharge perihepatitis, septicaemia, arthritis, or a rash.

Diagnosis is made by culture or the presence of intracellular Gram-negative diplococci on Gram-stained preparations from cervical, urethral, or rectal swabs.

Treatment. Amoxicillin 3 g with probenicid 2 g, ciprofloxacin 500 mg, or 1 g of azithromycin all given as a single dose. Treatment should also be given for chlamydia. Contact tracing and treatment of partners is essential prior to resuming intercourse. Confirmation of cure should be obtained by two sets of cultures following treatment.

Herpes

Herpes is caused by DNA viruses *Herpes simplex* types 2 (genital) and 1 (oral, cold sores). Of genital lesions, 50% are due to HSV1.

Presentation. Incubation period of 21 days. The first attack is the most severe with pain, vulvitis (may be severe enough to cause urinary retention), ulceration, lymphadenopathy, and discharge. It resolves after 3–4 weeks but may cause a secondary sacral radiculomyelopathy or meningitis. Recurrence can be triggered by stress, sex, or menstruation but subsequent attacks are normally shorter and less severe. There may be prodromal symptoms. Asymptomatic shedding of the virus may occur.

Diagnosis. Culture of serum collected from vesicles by aspiration or by swabbing the base of the ulcers. Serum anti-HSV antibody levels are increased with both types of infection.

Treatment is largely supportive with analgesia and the treatment of any secondary infections. Acyclovir 200 mg five times a day for 5 days if given within 5 days of onset of symptoms shortens the duration of the primary attack and may abort recurrent episodes if taken when prodromal symptoms occur. Condoms should be used unless both partners have a history of herpes.

Molluscum contagiosum, pubic lice, and scabies

- *Molluscum contagiosum* is a member of the poxvirus group.
  —*Presentation.* Papules up to 5 mm in diameter with central umbilication usually in the pubic area.
  —*Treatment* is by topical application of phenol or by cryotherapy.
- The *pubic louse* is a sexually transmitted parasite that lays its eggs on pubic hair.
  —*Presentation.* Itch secondary to reaction to its bite.
  —*Treatment.* Topical aqueous malathion (30–60 g) applied as a single application to all parts of the body for 12 hours or overnight and repeated after 7 days.
- *Scabies* is caused by *Sarcoptes scabiei*, a mite that burrows into the skin and lays eggs. There is both sexual and non-sexual transmission.
  —*Presentation.* Itch, rash over trunks and limbs.
  —*Treatment.* Topical aqueous malathion (30–60 g) applied as a single application to all parts of the body for 12 hours or overnight.

Syphilis

Treponemum pallidum is a treponemal infection (others include yaws and pinta). There is both sexual and vertical transmission. The incubation period 9–90 days.

- *Presentation.*
  —Primary infection usually presents 3–6 weeks after infection with chancre (painless genital ulceration) and inguinal lymphadenopathy. The most common site for chancre in women is the cervix and it may therefore be relatively asymptomatic. The primary infection will resolve after a few weeks if untreated.
  —Secondary syphilis may arise immediately after the primary disease or up to 6 months later. Signs include rash, fever, joint pains, condylomata lata (wart -like lesions), iritis, and hepatitis.
- *Diagnosis.* The organism can be identified in exudate obtained from the primary lesion mixed with saline using dark field microscopy. The most sensitive serological test is the fluorescent treponemal antibody test (FTA). In primary disease serology may be negative.
- *Treatment.* Intramuscular (IM) penicillin 1.2 million units for 12 days is the treatment of choice. Doxycycline 100 mg two times a day for 14 days or erythromycin 500 mg four times a day for 14 days are suitable alternatives. Contact tracing may need to involve partners from several years previously.

ichomonas

homonas vaginalis is a protozoan with four flagellae. It is sexually transmitted.
resentation. It may be asymptomatic. Symptoms are a mucopurulent,
ellow or green offensive vaginal discharge associated with vulvovaginitis.
The cervix may have a 'strawberry' appearance because of the presence of
unctate haemorrhages.
Diagnosis. Flagellate organisms can be seen on wet slide preparation or can
e cultured.
Management. Metronidazole 400 mg twice daily for 7 days (200 mg three
imes a day in pregnancy) or 2 g as a single dose. Treat partner and check
or other STDs (gonorrhoea).

arts (human papillomavirus)

most important serotypes are 6, 11, 16, 18, and 31 of which 6 and 11 are the
st common. Serotypes 16, 18, and 31 have been linked to the development of
vical cancer. There is an incubation period of weeks to months. The virus
y be carried (and shed) without any visible lesions being present. Infection is
ually acquired.
Presentation. The lesions are usually asymptomatic (any itch is usually due
o secondary infection). The appearance depends on the site. They are
associated with other STDs (25%).
Treatment.
—Visible lesions are treated with cryotherapy or topical application of
  podophyllin one to two times a week for 6 weeks. Surgical excision or
  ablation by laser or diathermy are alternatives.
—Relapse is common whatever the method of treatment used especially in
  immunocompromised patients.
—Sexual partners should be examined for warts and other STDs. Barrier
  contraception is usually advised during treatment.
—There is no need for women with warts to have more frequent cervical
  screening although patients with cervical warts should be referred for
  colposcopic assessment.

Pelvic pain

Acute pelvic pain

The common causes of acute pelvic pain are:
- Early pregnancy complications such as ectopic pregnancy and miscarriage.
- Pelvic inflammatory disease (PID).
- Appendicitis.
- Ovarian cyst 'accidents' or Mittelschmerz.

Other causes of acute pelvic pain include:
- Ovarian hyperstimulation syndrome.
- Haematometra and haematocolpos.
- Necrosis of uterine fibroids.
- Other non-gynaecological causes such as bowel or urinary disease.

Early pregnancy complications are discussed in Chapters 6 and 58 and PID discussed in Chapter 66.

Ovarian cyst accidents

These include the pain produced as a result of torsion (leading to occlusion the blood supply and necrosis) as well as bleeding into or from a cyst. This be the presenting symptom of ovarian neoplasia but is more commonly asso ated with functional ovarian cysts in younger women. Ovarian cysts may r ture causing an acute chemical peritonitis if they contain irritant material (s as endometriotic or dermoid cysts). Torsion presents with sudden onset of icky pelvic pain often located to one or other of the iliac fossae. The pain r become more constant after several hours or even disappear. During the few hours the patient is usually apyrexial, but later on necrosis can ca pyrexia. Dermoid cysts, teratomas, or simple cysts are more common cause torsion.

Mittelschmerz

Mittelschmerz (from the German *mittel* = middle and *Schmerz* = pain) is m cycle pain occurring at the time of ovulation more commonly in teenagers older women.

Chronic pelvic pain

Pelvic pain is deemed chronic when it is of more than 6 months durati
Chronic pelvic pain is the most common gynaecological problem affect
women of reproductive age.

Endometriosis and chronic PID are discussed in Chapters 67 and 66, respectiv

Pelvic adhesions

It remains unclear whether adhesion cause chronic pelvic pain. Adhesioly
results in pain relief in 60–90% of cases in uncontrolled studies. However, i
randomized controlled trial of adhesiolysis, only patients with severe, vascul
ized, and dense adhesions involving bowel benefited from surgery. Th
appears to be little benefit from adhesiolysis for simple pelvic adhesions.[1]

- *Ovarian remnant syndrome* or the trapped ovary syndrome refers to chro
  pelvic pain caused by dense fibrous adhesions around the ovarian tissue.
  This can be relieved by ovarian suppression or removal.[2]

Pelvic congestion

Pelvic congestion is characterized by dilatation of pelvic veins, which leads
cyclical dragging pelvic pain. The pain usually occurs during the premenstr
phase of the cycle and is worse on standing or walking. It varies in site and inte
sity and may be associated with deep dyspareunia after intercourse. The dila
pelvic veins may be demonstrated by laparoscopy, and sometimes by ultrasou
scan.

- *Treatment* is by using medroxyprogesterone acetate (MPA; 30–50 mg dail
  for 3 months). Side-effects include weight gain, amenorrhoea, and bloatin
  —Suppression of ovarian activity with gonadotrophin-releasing hormone
    (GnRH) analogues has been used to treat pelvic pain.
  —In severe cases hysterectomy with bilateral oophorectomy (with hormo
    replacement therapy afterwards) is curative.

Bowel-related pain

- *Irritable bowel syndrome* (IBS) is the most common bowel-related cause o
  chronic pelvic pain. It affects around 10–20% of the general population a
  is common in women of reproductive age. It is a functional disease. The
  diagnosis of IBS is based on the history of pain and bowel symptoms.
  Treatment is by high-fibre diet and antispasmodic drugs.
- *Constipation* is a common cause of bowel distension and chronic pelvic
  pain. Other conditions such as *inflammatory bowel disease* may present w
  pain, but other symptoms, such as bloody diarrhoea, are usually present.

Urological causes

- *Interstitial cystitis* (IC) is an inflammatory condition of unknown cause,
  which may cause pain and urinary symptoms such as urgency, frequency,
  and nocturia. The pain increases as the bladder fills and is relieved by
  passing urine. The diagnosis is made by cystoscopy with the characteristic
  appearance of submucosal oedema and petechiae. Dyspareunia is more
  common among women with IC.
- *Chronic urethral syndrome* is characterized by symptoms of irritation, pos
  voiding fullness, and incontinence.
- Other conditions such as urethral diverticulae, urinary calculi, bladder
  neoplasia, or radiation cystitis may also cause chronic pain.

usculoskeletal pain

n *sacroiliac dysfunction* pain may arise from the joints themselves or from he associated muscle spasm. The pain is typically worse with movement. Some patients with chronic pelvic pain have an *abnormal posture*, which may cause chronic muscle tension and strain on joints and ligaments, which then becomes a source of chronic pelvic pain.

Tension myalgia of the pelvic floor itself may be a cause of pelvic pain.

uropathic pain

e pain arises from a damaged nerve rather than tissue damage. Nerve entrap-nt in scar tissue or fascia may give rise to pain. The pain may be sharp or bbing in nature, or may be a constant dull ache. The diagnosis can be con-ned by injecting local anaesthetic at the site of maximal tenderness. Presacral rectomy has been used for patients with endometriosis with mixed results.

ychosocial factors

ronic pelvic pain may have a number of contributory factors: psychological, vsical, and social. The balance between the factors will vary from patient to ient and at different time of individual's disease. The presence of chronic vic pain may exacerbate or provoke difficulties in sleeping or depression. chological morbidity is more likely to be a consequence rather than a cause chronic pelvic pain. However, chronic pelvic pain is often associated with gative findings at clinical examination and laparoscopy and more than 50% patients have evidence of significant emotional disturbance. Pelvic pain may prove after reassurance following a negative laparoscopy. Women with onic pelvic pain have a higher incidence of past sexual abuse compared to se with other types of pain or no pain.[3]

Diagnosis

History
- Ask about the location of the pain, mode of onset, whether it is constant colicky in nature, radiation, and relation to the menstrual cycle.
- When was the last menstrual period?
- What contraception is she using?
- Is there any associated vaginal discharge or bleeding?
- Are there any bowel or urinary symptoms?[4]

Physical examination
- Is the patient able to move or crouched up in bed?
- Check blood pressure, temperature, and pulse.
- On abdominal examination, look for the location of the pain, rebound tenderness or guarding, and any mass or hernia.
- Carry out a pelvic examination (including speculum) to look for vaginal discharge or a pelvic mass and to assess pelvic tenderness.
    —If movement of the cervix elicits increased pain (cervical excitation) th may indicate the presence of blood in the peritoneal cavity (ectopic pregnancy) or inflammation of the peritoneum (PID).
    —Pelvic examination should not be done in ovarian hyperstimulation syndrome (risk of rupture of ovarian cysts) and is only carried out whe a diagnosis of ectopic pregnancy is suspected if facilities are available fe immediate laparotomy.

Investigations
- Triple swabs (high vaginal, cervical, and endocervical) should be obtaine to exclude sexually transmitted diseases such as chlamydia or gonorrhoea
- Send a midstream urine specimen to exclude urinary tract infection.
- Take blood samples for full blood count, group and save, and C-reactive protein.
- A urinary or serum β-hCG (beta human chorionic gonadotrophin) shou be checked to exclude pregnancy.
- Pelvic ultrasound scan—vaginal/abdominal to exclude pelvic pathology.
- Laparoscopy has an important place in the management of conditions th cause pelvic pain in women of reproductive age.[5] It is the 'gold standard' investigation for the diagnosis of ectopic pregnancy, endometriosis, and pelvic inflammatory disease.

65 Pelvic pain

References

1 Drife, J.O. (1993). The pelvic pain syndrome. *British Journal of Obstetrics and Gynaecology* **100**, 508–10.

2. Carey, M.P. and Slack, M.C. (1996). GnRH analogue in assessing chronic pelvic pain in women with residual ovaries. *British Journal of Obstetrics and Gynaecology* **103**, 150–3.

3 Collett, B.J., *et al.* (1998). A comparative study of women with chronic pelvic pain, chronic non-pelvic pain, and those with no history of pain attending general practitioners. *British Journal of Obstetrics and Gynaecology* **105**, 87–92.

4 Prentice, A. (2000). Medical management of chronic pelvic pain. *Best Practice and Research in Clinical Obstetrics and Gynaecology* **14**, 495–9.

5 Porpora M.G. and Gomel, V. (1997). The role of laparoscopy in the management of pelvic pain in women of reproductive age. *Fertility and Sterility* **68** (5), 765–79.

Pelvic inflammatory disease

Pelvic inflammatory disease (PID) is a common diagnosis for women presenting with lower abdominal pain. Although only a small proportion actually have pelvic infection, it is important to confirm the diagnosis because of the serious sequelae and associated problems of contact tracing.

PID is defined as an acute clinical syndrome associated with ascending spread of micro-organisms, usually unrelated to pregnancy or surgery, from the vaginal cervix to the endometrium, Fallopian tubes, and/or contiguous structures. PID may affect the pelvic peritoneum (pelvic peritonitis), the ovaries (oophoritis), the Fallopian tubes (salpingitis), or the uterus (endometritis).

Causal organisms

- *Chlamydia trachomatis* is the major aetiological pathogen in PID in Europe and the USA, although it may not be the same throughout the world. *Chlamydia* is an obligate intracellular 'parasitic bacterium'. The extent of damage caused by *Chlamydia* is variable, from being asymptomatic to causing severe pelvic infection.
- *Neisseria gonorrhoeae.* Gonococcal infections appear to be decreasing in frequency whilst chlamydial infections have increased. It is estimated that 15–20% of pelvic infection may be due to gonococci. Gonococci selectively invade the non-ciliated cells in the mucosa of the Fallopian tube, although it is the ciliated cells that are damaged.
- It is uncertain what role *mycoplasma* play in PID as they may be found in the flora of the genital tract of healthy women.
- *Bacterial vaginosis* (BV) causes a disturbance in the vaginal flora with an increase in the amount of anaerobic organisms. However, it is uncertain whether BV plays a role in the aetiology of PID.

Presentation

The spectrum of presentation for PID is very wide ranging from asymptomatic to severe.
- *Asymptomatic.* There may be no history at all of symptoms and the disease may be picked up incidentally at laparoscopy.
- *Mild.* Some women present with a vague lower abdominal pain with no vaginal discharge.
- *Moderate.* Moderate pain associated with dyspareunia and a vaginal discharge.
- *Severe.* In severe cases there may be evidence of high fever, rigors, peritonism, and a mass suggesting abscess formation.

Diagnosis

History

Because the spectrum of disease is so wide, the following features that raise the possibility of PID should be looked for in the history.

- Constant lower abdominal pain.
- Purulent vaginal discharge, sometimes offensive, sometimes irritating.
- Deep dyspareunia.
- Dysmenorrhoea.
- Menstrual irregularities.
- Current or previous intrauterine contraceptive device (IUCD) use.
- History of infertility or ectopic pregnancy.

Examination

The following features are associated with PID.

- Pyrexia.
- Lower abdominal pain.
- Cervical excitation pain.
- Tenderness on pelvic examination with a tender uterus and adnexae and reduced mobility of the pelvic organs.
- Adnexal enlargement (abscess or hydrosalpinges or tubo-ovarian mass).

Criteria for diagnosis

There is no proven ideal way to diagnose PID, but various criteria may be taken into account. Rolf's criteria for diagnosis of PID are the following.

- Lower abdominal tenderness.
- Bilateral adnexal tenderness.
- Cervical motion tenderness.
- No evidence of a competing diagnosis.

With these criteria antibiotic treatment should be started for probable PID. In more severe cases hospitalization will be necessary and further investigations may be required.

Investigations

If the history and examination are suggestive of PID the following investigations should be considered.

- Full blood count (FBC) and differential white count.
- Beta-human chorionic gonadotrophin (in appropriate patients).
- Midstream urine for microscopy, culture, and sensitivity.
- High vaginal swab.
- Endocervical swabs for *Chlamydia* and *Gonococci*.
- Blood cultures in patients with severe symptoms.
- Pelvic ultrasound scan.
- Laparoscopy.

Sequelae of PID

If it is treated inadequately or the diagnosis is unrecognized, PID may result in:

- Infertility. Following one episode of PID, 8% of women will have tubal factor infertility, 20% will be affected after two infections, and 40% after three or more infections.
- Recurrent PID. After initial PID 25% of women will develop a second infection
- Ectopic pregnancy. There is a sixfold increase in the risk of an ectopic pregnancy after pelvic infection.
- Chronic pelvic pain and dyspareunia.
- Tubo-ovarian abscess.

Treatment

Treatment depends on the severity of the disease. Patients with severe disease (e.g. pyrexia, pelvic peritonitis, severe pain and unable to do normal work, tender adnexal masses) should be admitted to hospital, whereas milder infections may be treated in the community.

- Antibiotic treatment should involve broad-spectrum antibiotics, initiated before the pathogens have been identified. A useful combination for treatment will include a second- or third-generation cephalosporin or amoxycillin with probenecid, a tetracycline, and metronidazole.
  - In severe cases treatment is usually intravenous (IV) initially and should continue for up to 14 days.
- In severely ill patients, analgesia and IV fluid replacement should be given.
- Laparoscopy is indicated if symptoms do not improve within 24–48 hours, and laparotomy and surgical drainage are usually necessary for pelvic abscesses.

Prevention

Successful strategies have been employed in Sweden to control genital chlamydia and gonorrhoea and this has led to a significant reduction in the occurrence of symptomatic pelvic infection. Education is important, particularly for the young. This needs to be culturally sensitive and local practice will determine the age at which it should be started. Contact tracing should be rigorous for all patients with proven genital tract infection with treatment and eradication of disease in sexual partners.

Endometriosis

This painful inflammatory condition is characterized by *the presence of endome* *trial tissue at ectopic sites*. Endometriosis is diagnosed at laparoscopy, and shoul then be classified using the American Fertility Society system of classification. I is highly likely that women with this condition have a genetic predisposition t both implantation of the ectopic endometrium and, more importantly, to th inflammatory response that occurs with cyclical endometrial changes.

Prevalence is estimated as 1–20% during reproductive years. Up to 25% o women presenting with gynaecological symptoms are found to have endometri otic lesions at thorough laparoscopic assessment.

Pathogenesis

A number of theories have been proposed—the 'disease of theories'. Retrograde menstruation, although probably universal, is the most likely cause. Endometriosis is certainly oestrogen-dependent and regresses after bilatera oopherectomy. Distant sites can be explained by coelomic metaplasia, but in al cases a genetic and immunological basis is emerging from immunohistochemi cal studies. There is now extensive evidence of altered immune function ir endometriosis. A large proportion of women have retrograde menstruation, bu only a minority of those develop endometriosis. In this condition peritoneal cel populations are increased and activated. This in turn leads to a chronic inflam matory response also seen in other autoimmune disorders with local release o prostanoids and cytokines, and subsequent peritoneal scarring.

Clinical presentation

The classic form of pelvic pain in endometriosis usually takes the form of sec ondary dysmenorrhoea (32% of women) becoming apparent after a lapse o years following menarche and starting before the onset of a period and contin uing throughout. With increasing tissue damage and scarring, the duration o the chronic pelvic pain (16%) increases to occur outside and seemingly with les relation to menstruation.

The uterosacral ligaments and ovaries are a very common site for endometrioti deposits, leading to deep dyspareunia, which is a complaint in 26% of womer with endometriosis.

Pain in endometriosis is caused by:
- Local peritoneal inflammation.
- Deeply infiltrating deposits.
- Formation of adhesions and fibrosis limiting movements.
- Traction on tissues.

In this enigmatic condition severe pelvic pathology is often seen in women with no symptoms and, overall, studies have not detected any correlation between severity of endometriosis and pelvic pain symptoms.

The role of endometriosis in the pathogenesis of infertility remains unclear. It is easy to see how *severe* endometriosis can affect fertility by mechanical distortion of the tubes and ovaries and the formation of adhesions. It is uncertain to what extent *minimal* to *mild* endometriosis affects fertility, and medical treatment of these women does not enhance their fertility if they are clearly subfertile.

Possible mechanisms of endometriosis associated with subfertility include the following.

- Tubal dysfunction.
- Failure of oocyte collection.
- Ovulation dysfunction.
- Lutenized unruptured follicle syndrome.
- Peritoneal inflammation with local immune activation.
- Dyspareunia, if present, often as part of pelvic pain, can also affect fertility by reducing sexual activity.

Diagnosis

This depends on the sites involved, and endometriosis can be detected on clinical examination. Commonly, involved ovaries enlarge with endometrioma or uterosacral ligaments become nodular and tender and can be felt on bimanual pelvic examination. A fixed retroverted tender uterus indicates disease in the pouch of Douglas.

- *Ultrasound* is useful for distinguishing between different adnexal enlargements. Endometriomas are highly echogenic and cystic, as opposed to a tubular hydrosalpinx.
- *Adenomyosis*—myometrial endometriosis—causes uniform enlargement of the uterus unlike uterine fibroids.
- *Tumour markers.* CA 125 (carcinoma antigen 125) can be used as a marker for extensive disease, but is also found to be elevated in 2.6% of healthy women and up to 20% of those with other benign gynaecological conditions. CA 125 is not very helpful in monitoring results of medical treatment. Other markers, such as placental protein 14, are less helpful.
- *Laparoscopy* is essential to confirm the diagnosis suspected on clinical grounds, or to exclude the diagnosis in women with pelvic pain or subfertility. This invasive diagnostic tool enables description and staging of the disease by visual inspection.
- *Ovarian endometrioma* is seen on the ovarian surface as pigmented and retracted areas, often with adhesions to the ovarian fossa. Small endometriomas can easily be missed unless the full ovarian surface is inspected.
- *Peritoneal lesions* are seen to be papular or vesicular, containing red haemorrhagic fluid in the early stages, becoming more puckered black 'powder-burn' lesions or whitish scar tissue, which probably indicates old deposits. Nodular lesions are more often seen on the uterosacral ligaments.[2]

The American Fertility Society (AFS 1985) revised system of classification is currently used to stage pelvic endometriosis. This involves an estimation of the size and depth of peritoneal and ovarian lesions, the extent and type of adhesions, and the degree of obliteration of the pouch of Douglas with surrounding tissue scarring.

Treatment

Many aspects remain unclear, but in all cases treatment must be individualized based on:

- Age.
- Presenting symptoms.
- Desire for future fertility.
- Severity of condition based on the AFS classification.

Ongoing subfertility
Minimal to mild endometriosis

- There is no evidence to show that the successful medical treatment of minimal to mild endometriosis without mechanical distortion of tubes and ovaries enhances fertility in subfertile women.[3]
- Surgical ablation, best performed at the time of the initial laparoscopy, does improve fertility. This might also slow the progress of the condition subsequently causing pain. If pregnancy then fails to occur, and the patient remains asymptomatic after expectant management, resumption of treatment is then along the lines of 'unexplained infertility'.
- *Ovarian stimulation with intrauterine insemination* (IUI) is more effective than either no treatment or IUI alone.
- The presence of minimal to mild endometriosis does not adversely affect pregnancy rates in *in vitro* fertilization (IVF)/gamete intrafallopian transfer (GIFT).

Medical therapy is to inhibit endometrial growth, e.g. with the use of continuous hormonal contraceptives. However evidence suggests that the effect of medical therapy on the appearance of the disease may be temporary.

Moderate to severe endometriosis

Moderate to severe endometriosis with coexisting mechanical pelvic subfertility should have further surgery if the anatomical problems can be corrected. This can be done after an episode of medical treatment, and can be performed with either open surgical techniques, or better approached endoscopically. There are *no* controlled studies and *no* comparison of the success of this treatment with assisted reproduction techniques. Iatrogenic postsurgical adhesions remain a problem, and assisted reproduction techniques should be considered as an alternative to or following unsuccessful surgery. Large ovarian endometriomas are best treated surgically prior to assisted reproduction to facilitate egg collection and, subsequently, to improve pregnancy rate. Presurgery medical treatment can be considered, but will further delay treatment cycles.[4]

Symptomatic endometriosis

Definitive surgery in the form of a hysterectomy and bilateral salpingo-oophorectomy for pain can only be considered after completion of family or if pregnancy is not a requisite. Otherwise, surgery is conservative and used in tandem with or as a supplement to medical treatment.

- *Danazol*, an androgenic steroid, is used in increasing doses to achieve amenorrhoea, starting with 200 mg and increasing to 800 mg. The treatment is continued for 6 months. Long-term follow-up studies have shown a recurrence of 37% for minimal and over 60% for severe disease. The side-effects are mostly androgenic, such as acne, seborrhoea, hirsutism, and weight gain. All these side-effects are reversible on cessation of therapy, apart from reported voice changes, as recorded by audiology measurements. Compliance can be poor because of side-effects.

Initial laboratory investigations

- Semen analysis (please refer to Chapter 69).
- Mid-luteal phase progesterone. If cycles are longer than 28 days the serum progesterone is estimated 7 days before the onset of menstruation.
  —If > 30 nmol/L there is adequate ovulation.
  —If < 30 nmol/L repeat in another cycle.
  —If level is consistently low, couple should be referred to a gynaecologist.
- Rubella status.
- Luteinizing hormone (LH)/follicle-stimulating hormone (FSH), prolactin, and thyroid function test prior to early referral in women with oligo/amenorrhoea.

Management in secondary care

- All the information accrued during the couple's primary care management must be communicated to the secondary care team. This will greatly hasten the subsequent investigations and management of the couple.
- The secondary management of infertility should preferably take place in a dedicated clinic run by trained staff who are readily accessible to help couples make their choices and orientate the management of their subfertility.
- Both partners should be seen together, but care is required to maintain individual's confidentiality if prompted by the referral letter.
- Full histories and examinations of both partners are performed if this has not been done previously, but is best delayed to the second visit in certain circumstances.
- The initial set of investigations requested will be dependent on those already performed by the GP, and points raised from the history and examination. If no abnormalities are identified after the initial investigations, tubal function is then investigated with the purpose of achieving a diagnosis prior to treatment and to avoid empirical non-evidence based treatments. Table 68.1 lists the diagnostic groups and the estimated prevalence of each diagnosis. Many couples have more than one problem leading to their joint subfertility.

Male factors and endometriosis are discussed in Chapters 69 and 67, respectively. Ovulation disorder will only be briefly discussed here. (See Chapters 55 and 62.)

Ovulation disorder

Anovulation may present with amenorrhoea, oligomenorrhoea, or rarely with regular menstrual cycles but low serum progesterone in previously investigated cycles. Some causes of anovulation are listed in Table 68.2.

- Investigations to be performed, if not already available, should be serum FSH (high in primary ovarian failure) and serum LH (high in polycystic ovary syndrome (PCOS)) in the early 'follicular' phase of a menstrual cycle.
  —Serum prolactin and thyroid function tests (TFTs) are mandatory in women with secondary amenorrhoea (for further investigations see Chapter 55).
  —Serum oestradiol concentration varies widely and a single measurement is rarely of value. Assessment of endogenous oestrogen production can be performed using a *progestogen challenge test* after a negative pregnancy test (medroxyprogesterone acetate 10 mg three times a day for 1 week).
- *Ultrasound scan* of the pelvis is helpful to identify polycystic ovaries and exclude large endometriomas. As part of later investigations tracking of follicular growth and rupture using serial scans is used for the rare diagnosis of the *lutenized unruptured follicle syndrome* where a pre-ovulatory follicle fails to rupture.

Table 68.1 The diagnostic groups and the estimated prevalence of each diagnosis

Diagnostic groups	Estimated prevalence (%)
Ovulation disorders	20–30
Endometriosis	5–15
Tubal factor	20–35
Cervical factor	5
Male factor	25
Unexplained	27
Sexual dysfunction	5

Table 68.2 Causes of anovulation

Primary ovarian failure

Autoimmune

Genetic, e.g. Turner's syndrome

Secondary ovarian disorders

Polycystic ovary syndrome

Abnormal gonadotrophin regulation

  Specific

    Hyperprolactinaemia

    Kallman's syndrome

Functional

    Weight problems

    Excessive exercise

    Idiopathic

Gonadotrophin deficiency

  Pituitary tumour

  Previous pituitary surgery

Management in secondary care (*continued*)

Induction of ovulation

Induction of ovulation regimes are chosen based on a diagnosis of the cause of the anovulation. All patients must be given clear information about the risks of multiple pregnancy and ovarian hyperstimulation (see Chapter 62). The aim of an ovulation induction programme is to achieve a unifollicular ovulation.

- Dopamine agonist, bromocriptine, is effective treatment for women with hyperprolactinaemia (normal or low FSH and raised prolactin). Those patients should ideally be managed in a gynaecology/endocrinology joint clinic run by an endocrinologist and gynaecologist. The same applies to women with coexisting thyroid dysfunction.
- In anovular women with normal FSH and normal endogenous oestrogen levels, the first-line management to induce ovulation should be an anti-oestrogen like clomiphene starting at 50 mg on days 2–6 of the menstrual cycle. This should only be performed if monitoring of response to therapy using endocrine and ultrasound means is readily available. Treatment is thereafter changed according to the monitored response and up to 12 cycles of treatment should be considered after informed counselling of couples regarding the risks of ovarian cancer associated with ovulation induction therapy.
- Women with low oestrogen levels and normal/low FSH can have ovulation successfully induced with exogenous gonadotrophins or pulsatile gonadotrophin-releasing hormone (GnRH). A regular or low-dose gonadotrophin regime is used in PCOS.
- There is no evidence that ovulation induction is effective in women with clear primary ovarian failure or with persistently raised FSH levels in the early follicular phase. Assisted reproduction with egg donation is now an effective option.

Tubal factor

The 'gold standard' basic investigation remains a diagnostic laparoscopy and dye insufflation, but a hysterosalpingogram (HSG) is an effective initial screening investigation for women without significant past history and ongoing symptoms.

- HSG provides an outline of both the uterine cavity and the Fallopian tubes. This investigation can occasionally produce severe pain and antibiotic cover should be used where there is a past history of pelvic inflammatory disease (PID).
- The false-positive likely tubal factor subfertility diagnosed at HSG is corrected by subsequent laparoscopy, which is indicated whenever the HSG is abnormal.
- HSG using ultrasound and a galactose-containing contrast medium (HyCoSy) is now available and yields similar information to a conventional HSG, without radiation exposure.
- *Laparoscopy and dye* is also indicated prior to a diagnosis of unexplained infertility, despite a normal HSG. The pelvis should be systematically examined prior to methylene blue being injected transcervically.

- The findings and extent of pelvic pathology—line drawings in the notes—should lead to a management plan. The options are selective salpingorrhaphy/tubal catheterization (only available in a few centres), surgery, or assisted reproduction in the form of IVF.
- Peritubular adhesions interfere with ovulation and ovum pick-up, so laparoscopic adhesiolysis when tubes are patent results in good cumulative conception rates. A microsurgical approach for women with tubal proximal disease is appropriate for mild tubal disease (grade I or II). If pregnancy has not occurred within 12 months of surgery, *in vitro* fertilization (IVF) should be considered. The latter should be considered as first-line treatment for all other women with tubal disease.

Unexplained infertility

This is a diagnosis of exclusion reached when investigations have been completed, and no clear explanation reached for the couple's ongoing inability to conceive after 2 years of unprotected sexual intercourse.

- Cervical factor subfertility is first excluded by an *in vivo* postcoital test (PCT) with or without further *in vitro* sperm–mucus interaction studies.
- Without a formal underlying cause, treatment is empirical but counselling of couples is essential pre-treatment. Expectant management, after counselling, depends on the duration of subfertility and the age of the women. Spontaneous pregnancy is still likely for couples with 2 years unexplained infertility.
- Ovarian stimulation with intrauterine insemination is an effective form of treatment—monthly fertility of 9.5% versus 3.3% in controls—but treatment with ovulation induction alone is of no benefit. Gamete intrafallopian transfer (GIFT) carries similar outcome results when compared to intrauterine insemination with ovulation induction (IUI + OI). IVF provides further therapeutic options for this group of couples, and is now the next step after failed IUI cyles.

Counselling in subfertility

This should be available to all couples and backed up by detailed and regularly reviewed information leaflets. Counselling, although part of general clinical management, should be provided by an independent qualified counsellor. This takes the form of information, discussion of implications, support, and therapeutic counselling.

Male subfertility

Male infertility affects about 25% of subfertile couples. In the majority of these, the male partner is subfertile and, in a small number, infertile.

Andrology is the branch of science and medicine that deals with the reproductive functions of the male, of which nowadays subfertility and hypogonadism with desired paternity are central topics. At the core of andrology is semen analysis (seminology), which determines management lines in reproductive medicine.

The organs of reproduction

These consist of two testes in which normal spermatogenesis takes place in the seminiferous tubules and efferent duct system and a number of accessory glands. The duct starts as an extremely coiled tube lying on the surface of the testis—the epididymis—which then straightens out to become the ductus deferens or 'vas'. The vas empties into the prostatic urethra, which is continuous with the penile urethra. The accessory glands, of which the epididymis acts as one, are the seminal vesicles, the prostate, and the urethral glands, all of which empty into the prostatic urethra. The penis has tubes of erectile tissue—corpora cavernosum and spongiosum.

Sperm production and control

The testes have two functions—production of spermatozoa and production of male sex hormones. Each function is complementary to the other, and the two functions take place in different compartments. Some 2×10^{12} spermatozoa are produced in a lifetime, and the main regulators of spermatogenesis, follicle-stimulating hormone (FSH) and testosterone, act on the Sertoli cells and spermatogenic (germ) cells, both being within the tubular compartments of the testes.

In the absence of these hormones, spermatogenesis eventually stops. Sertoli cells are thought to control the proliferation and development of spermatogonia, leading to spermatozoa. This process takes 74 days.

In the intertubular compartment of the testes, testosterone is synthesized from cholesterol within the Leydig cells. This is regulated by luteinizing hormone (LH). There are known to be specific receptors to LH and FSH in the Leydig and Sertoli cells, respectively.

Similarly to other endocrine control mechanisms, testosterone and inhibin, produced from Leydig cells, exert negative feedback regulation on the release of pulsatile pituitary LH and FSH. The end product of this process, a spermatozoon, has four features that make it unique when compared to other body cells. It is devoid of cytoplasm, has a mobile tail, functions independently of other spermatozoa, and is haploid. Spermatozoa form 10% or less of the volume of seminal fluid ejaculated.

Sperm transport

Penile erection and ejaculation are under the control of the autonomic nervous system. During sexual arousal parasympathetic impulses cause vasodilatation of the pudendal arteries. The distal branches of the pudendal arteries are coiled in the corpora cavernosum, and with vasodilatation these penile arteries straighten out and fill the sinus of erectile tissues with blood. This compresses venous outflow and leads to erection.

aculation or delivery of the seminal fluid into the prostatic urethra is under mpathetic control. Adrenaline (also called epinephrine) causes contractions local smooth muscles. Coagulated semen is then released.

the female, millions of sperms are deposited around the cervical external os. perm penetration and passage through the cervical mucus is dependent on erm motility and the quality of the mucus. Myometrial contractions transport e sperm from the cervix to the uterotubal junction. In the human female, gasm is thought to aid this process. In the Fallopian tube cilial activity and erm motility lead to progress towards the middle third of the tube, where fer- ization usually occurs.

Diagnosis of male infertility

Ideally, history-taking and examination should precede semen analysi
However, in clinical practice this often only takes place if the initial analysis
not entirely normal. This is slowly changing. A thorough case history and exam
ination can yield important information and allow meaningful interpretation
the analysis.

History
- A medical history must include details about onset of puberty, any
  testicular maldescent and timing of surgery, hernia repair, and ongoing
  general medical conditions (diabetes mellitus). Past history of mumps and
  other causes of orchitis (recurrent trauma) or sexually transmitted disease
  (STD) is also important.
- Family history should include enquiries about cystic fibrosis and other
  possible genetic cause of hypogonadism.
- Many drugs can affect spermatogenesis and sexual function including the
  use of anabolic steroids.
- Certain occupations with inherent exposure to heat, chemical, dyes, and
  toxins can cause infertility.
- Finally, smoking, excessive alcohol intake, and excessive athletic activities
  are also important.

Examination
- Physical examination should include body proportions and fat distribution
  as well as other clinical features of androgenicity—voice, hair, and skin.
  Anosmia is diagnostic of Kallmann's syndrome.
- Testicular size is then determined by palpation with or without the use
  of a Prader orchidometer. The normal range is 12–30 mL (average volume
  18 mL). Normal volume with azoospermia is suggestive of an obstruction,
  and small soft testicles are indicative of low gonadotrophins.
- Undescended or maldescended testis, swelling of the epididymis
  (spermatocele), and distension of the pampiniform plexus (varicocele)
  must be looked for.[2] Congenital absence of the vas deferens is seen in abou
  2% of patients. The urethral opening should be at the end of the penis.

Semen analysis
Semen analysis forms the cornerstone of the assessment of the subfertile coupl

Collection of the sample
An instruction sheet should be given to the patient. The specimen should
produced by masturbation. Condoms should not be used as they contain spe
micides. Abstinence from coitus for 48–72 hours is suggested. This improves t
standardization of the test, and may increase the total count. Prolonged abst
nence beyond 5 days is associated with a decrease in motility.

Wide-mouth sterile plastic containers should be used and labelled with the da
and time of production. Most fertility units have a dedicated room for produ
tion on site—this allows optimum analysis once liquefaction has taken plac
Otherwise, the sample should be delivered to the laboratory within 30 minut
of production.

Normal values for semen analysis

Laboratories reporting semen analysis results should establish normal ranges for their own population, and indicate these on the report. Table 69.1 gives the World Health Organization (WHO) standards for 'normal' semen samples.[3]

Recently ejaculated spermatozoa are actively motile and normally are able to swim with a forward progressive motion (grade I, fast; grade II, slow). Low motility and minimal forward progression (grade III) and no motility (grade IV) in a freshly ejaculated sample might indicate the presence of auto-antibodies in the sperm. Further specific investigations are then indicated. Samples with high white cell count should be screened for infection.

Further investigations

- The evaluation of serum levels of LH, FSH, and testosterone and prolactin provides important information for specifying the cause of subfertility and hypogonadism.
- High gonadotrophin levels with low testosterone indicate a testicular origin of hypogonadism—primary testicular failure.
- Chromosome analysis should be performed if testicles are also small and firm—Klinefelter's syndrome.
- Low gonadotrophin and testosterone levels usually indicate a central cause. Other investigations occasionally needed to complete the investigation of the male factor are ultrasound of the scrotum, magnetic resonance imaging (MRI) of the pituitary gland, and pituitary stimulation tests.
- Azoospermia with a normal endocrine profile raises the possibility of an obstruction. Vasogram and testicular biopsy are then best performed in units where there are facilities for sperm recovery and cryostorage.

Table 69.1 WHO[3] standards for 'normal' semen samples

Parameter	Normal range
Volume	2–5 mL
Liquefaction time	Within 30 minutes
Concentration	20–200 million/mL
Motility	Greater than 40% motile (grades I and II)
Morphology	Greater than 40% normal forms
White blood cells	Less than 1 million/mL

Treatment of male subfertility

Concern has been expressed that with assisted reproduction techniques (ART) most treatments are now designed to enhance sperm quality *in vitro* rather than to treat the underlying problem. These, techniques, including gamete donation are discussed in Chapter 71.

Specific dysfunctions can be treated successfully.
- Infection in the male genital tract should be treated if present, although there is no evidence that fertility is improved.
- Where a diagnosis of hypogonadotrophic hypogonadism is made in the male partner, the use of gonadotrophin is effective.[4]
- Similarly, the use of bromocriptine is effective if hyperprolactinaemia is diagnosed.
- The use of systemic corticosteroids for the treatment of antisperm antibodies[5] and the surgical correction of varicocele remain controversial.
- The use of antioxidants, mast cell blockers, zinc, and certain vitamins[6] (for the treatment of men with abnormalities of semen quality) needs further evaluation before they can be used in clinical practice.

eferences

Glover, T.D., Barrat, C.L.R., Tyler, J.P.P., and Hennessey, J.F. (1990). *Human male fertility and semen analysis.* Academic Press, London.

Nieschlag, E. (1998). Update on treatment of varicocele: counselling as effective as occlusion of the vena spermatica. *Human Reproduction* 13, 2147–50.

World Health Organisation (WHO) (1992). *WHO laboratory manual for the examination of human semen and sperm–cervical mucus interactions,* 3rd edn. Cambridge University Press, Cambridge.

Buchter, D., Behre, H.M., Kliesch, S., and Nieschlag, E. (1998). Pulsatile GnRH or human chorionic gonadotrophin/human menopausal gonadotrophin as effective treatment for men with hypogonadotrophic hypogonadism: a review of 42 cases. *European Journal of Endocrinology* 139, 298–303.

Abshagen, K., Behre, H.M., Cooper, T.G., and Nieschlag, E. (1998). Influence of sperm surface antibodies on spontaneous pregnancy rates. *Fertility and Sterility* 70, 355–6.

Suleiman, S.A., Ali, M.E., Zaki, Z.M., el-Malik, E.M., and Nasr, M.A. (1996). Lipid peroxidation and human sperm motility: protective role of vitamin E. *European Journal of Andrology* 17, 530–7.

Chapter 70

Gonadotrophin-releasing hormone (GnRH) in gynaecology

GnRH agonists available for clinical use are derived from the naturally occur ring GnRH decapeptide but are over 100 times more potent than the natura endogenous hormone. The molecule is altered to decrease enzyme breakdow and therefore has increased half-life.

Mode of action

During the luteal phase, endogenous GnRH pulses are large and relatively infre quent leading to a similar pattern of luteinizing hormone (LH) secretion. In th follicular phase, GnRH pulses increase in frequency, causing similar increases c LH production.

With pharmacological GnRH agonist, the majority of GnRH receptors i the pituitary glands are occupied resulting in an initial surge of plasm gonadotrophin levels. After the initial stimulation, continued receptor occu pancy downregulates pituitary gonadotrophin production resulting in the sup pression of gonadotrophin secretion. A reversible 'menopause' is activated b prolonged GnRH agonist treatment.

Indications for GnRH agonist use in gynaecology

- Precocious puberty.
- Endometriosis.
- Fibroids.
- Premenstrual syndrome.
- Induction of ovulation in women with polycystic ovary (PCO), and for controlled hyperstimulation in assisted reproduction.

Precocious puberty

This can be treated with GnRH agonist when no cause can be found, or when a cause cannot be removed. Pubic hair will not disappear, but further menstruation, the growth spurt leading to premature epiphyseal closure, and breast development will be inhibited. Normal adult height can be achieved by delaying bone maturation until adrenarche.

Endometriosis

Treatment with GnRH agonist is usually limited to 6 months.[1] The initial surge of gonadotrophins can cause a transient deterioration of symptoms. To avoid disturbing hypo-oestrogenic symptoms, and to prevent loss of bone mineral content, long-term therapy with GnRH agonist is combined with 'add-back' therapy. The additional oestrogen and progestogen can be used sequentially or continuously. Two preparations commonly used are Cyclo-Progynova or Tibolone. It is preferable to start the 'add-back' replacement after the downregulation is well established.

The *side-effects* of GnRH agonists, which include bone loss associated with prolonged use, are all those that occur in menopausal women, i.e. bone loss, vasomotor symptoms, reduced libido, vaginal dryness, and irritability and are relieved by the use of 'add-back' oestrogen (and progestogen). The oestrogen effect of 'add-back' therapy is much less than that due to oestrogen in the natural cycles and hence does not stimulate endometriosis.

Fibroids

Not all GnRH agonists are licensed for use to shrink fibroids in the UK, but they are widely used in clinical practice in certain circumstances[2] because the benefits of therapy only last for as long as it is continued.

In cases needing myomectomy some use GnRH analogues preoperatively for the following reasons.
- Reduced intraoperative blood loss.
- Relief of symptoms.
- Relief of anaemia and reduced need for transfusion.
- May enable use of lower transverse incision.
- Reduction of tissue trauma at myomectomy.

Ultrasound scans should be used during therapy, to measure reduction in size of uterus/fibroids. Loss of tissue planes and being unable to identify smaller fibroids at myomectomy are disadvantages that are outweighed by the benefits of therapy. This is, however, an expensive approach, and the use of add-back oestrogen to relieve vasomotor symptoms and avoid bone loss remains uncertain for this indication.

Premenstrual syndrome

This has been effectively treated by GnRH agonists,[3] but treatment should be limited to 6 months or less. Symptoms often gradually recur after cessation of therapy, which is therefore best used as a diagnostic test of the long-term benefits of bilateral salpingo-oophorectomy in severe cases of premenstrual syndrome.

Induction of ovulation

There are two areas where GnRH agonists are used in regimes to stimulate folliculogenesis.

- Ovulation induction in women with anovulatory subfertility.
- Stimulation for assisted reproduction.

Over 20% of anovulatory women, especially those with PCO, do not respond to clomiphene, which is the first line of therapy. Gonadotrophins are therefore used in this group. This carries a high rate of multiple pregnancy, and a high risk of ovarian hyperstimulation syndrome. These are not improved by the *routine* use of GnRH agonist, and neither is the pregnancy rate improved. Downregulation in this group reduces the risk of premature LH surge before follicular maturation is complete, and can improve human chorionic gonadotrophin (hCG) injection timing.

There is no one ideal programme for ovulation stimulation in assisted reproduction, but the use of GnRH agonists, together with gonadotrophins, prevents spontaneous LH surges and improves egg collection rate and subsequent fertilization and implantation. This leads to an improved pregnancy rate per cycle.

- A recent meta-analysis has shown that, with the use of GnRH agonists in assisted reproduction, cycle cancellation rates are clearly reduced, oocytes recovered are increased, and the pregnancy rate per embryo transfer is improved.[4]
- Two basic protocols are widely used.
   —In the *short* protocol, no downregulation is induced, and GnRH agonist and gonadotrophins are used in parallel.
   —The *long protocol*, in which stimulation of the ovary only starts after complete pituitary downregulation, results in higher pregnancy rates but is more expensive and time-consuming.

Preparations

A number of GnRH agonists are now available, two as nasal spray and two as injection/intramuscular or biodegradable implant (Table 70.1).

Table 70.1 GnRH agonist preparations currently available

Preparation	Mode of use	Dosage	Frequency
Buserelin	Nasal spray	150 μg	3 doses a day
Nafarelin	Nasal spray	200 μg	2 doses a day
Goserelin	Implant	3.6 mg	28 days
Leuprorelin	Subcutaneous	3.75 mg	28 days

GnRH antagonists

New analogues have been synthesized that also bind to the pituitary GnRH receptors, but do not induce an initial release of gonadotrophins. These analogues are much more complex than GnRH agonists. Their mode of action is different. They do not act through downregulation of receptors, and desensitization of gonadotrophins, but by competitive binding to the receptor and therefore reducing the secretion of gonadotrophins within hours. Suppression is then maintained by continuous treatment without initial stimulatory effect.

- Two such compounds are available—cetrorelix and ganirelix—and both have been successfully used in ovulation induction protocols in assisted reproduction.[5]
- Cetrorelix is for use in single dose (3 mg subcutaneous (SC) injection) or multiple dose (0.25 mg SC daily injections) regimens. Limited reports suggest that it is well tolerated with reduced risks of ovarian hyperstimulation when compared to agonists.

GnRH antagonists open new treatment options that require more clinical data.

References

1 The Nafarelin European Endometriosis Trial Group (NEET) (1992). Nafarelin for endometriosis: a large-scale, danazol controlled trial of efficacy and safety with 1 year follow-up. *Fertility and Sterility* 57, 514–22.

2 West, C.P., Lumsden, M.A., and Baird, D.T. (1993). Gozerelin (Zoladex) in the treatment of fibroids. *Reproductive Medicine Review* 2 (18), 1–97.

3 Hussain, S.Y., Massil, J.H., Matta, W.H., *et al.* (1992). Buserelin in premenstrual syndrome. *Gynecological Endocrinology* 6, 57–64.

4 Tom, S.L., Maconoachie, M., Doyle, P., Campbell, S., Balen, A., Bercir, J., *et al.* (1994). Cumulative conception and live-birth rates after in vitro fertilization with and without the use of long, short and ultrashort regimes of the gonadotrophin-releasing hormone agonist buserelin. *American Journal of Obstetrics and Gynecology* 171, 513–20.

5 Felberbaum, R.E., Ludwig, M., and Diedrich, K. (1998). Are we on the verge of a new era in ART. *Human Reproduction* 13, 1778–80.

Chapter 71

Assisted reproductive techniques (ART)

The first test-tube baby was born in the UK in 1978. Since then *in vitro* fertilization (IVF) has been 'finely tuned', and many other forms of ART have been developed for specific clinical indications. IVF remains the most widely used ART to treat all categories of subfertility and the number of IVF cycles has increased tenfold over the last 10 years. The take-home baby rate per cycle of IVF during 1997–98, based on 27 282 cycles of treatment for all ages, was 17.4%.[1] The success of ART is very dependent on the skill and expertise of staff of individual units, as shown by wide interunit variations (take-home baby rate per IVF/intracytoplasmic sperm injection (ICSI) cycle is 11.8–36% for all ages).

Overall, only about 1 in 6 IVF cycles is successful. Based on the 27 282 cycles reported, 76% were unsuccessful, 12% single births, 7% multiple births, and 5% were adverse outcomes (ectopics, spontaneous miscarriages, stillbirths, and neonatal deaths).[1]

Features affecting outcome

- *Age*. Female fertility reduces with advancing age. Similarly, IVF outcome is affected by age. IVF pregnancy rates are highest between the ages of 25 and 35, with a steep decline thereafter. Predicted live birth rate for a 30-year-old is 16.1% and it is down to 7.3% at 40.[2]
- *Duration of subfertility*. This has a major effect on the outcome of ART treatment cycles. At under 3 years of subfertility the live birth rate per cycle is 15% as compared to 8% after 12 years' subfertility.
- *Previous cycles of treatment*. The best chances of conceiving are in the first ART cycle (14% live birth rate), with reduced outcome for each subsequent cycle—8.9% with four cycles of treatment.
- *Previous pregnancies*. Women who have had a previous successful pregnancy, either spontaneous or following an ART cycle, have a higher chance of conceiving with IVF treatment.

In vitro fertilization (IVF)

The recommendation for IVF now includes a wide range of indications.
- *Tubal disease* if not amenable to surgery or if pregnancy fails 12 months after successful surgery.
- *Unexplained infertility* after failed intrauterine insemination and ovulation induction (IUI + OI) using partner's sperm.
- *Male factor* with satisfactory sperm function. The chance of fertilization can be improved using a high insemination concentration (IVF-HIC), but this is now being replaced by ICSI.
- *Endometriosis*—moderate and severe disease.
- *Ovulation disorders*. If conception fails to occur after 6–12 cycles of successful ovulation induction.
- *Donor insemination*. Failure to conceive after 10–12 cycles of donor insemination with or without ovulation induction.
- *Egg donation* for women with premature ovarian failure, gonadal dysgenesis, iatrogenic menopause, carriers of a genetic condition, and raised follicle-stimulating hormone (FSH) levels in older women.
- *Surrogacy* for women with absent uterus, but with functional ovaries.

Steps of IVF cycle

- Downregulation of ovaries for 10–14 days started during the luteal phase of the previous cycle.

- Gonadotrophins (FSH or human menopausal gonadotrophin) generally in higher doses than those used in patients undergoing ovulation induction to cause superovulation. Short or long treatment protocols are widely used.
- Monitor treatment and measure follicular response and growth. This is essential to prevent serious side-effects.
- Oocyte collection is carried out under ultrasound guidance, through the vaginal wall. The follicles are aspirated by gentle suction from a vacuum pump. Up to 90% of follicles yield an oocyte. In a minority of women collection is performed at laparoscopy.
- Sperm sample is provided on the same day as oocyte collection.
- Oocyte and sperm are cultured overnight and, if fertilization has occurred, the embryos are further cultured. In some centres ICSI is performed as a routine to assist fertilization.
- Embryo transfer performed using a fine catheter through the cervix and into the uterine cavity 2–3 days postfertilization. A maximum of three embryos are returned in the UK.[3] The rest are cryopreserved for use in future cycles.
- Luteal support using progesterone is followed by pregnancy testing.

Intracytoplasmic sperm injection (ICSI)

This is a newer technique in which a single sperm is injected directly into the oocyte. It is used for severe male-factor subfertility.[4] It involves a conventional IVF treatment cycle and, as with IVF, a maximum of three embryos can be transferred into the uterus. The outcome with ICSI has improved the success rate for severe male-factor subfertility and the success rate of ICSI is now higher than that of IVF.

There are still concerns about the use of potentially abnormal sperm and screening for cystic fibrosis is often performed pre-ICSI treatment cycles, which have now replaced SUZI (sub-zonal insemination) and PZD (partial zonal dissection).

Sperm can be surgically recovered from the testis (testicular/epididymal sperm aspiration; TESA) or the epididymis (percutaneous epididymal sperm aspiration; PESA) in men with vas deferens obstruction (past infection or after vasectomy) or congenital absence of the vas. The extracted sperm can be frozen initially and used for injection into the oocyte using ICSI.

Gamete intrafallopian transfer (GIFT)

This is only effective with functional Fallopian tubes in couples with unexplained subfertility. The oocytes are collected at laparoscopy, mixed with washed and re-suspended sperms, and returned into the tubes. This is now used less frequently.

Intrauterine insemination and ovulation induction (IUI + OI)

This involves replacing carefully washed sperm into the uterine cavity at the time of ovulation. IUI requires ovulation induction[5] with follicular growth monitoring using ultrasound to determine the day of insemination. Both Fallopian tubes must be patent. The main indications are unexplained, male- and cervical-factor subfertility.

Donor insemination (DI)

This treatment is offered to couples when the male partner has azoospermia or the semen analysis is such that a pregnancy is unlikely—severe oligozoospermia, gross teratozoospermia, and severe asthenozoospermia. Otherwise, DI can be appropriate for couples who have a past history of severe rhesus isoimmunization with a homozygous husband or if genetic counselling suggests a high risk of major genetic problems.

- DI requires careful consideration, and all couples are advised to have formal counselling. It should be pointed out that the male partner's name will appear on the birth certificate, but informing the child later on in life must be strongly considered.
- The female partner should be investigated prior to starting DI, including tubal investigations. To maximize outcome, accurate timing of insemination is essential. Ovulation is therefore closely monitored using ultrasound following ovulation induction.
- The frozen donor sperm is thawed and placed in the cervix or, after preparation, IUI is performed.[6]
- Couples are offered 4–6 cycles, and failure must be followed by a formal review.
- *The donors*: Men between 18 and 55, with a normal sperm count. After detailed family, social, and medical history, potential donors are also counselled. All donors are screened for hepatitis and sexually transmitted disease, including HIV. The sperm straws are then frozen and quarantine for 6 months or more, after which the donors are retested for HIV before the straw is released for use. Clinics do their best to use a donor who has physical characteristics similar to those of the male partner.
- *Outcome for women below the age of 38.* The live birth rate is currently 10% and is 6% per treatment cycle started (National Data 1999). Chances of success decrease with age.

Donor oocyte within an IVF/ICSI cycle

This has been successfully used since 1984. The main indication for egg donation is women with premature ovarian failure, or others with persistently raised gonadotrophins in the early follicular phase of the menstrual cycle, where success with own eggs is extremely poor.

Counselling in subfertility

In the UK all clinics offering ART to treat subfertility couples are required in law to offer independent counselling. This is because such therapy creates a great deal of stress for the majority of couples who, often as a consequence of the subfertility and failure of treatment, experience a deep bereavement. This counselling takes the form of information, implication, and support counselling. Confidentiality is paramount as part of counselling, but also in all aspects of subfertility management.

References

1 Human Fertilisation and Embryology Authority (HFEA) (1999). *HFEA annual report*. HFEA, London.

2 Templeton, A., Morris, J.K., and Parslow, W. (1996). Factors that affect outcome of *in vitro* fertilization treatment. *Lancet* **348**, 1402–6.

3 Templeton, A.A. and Morris, J.K. (1998). Reducing the risk of multiple births by transfer of two embryos after IVF. *New England Journal of Medicine* **339**, 573–7.

4 Alikani, M., Cohen, J., and Palermo, G.D. (1995). Enhancement of fertilization by micromanipulation. *Current Opinion in Obstetrics and Gynaecology* **7**, 182–7.

5 Hughes, E.G. (1997). The effectiveness of ovulation induction and intrauterine insemination in the treatment of persistent infertility: a meta-analysis. *Human Reproduction* **12**, 1865–72.

6 Zayed, F., Lenton, E.A., and Cooke, I.E. (1997). Comparison between stimulated in-vitro fertilization and stimulated intrauterine insemination for the treatment of unexplained and milk male factor infertility. *Human Reproduction* **12**, 2408–13.

Chapter 72

Recurrent miscarriage

A *miscarriage* is loss of a pregnancy before viability. *Recurrent miscarriage* is defined as three consecutive pregnancies ending spontaneously before the 20th week of gestation.[1] This is a rare condition, with an expected chance of three consecutive pregnancy losses of 0.4%, and an observed risk of 1% of couples suffering from recurrent miscarriage. Overall, over 15% of diagnosed pregnancies will miscarry.

Couples who have recurrent early pregnancy losses are usually extremely distressed and hope for a diagnosis and therefore preventative measures for the future. Identification of a specific cause for the miscarriages is rarely the case, and very few specific effective therapies exist. Some have been discredited, and studies of new modalities of treatment must take into account the overall spontaneous 'cure rates' of over 50%.

Causes

More than one factor may exist within one individual, but couples must be warned prior to the onset of investigations that a cause is rarely identified. Only in special circumstances should women be investigated after two or fewer losses.

Anatomical causes

Prior to performing corrective surgery, which carries inherent potential postoperative infertility risks, the causal relationship between the anatomical abnormality and recent pregnancy losses must be very clear.

- *Uterine retroversion* as an aetiological factor leading to recurrent miscarriage is now thought not to be relevant.
- *Intrauterine adhesions* and *submucous fibroids* are unlikely to cause infertility, although the latter could cause very early miscarriage if implantation occurs on the fibroid. Myomectomy or endoscopic resection of fibroids carry the risk of adhesion formation.
- *Cervical incompetence* causes mid-trimester pregnancy loss, with typical spontaneous rupture of membranes and painless cervical dilatation. Incompetence is *overdiagnosed*. The use of cervical cerclage in suspected cases leads to a modest reduction in the incidence of pre-term deliveries, but no significant improvement in fetal survival.[2]
- *Congenital malformation* of the uterus, usually caused by abnormal fusion of the Müllerian ducts, is rare. The reported incidence varies between 0.1% and 3%. Implantation problems are thought to be more frequent in women with a single uterine horn or a bicornuate uterus. Restoring the uterine cavity to normal should only be considered as a last resort, and is best performed by experienced surgeons.

Infections

Many organisms have been put forward as causing recurrent miscarriages. Severe infection causing a high pyrexia, e.g. malaria, can lead to a *sporadic* pregnancy loss. The TORCH group of organisms (toxoplasma, rubella, cytomegalovirus, and herpes) are now thought to be unlikely causes of recurrent miscarriage; the same applies to bacterial vaginosis, which is still being investigated.

Genetic causes

A high percentage of *sporadic* spontaneous miscarriages are chromosomally abnormal and in a few cases this may be the cause for the recurrent condition. It is, however, important to evaluate the chromosome complement of both partners. An abnormal karyotype will be diagnosed in one of the partners in 3–5% of couples with recurrent miscarriage. The most common abnormality—over 60%—is a balanced reciprocal translocation, with 30% being a Robertsonian translocation. All such couples should be referred for formal genetic counselling.

Hormonal causes

It is clear that oestrogen and progesterone are important in the support of early pregnancy, but deficiencies of either have never been clearly identified, and the use of exogenous progesterone and human chorionic gonadotrophin (hCG) after the onset of pregnancy does not reduce the risk of recurrent losses. In assisted reproduction pregnancies both are started at time of conception, as part of artificial cycles.

Polycystic ovaries (PCO) are seen more frequently in patients with recurrent miscarriage (58%), as opposed to the general population (20%). This is possibly caused by the high luteinizing hormone (LH) levels seen in PCO, but downregulation and lowering overall LH levels does not improve the pregnancy outcome. Women with PCO should be informed of the higher early pregnancy losses when embarking on an ovulation induction programme.

Immune causes

The mechanism that stops fetal rejection by the mother remains unidentified. This may reflect either active maternal immunosuppression, or a failure of maternal immune system response. The theory that women who have recurrent miscarriages share a higher proportion of HLA antigens with their partners and hence are unable to initiate the above mechanisms leading to fetal rejection, has now been discredited. Similarly, prospective data using partner's lymphocyte infusions were initially promising, but have not been confirmed.[3]

Immunopathology studies of an endometrial biopsy in women with recurrent miscarriage looking for natural killer cells are in progress.

Autoimmune factors

Thrombophilic defects are now known to be an important cause of recurrent miscarriage. The initial association between recurrent miscarriage and antiphospholipid antibodies, lupus anticoagulant, and anticardiolipin antibodies has now been extended to include activated protein C resistance and antithrombin III and factor XII deficiencies. Low levels of the naturally occurring anticoagulants protein C and protein S have now been associated with this problem.

The common mechanism leading to pregnancy loss and other pregnancy problems is likely to be uteroplacental microthrombosis.

- Low-dose aspirin, heparin, and steroids (prednisolone/dexamethasone) have been used either in combination or singly to treat women with autoimmune thrombophilic defects and associated recurrent miscarriage. Cyclosporin, a drug that decreases the development of stem cells in the bone marrow and is used for transplant patients, has been proposed for use in early pregnancy—up to 10 weeks gestation. Controlled data are awaited.
  —Treatment with corticosteroid is associated with significant maternal and fetal morbidity, and does not seem to improve the live birth rate.
  —The treatment of choice is low-dose aspirin alone (75 mg daily) or with added low-dose heparin (5000 IU subcutaneous (SC) 12-hourly).[4]

Unexplained cause

This is a significant group who require explanation, support, and reassurance. The prognosis for future successful pregnancy is good—over 75% in the future. It is important to resist empirical treatment of this group.[5]

Investigation

History, examination, and investigations may help to identify a possible aetiological factor.

Investigations for all:
- Karyotyping for both partners.
- Pelvic ultrasound.
- Day 2 LH/follicle-stimulating hormone (FSH).
- Antiphospholipid antibodies.
- Activated protein C resistance.
- Antithrombin III.
- Protein C and S

Treatment

Couples who have a first or second miscarriage should be reassured and not investigated unless there is a specific reason to do so. Couples with three or more miscarriages should be fully investigated according to a protocol and, ideally, managed in a dedicated miscarriage clinic,[6] but warned at the outset that in the majority of couples no explanation will be found. Empirical treatment in this large group must be resisted. In situations when surgical treatment is available, the benefits must be thoroughly weighed against the drawbacks with the couple. Similarly, treatment of thrombophilic defects can be associated with maternal and fetal morbidity, but remains promising with increasing live birth rates with combination treatment.

References

Stirrat, G.M. (1990). Recurrent miscarriage I: definitions and epidemiology. *Lancet* **336**, 673–5.

MRC/RCOG Working Party on Cervical Cerclage (1993). Final report of the Medical Research Council/Royal College of Obstetricians and Gynaecologists multicentred randomized trial of cervical cerclage. *British Journal of Obstetrics and Gynaecology* **100**, 516–23.

Mowbray, J.F. (1994). Genetic and immunological factors in human recurrent abortion. *American Journal of Reproductive Immunology* **15**, 261–74.

Sher, G., Matzner, W., Ferviman, M., Maassarani, G., Eonves, C., Chong, P., *et al.* (1998). The selective use of heparin/aspirin therapy, alone or in combination with intravenous immunoglobulin G, in the management of antiphospholipid antibody positive women undergoing in vitro fertilization. *American Journal of Reproductive Immunology* **40** (2), 74–82.

Clifford, K., Rai, R., Watson, H., and Regan, L. (1995). An informative protocol for the investigation of recurrent miscarriage: preliminary experience of 500 conservative cases. *Human Reproduction* **9**, 1328–32.

Li, T.C. (1998). Guides for practitioners. Recurrent miscarriage: principles of management. *Human Reproduction* **13** (2), 478–82.

Chapter 73

Psychosexual problems and sexual dysfunction

Sexual problems within a relationship are not uncommon and more women and men now feel able to seek advice about them. The recognition of a problem as a psychosexual disorder will be influenced by the expectations of society and the individual or couples concerned, as well as by those of their professionals. The prevalence of sexual dysfunction in a study of 4000 randomly selected patients in four general practices was reported to be 44% among men and 36% among women. The prevalence varies according to how people are surveyed and what definition of sexual dysfunction is adopted.

Physiology of human sexual function

The physiology of human sexual response was described in the 1960s by Masters and Johnson. They described the five phases of human sexual response as sexual desire, sexual arousal or excitement, plateau phase, orgasm, and resolution. The physiological changes observed during sexual response are mediated by psychic and/or physical sexual stimulation but can be inhibited, to a greater or lesser extent, by subconscious influences.

- *Sexual desire* is stimulated by the thought, sight, smell, or touch of another person. It may be suppressed or merge into the arousal phase.
- The *arousal or excitement phase* is the initial response to sexual stimulation—physical or psychological. It is characterized by reflex vasodilatation in the genitalia. There is an associated systemic component characterized by a rise in pulse and respiratory rate and blood pressure. Arousal at this stage remains vulnerable to distracting influence (thoughts, noise) and may also be affected by fatigue, alcohol, or worry.
- *Plateau phase.* During this phase the changes in the arousal phase are consolidated and further enhanced, as is the sexual pleasure and the partners' desire for penetrative intercourse. Lower genital tract and breast changes reach a maximum while continuing stimulation may build up sexual excitement to the intensity required to achieve orgasm.
- *Orgasm* provides an intense feeling of pleasure associated with the discharge of sexual tension built up in the preceding phases. In both sexes it is associated with rhythmic contractions of the genital muscles.
  —Following ejaculation, the male experiences a refractory period that may vary in length and increases from a few minutes in the teenager to several hours in the elderly.
  —Many women and a minority of men do not have a refractory period with further stimulation leading to further orgasms in this group.
- *Resolution.* Following orgasm the body returns to the non-aroused state unless stimulation is continued. In the initial moments after orgasm the penis and clitoris are exquisitely sensitive but this is very transient with rapid decongestion of the tissues in the lower genital tract in both sexes.

73 Psychosexual problems

The phases of sexual response leading up to orgasm are mediated by the parasympathetic nerves and lead to vasodilatation and vasocongestion of the genital organs. Failure of sexual arousal and therefore of these changes to occur results in erectile failure in a man and general sexual dysfunction in a woman. The orgasmic phase is mediated by the sympathetic nervous system, leading to the clonic contractions of the pelvic and other muscles. Where the sympathetic component fails to occur in an orderly fashion, there is premature or retarded ejaculation as a result. The feeling of pleasure experienced by both sexes appears to have its origin in the sex centre in the thalamic and limbic areas of the old cortex. Failure to achieve orgasm in women is often a result of a failure of the sensations invoked in the clitoris and vagina being transmitted to the brain.

Assessment of the patient

Presentation

Problems may be hidden behind a variety of 'opening gambits'. Sexual difficulties underlie many cases of vague ill health in women that defy diagnosis until repeated attempts at communication are made. Lack of energy, backache, and irritability along with anxiety and depression may be the presenting symptoms. Similarly, patients may present in family planning clinics focusing their problems on contraception but where the hidden agenda is 'permission' or 'approval' that sexual intercourse is respectable when the aim is pleasure and love rather than procreation. Every one of the basic gynaecological symptoms may be wholly or partially determined by organic pathology or psychogenic distress.

Obtaining a sexual problem history

A good fundamental knowledge of human sexual functioning as well as experience in interviewing and counselling skills is paramount. It is essential to be guided by the patient, using the information offered by the patient to focus on establishing what the current problem is rather than taking a more general sexual history. Once the main problem has been defined, then a history of the development and progression of the problem should be obtained. This information should include the duration, nature of onset, whether improving or deteriorating, whether situational (i.e. present in one relationship but not another, one position and not another, etc.), and any factors that exacerbate or ameliorate the problem. It is also helpful to explore the patient's own assessment of the cause of the problem.

The consultation has to determine whether the problem is primary or secondary, by ascertaining when the problem started and whether it is causally associated with any other event occurring at the time the problem came to surface. It is also important to determine what prompted the patient to present at this point in time. One of the goals of the consultation is also to exclude any possible underlying organic factor.

Clinical examination

The role of clinical examination is to exclude developmental abnormalities that may interfere with sexual function. This includes detection of potential causes of dyspareunia and evidence of other medical conditions that may interfere with sexual function. Vaginal atresia and imperforate hymen in the female and undescended testes or hypospadias are among causes that would be identified on clinical examination.

In cases of *dyspareunia* a clinical assessment is imperative.
- Spasm of the pubococcygeus muscle may be detected during pelvic examination leading to a possible diagnosis of vaginismus while deep pelvic pain elicited on bimanual examination may be similar to discomfort experienced on intercourse.
- Acute infections such as candidiasis, herpes, and trichomoniasis along with acute or chronic inflammation of the Bartholin's gland or vestibular glands may lead to vulvovaginal irritation and superficial dyspareunia.
- Pelvic examination may detect evidence of pelvic inflammatory disorder (PID) or endometriosis as a cause of deep dyspareunia. A normal anatomical variant of a retroverted uterus and ovaries prolapsing into the pouch of Douglas may be a further cause of deep dyspareunia.

Medical conditions such as respiratory or cardiac disease may interfere with sexual activity as would osteoarthritis and limited mobility of the hips. Loss of sensation or reflexes in the perineal area, as may be associated with multiple sclerosis (MS) or damage to pelvic nerves through extensive pelvic surgery and associated scarring are other causes that may interfere with sexual function.

Any investigations should be guided by the suspected underlying pathology, but great care should be taken not to ascribe the cause of a sexual problem to an incidentally discovered abnormality.

Sexual dysfunction in the female

The majority of sexual dysfunctions do not have an organic basis to them. Many stem from:
- Poor relationship with partner.
- Low or mismatched sexual drive between partners.
- Ignorance about sexuality or sexual technique.
- Performance anxiety.
- Changing age affects sexual drive, desire, and response.
- Illness or treatment side-effects.
- Fear that sex may aggravate an existing medical condition.
- Depression.
- Excess alcohol.

The main sexual dysfunctions in women can be viewed under the headings:
- Inhibited sexual desire.
- Failure to achieve orgasm.
- Dyspareunia.
- Apareunia/vaginismus.

Inhibited sexual desire (hypoactive sexual desire disorder or general sexual dysfunction)

This may have a prevalence as high as 10% affecting women more than men. It is characterized by the absence of sexual fantasies and the desire for sexual activity. It may have its onset at puberty or may occur some months or years after normal sexual activity. Inhibited sexual desire may be a manifestation of clinical depression or of a deteriorating relationship but may present as a mismatch between the sexual desires of the partners. Although the woman may not be aroused by or reject her partner's sexual advances, she derives little or no enjoyment from them. A variety of factors may contribute to this lack or loss of desire. These include guilt about sexual activity acquired through upbringing, fear of pregnancy, or infection or injury, e.g. following surgery or a myocardial infarction. Relationship difficulties and the boredom of routine along with pressures of life and work may all have detrimental effects on sexual desire.

Management of inhibited sexual desire needs to involve both partners as the difficulties may arise from poor communication between the couple. Intensive therapy involves some level of compromise between the psychoanalytic and behavioural approaches and is loosely based around the work of Masters and Johnson and Annon and Kaplan. One of the most commonly used approaches is the use of graded 'tasks' that the couple perform at home in a relaxed atmosphere.

Failure to achieve orgasm

In 90% of women, the thrusting of the penis in the vagina or digital or oral stimulation of her clitoral area directly leads to orgasm. Half the sexually active women achieve orgasm when the clitoral area is directly stimulated, while a quarter reach it during penile thrusting in the vagina. One in six women are able to achieve multiple orgasms, while one in ten is unable to achieve orgasm.

Orgasmic dysfunction may be associated with a general inability to become aroused or, alternatively, may be a failure to climax after normal arousal and plateau phases. Most experts would agree that inability to achieve orgasm by intercourse alone is sufficiently common not to constitute a dysfunction if the woman is able to achieve climax by masturbation or oral/finger stimulation by

er partner. Despite this, among the lay public, the common but erroneous
belief is that, unless a woman reaches orgasm during penile thrusting preferably
simultaneously with the man, she is sexually dysfunctional. A number of techniques are available for a woman who wishes to achieve orgasm. The most successful of these is masturbation and learning to achieve orgasm by masturbation supplemented by discussion and counselling from a trained practitioner often cures anorgasmia.

Dyspareunia

Dyspareunia is defined as recurrent or persistent pain during or after intercourse. It is traditionally divided into superficial (when the pain is solely at the vaginal introitus) or deep (when the pain is felt deep in the pelvis). There may be an organic component to the pain and therefore organic causes need to be excluded before it can be classed as psychosomatic. It is important to elicit whether the pain is sufficient to prevent intercourse, whether it is continuous or intermittent, and whether it persists after attempts at intercourse have ceased.

It is essential to enquire about the basic features that are assessed with any pain such as onset, duration, radiation, associated features, and ameliorating and exacerbating features. Organic causes of superficial dyspareunia include vulvovaginal infections, atrophic changes of the lower genital tract, and conditions such as lichen sclerosus and painful episiotomy scars along with atrophic changes of the lower genital tract along with inadequate lubrication associated with inadequate sexual stimulation. Deep dyspareunia may be associated with PID, endometriosis, ovarian cysts, and pelvic tumours along with a retroverted uterus and ovaries prolapsing in the pouch of Douglas. After a total hysterectomy, where a vaginal cuff has been removed, deep dyspareunia is more common due to thrusting against a scarred vault that no longer has the capacity to balloon on arousal. Furthermore, a hysterectomy will in a proportion of women result in earlier than usual ovarian failure and continued sexual enjoyment may well require oestrogen replacement therapy. Vaginal repair operations for prolapse may also result in vaginal narrowing and dyspareunia.

Psychosomatic disorders are more likely to be longstanding. The causes of psychogenic dyspareunia may include lack of sexual knowledge, guilt about sexuality, childhood sexual abuse, or history of sexual assault.

Patients who have undergone gynaecological cancer treatment (surgery and/or radiotherapy) may have an organic and psychosomatic component to sexual dysfunction. Thus libido may be affected by depression occurring as part of the illness process or the reaction to the diagnosis while radical surgery may be mutilating leading to deterioration of body image and consequently of sexual relationships. Radiotherapy, especially in the setting of cervical cancer, may lead to cervical stenosis, reduced lubrication, and soreness and therefore is best prevented by the prophylactic use of dilators.

Sexual dysfunction in the female (*continued*)

Vaginismus/apareunia

In apareunia the woman is unable to have penetrative intercourse. This is usually a result of involuntary spasm of the pubococcygeus muscle surrounding the introitus and lower one-third of the vagina. Attempts at penetration cause pain in the clenched muscle, thus aggravating the situation. In its most severe form the patient is not even able to tolerate the examiner's finger in the vagina due to the marked muscle spasm. Vaginismus may affect up to 3% of women of reproductive age group.

In the majority of cases the problem is psychosomatic but organic causes such as vaginal atresia, vulvovaginal infection, and erectile failure in the man need to be excluded. Occasionally, vaginismus may be traced to a sexual assault during childhood or a painful or brutal initial experience of sexual intercourse or simply an inadequate or faulty sex education. Primary vaginismus is usually due to fear and as such is similar to a phobic disorder.

Management evolves around identifying and if possible, treating any underlying physical cause. If a treatment is not possible than alternative techniques may be suggested to enable her to enjoy her sexuality. A therapist may be able to 'educate' the patient to relax her perineal muscles and reinforce the idea that there is no physical abnormality and that her genital structures are normal and no small made. A series of graded exercises such as inserting a lubricated finger in the vagina progressing gradually to two and three fingers may be helpful. Alternatively, metal or glass dilators may serve the same purpose.

Special circumstances

Sexual assault

Defined as 'carnal knowledge/intercourse/sexual contact with a woman without her consent by force, fear, or fraud'; it includes rape and incest. The epidemiology of rape suggests that, while only fewer than one-third of rapes get reported, in three-quarters of cases the perpetrator is known to the woman. Furthermore, about one woman in 200 has been raped or suffered attempted rape in the preceding year.

Women who have been subjected to rape need to be listened to non-judgementally and sympathetically, addressing both emotional and physical issues. Physical examination will need to be performed and its significance and nature need to be discussed with the woman. During the examination careful documentation needs to be made of all findings including scratches and bruises on the arms and legs. The vulva and vagina need to be inspected for evidence of bruising, blood or seminal staining, while a vaginal smear is examined for spermatozoa. Screening should also be offered for sexually transmitted diseases and postcoital contraception offered if there is a risk of pregnancy.

Pregnancy

During pregnancy there is a wide variation between couples with regard to interest and responsiveness to sexual activity. In general, there is a trend towards reduction in frequency and satisfaction as pregnancy advances. Postnatally, dyspareunia is common but underreported with a recent survey indicating that 8% had painful intercourse at 3 months with the problem persisting in almost 9% at 9 months. Vaginal dryness may also be a problem, especially in the breastfeeding group.

Summary

The management of sexual dysfunction involves:

Obtaining a comprehensive general and sexual history.

Paying particular attention to physical and psychiatric problems.

Identifying and homing in on the current problem.

Ruling out the presence of physical or pharmacological factors.

Exclusion of psychological factors (sexual fears, shame, guilt, fear of injury).

Looking out for hidden clues in the history whilst exploring the patient's attitudes to her sexuality and responses.

Provision of more information about normal sexual response and how this may be affected by, for example, pregnancy, puerperium, or the peri- and postmenopausal states.

Chapter 74

Imaging in gynaecology

Ultrasound

Ultrasound is the most widely used method of imaging in gynaecology. As in obstetrics, it has revolutionized the management of some clinical problems such as the complications of early pregnancy. Ultrasound is based on the transmission of sound frequencies between 3 and 8 MHz and the detection of the echoes that this generates in tissue when it meets interfaces of different densities. Transvaginal scanning gives better imaging of the pelvic organs and avoids the need for a full bladder. Doppler ultrasound gives information about the blood flow around the pelvic organs.

Estimation of gestational age

This is made by measurement of the crown–rump length in the first 90 days of pregnancy or biparietal diameters in the second trimester. Observer error as a proportion of the total distance measured decreases with increasing gestation but variation about the mean in the normal population increases. The optimum gestation for estimating gestational age is between 8 and 12 weeks.

Early pregnancy assessment

- In normal pregnancy an intrauterine gestation sac should be visible on transvaginal ultrasound by 6 weeks gestation or when the human chorionic gonadotrophin (hCG) is more than 1000 IU/L.
- Ectopic pregnancy may occasionally be seen as fetal heart activity outside of the uterus but is more commonly suggested by an empty uterus, a non-specific adnexal mass, or the presence of free fluid in the pouch of Douglas.
- Ultrasound can be invaluable in the diagnosis of miscarriage, especially early embryonic demise or anembryonic pregnancy.
- Fetal heart pulsation can normally be seen from 6 weeks. The absence of detectable fetal heart activity in a fetal pole of more than 7 mm or in a gestation sac greater than 20 mm is diagnostic of pregnancy failure, but a repeat scan should be performed in early pregnancy after 7–10 days to confirm the diagnosis.
- Trophoblastic disease is associated with multiple echoes within the uterus giving a snowstorm appearance.
- Retained products of conception may be suspected in incomplete miscarriage from the presence of echogenic material within the cavity but this may be difficult to distinguish from blood and the diagnosis should be made on clinical grounds.

Assessment of a pelvic mass

Ultrasound is used to distinguish cysts (usually ovarian) from solid pelvic tumours such as fibroids. Occasionally, a pedunculated fibroid may be mistaken for an ovarian tumour. Functional ovarian cysts (follicular cysts, corpus luteum) are usually simple, unilocular areas less than 5 cm in size that disappear when the scan is repeated after 6 weeks. The internal morphology of ovarian cysts can be used to give an indication of the likelihood of malignancy, although surgical removal is required for confirmation. Malignant change is also associated with changes in blood flow (angiogenesis) around ovarian cysts. Transvaginal scanning can be used for the detection of asymptomatic early-stage ovarian cancer.

Postmenopausal bleeding

Endometrial thickness is increased in postmenopausal women with endometrial carcinoma. Using a cut off of 5 mm, 96% of such carcinomas can be identified by transvaginal ultrasound although up to 55% of women with no disease will also have a positive result.[1] Benign endometrial lesions such as polyps can be detected as localized thickenings of the endometrium. Instillation of saline into the endometrial cavity increases the sensitivity for local pathology but is more invasive.

Infertility

In addition to its role in the diagnosis of conditions such as polycystic ovarian disease and hydrosalpinx, ultrasound is used to track follicular growth and rupture during normal and stimulated cycles in infertility treatment. It is used to determine the timing of hCG administration and whether hCG should be withheld to avoid high-order multiple gestation. Oocyte retrieval for assisted conception can be performed under ultrasound guidance. Ovarian hyperstimulation syndrome is assessed by ultrasound.

Pelvic pain

Ultrasound examination is unlikely to be informative in the non-pregnant women with normal pelvic examination findings who present with pain. However, a diagnosis of endometriosis may be suggested by the presence of characteristic haemorrhagic cysts (endometrioma) on the ovaries. Adenomyosis is associated with a thickening of the myometrium with areas of reduced and increased echogeneicity. In patients with acute symptoms ultrasound may be of value in the detection of tubo-ovarian masses in pelvic inflammatory disease or the diagnosis of haemorrhage into a functional ovarian cyst.

Radiological imaging

Radiological imaging in gynaecology has been largely replaced by ultrasoun
but still has a role in the diagnosis and assessment of malignancy and infertilit

Plain radiography

- Plain radiography of the abdomen may occasionally give additional
  information about a pelvic tumour. Dermoid cysts often contain
  radio-opaque material such as teeth or bone that distinguishes them
  from other ovarian tumours.
- Fibroids may be detected on abdominal X-rays if they become calcified.
- Erect and supine abdominal films are indicated in the assessment of
  suspected ileus or bowel obstruction.
- Lost intrauterine contraceptive devices that have perforated the wall of the
  uterus can be located on X-ray.
- Metal clips used for sterilization are occasionally seen outside of the pelvis.
  This does not indicate failure of the procedure as it is not uncommon for
  the clips to cause necrosis of the underlying tube and then become
  detached but leave the tube occluded.
- Chest X-rays form part of the routine assessment of patients with suspecte
  malignancy.
  —The presence of pleural effusions suggests stage IV ovarian carcinoma
    but pleural effusions also occur in ovarian hyperstimulation and
    occasionally with ovarian fibromas (Meig's syndrome).
  —Choriocarcinoma is associated with cannon-ball metastases in the lungs.

Intravenous urography

Renal colic is one of the causes of acute abdominal pain. Ureteric obstruction i
a patient with cervical carcinoma indicates stage III disease. Continuous urinar
incontinence following childbirth, radiotherapy, or gynaecological surgery ma
be due to fistula formation between the ureters or bladder and genital trac
Contrast studies of the renal tract should be considered when congenital mal
formations of the reproductive tract are diagnosed, as approximately 15% o
cases are associated with abnormalities of the urinary tract. Contrast imaging o
the bladder neck is used in the assessment of stress incontinence.

Hysterosalpingography

Hysterosalpingography is the injection of water-soluble contrast medium
through the cervix into the uterine cavity. It is used to visualize the uterine cav
ity and Fallopian tubes in the investigation of patients with infertility or recur
rent miscarriage. 2–3 mL of dye is injected using a Leech–Wilkinson cannula.

- Polyps or submucous fibroids produce rounded filling defects.
- The presence of intrauterine synechiae and congenital abnormalities of the
  uterine cavity (septate or bicornuate uterus) can also be identified.
- If the Fallopian tubes are patent, dye will be seen spilling into the peritonea
  cavity. The site of any tubal obstruction can be identified and this is
  important in determining the feasibility of tubal surgery. If dye remains
  localized at the end of the tube this suggests peritubal adhesions.

Hysterosalpingography is an alternative to laparoscopy for assessing tubal patenc
and avoids the risks associated with the latter but gives more limited informatio
about pelvic pathology. Tubal spasm may cause artefactual obstruction of th
tubes.

Computerized tomography (CT scan)

CT scans of the pelvis are used mainly in the assessment of malignancy. CT's role in diagnosis is limited in primary ovarian tumours as laparotomy is usually required to establish the diagnosis. Its value is mainly in the postoperative identification of residual disease and as a method to assess response to treatment. In patients with recurrent disease it may be used to localize the site of disease when palliative or second look surgery is being considered. In patients with carcinoma of the cervix it can be used in disease staging and planning radiotherapy, although magnetic resonance imaging (MRI) is now probably the method of choice for imaging the disease.

633

Magnetic resonance imaging (MRI)

MRI is an alternative method of soft-tissue imaging that avoids the need for ionizing radiation. A strong magnetic field is used to polarize the hydrogen ions in tissue so that they emit radiofrequency energy of an appropriate frequency. In gynaecology MRI is of particular value in the imaging and staging of pelvic tumours and is the method of choice for identification of local spread of cervical and endometrial carcinoma when surgery is contemplated.

Immunoscintigraphy

This involves the injection of radiolabelled monoclonal antibody or fragments. The antibody binds to antigens that are expressed preferentially by tumour and the site of the disease is then identified as a hot spot on external gamma camera imaging. Although its sensitivity and specificity are comparable to those of conventional imaging, it has failed to become established in routine clinical care and its main value is the detection of distant metastases and localized recurrence in ovarian cancer.

Reference

1 Smith-Bindman, R., Kerlikowske, K., Feldstein, V.A., *et al.* (1998). Endovaginal ultrasound to exclude endometrial cancer: a meta analytic review. *Journal of the American Medical Association* **280**, 1510–17.

Chapter 75

Contraception (hormonal, intrauterine devices, emergency)

The use of contraception is widespread in the UK. Over 95% of sexually active women wishing to avoid pregnancy use contraception. There has been a significant rise in the use of contraception world-wide but contraceptive use is much lower in less developed countries, falling to less than 15% in some parts of Africa. Even in the UK adolescents and women over 40 are less willing to use contraception despite not wishing to get pregnant. This is partly responsible for the estimated 30% of babies that are delivered whose conception is unplanned. The vast majority of unplanned pregnancies end in termination. Contraceptive methods and their frequency of use are shown in Table 75.1. This chapter will deal with hormonal contraception, intrauterine contraceptive devices (IUCDs), and emergency contraception.

Combined oral contraceptives

The combined oral contraceptive pill (COCP) was approved for use in the UK in 1961. The usual combination is of ethinyloestradiol and a synthetic progesterone (progestogen). Ethinyloestradiol (a highly potent oestrogen compared to naturally occurring 17 beta-oestradiol) is the usual oestrogen. This is given in a dosage of 20 to 50 μg daily, the most common dosage being in the 20 to 35 μg bracket.

Second-generation progestogens (norethisterone, levonorgestrel, ethynodiol diacetate) are the commonly used progestogens, with the 'third generation' (gestodene, norgestimate, desogestrel) in some of the newer preparations.

The third-generation progestogens appear to have a less atherogenic lipid profile (lower low-density lipoprotein cholesterol (LDL-C) and a higher high-density lipoprotein cholesterol (HDL-C)). This lipid profile should in theory give rise to less myocardial infarction. However, this is a very rare complication. In 1995, the UK Committee on Safety of Medicines (CSM) reviewed evidence from three research studies suggesting increased risk of venous thrombosis associated with third-generation progestogens and this has been backed up by further studies. However, the risk is smaller than that associated with pregnancy. The spontaneous incidence of venous thromboembolism (VTE) in healthy non-pregnant women is 5 per 100 000, with second-generation pills it is 15 per 100 000, and with third-generation pills it is 25 per 100 000.

Mode of action
The COCP acts to inhibit ovulation. The ethinyloestradiol suppresses follicle-stimulating hormone (FSH) whilst the progestogen suppresses the luteinizing hormone (LH) surge. There is also some effect on cervical mucus, which is thicker and less penetrable by sperm.

Dosages and regimen
The pill is usually given at a dosage of 20–35 μg daily. Better cycle control is achieved with the higher oestrogen dosages, although all seem to be similarly effective. In older women the lower dosages are preferred, reducing the risk of side-effects. The COCP is taken for 3 weeks, with a 1-week gap when menstruation occurs. The dosage is either the same throughout the cycle (monophasic) or alters with increasing dosages mid-cycle (triphasic). If used properly, the failure rate is very low (see Table 75.2). The riskiest pills to miss are the first or last of the 3-week cycle.

Table 75.1 Contraceptive methods and their frequencies of use

Method	Frequency of use (%)
Combined oral contraceptive pill (COCP)	36
Barrier methods	20.8
Vasectomy	16
Female sterilization	10.1
Intrauterine contraceptive device (IUCD)	7.3
COCP and barrier	3.3
Natural family planning (NFP)	1.5
Withdrawal (coitus interruptus)	1.1
No method	3.6

Table 75.2 Efficacy of various methods of contraception

Method	Failure rate (%)*
No contraception (young women)	80–90
Male condom	2–15
Copper IUCD	0.3–1
Mirena IUS	< 0.5
POP	0.3–4
COCP	0.2–3
Injectable	0–1
Implanon/Norplant	0–1
Sterilization (female)	0–0.5
Sterilization (male)	0.02

*Failure rate per 100 women years of use.

Combined oral contraceptives (*continued*)

Contraindications to the COCP
- A current or past history of cardiovascular disease.
- Migraine: focal migraine, crescendo migraine, first attack of migraine on the COCP, severe migraines requiring the use of ergotamine.
- A personal history of venous thrombosis.
- Gross obesity.
- Heavy smoking in women over the age of 35.
- Oestrogen-dependent cancer.
- A family history of venous thrombosis in women under 45. May need activated protein C resistance testing.
- Varicose veins if severe.
- Various liver conditions.

Side-effects
Side effects are common in the first few months of use and may lead to discontinuation of the method. However, many will settle with time. It may be worth changing the COCP after 3–4 months if side-effects persist.
- *Weight gain.* A weight gain of 2 to 3 kilograms is common in the early months of treatment, but this weight will often be lost later on.
- *Hypertension.* Approximately 2% of women may become hypertensive after commencing the pill.
- *Headaches* are common in the early months of treatment but will often resolve. They need to be differentiated from migraines (see 'Contraindications').
- *Breakthrough bleeding.* Check compliance; try alternative progestogen or triphasic pill. If it persists, it is necessary to exclude local pathology.

Advantages
- Menstruation is regular, lighter, and less painful and there is less premenstrual tension (PMT).
- Reduced incidence of ovarian cysts.
- Reduced incidence of fibroids.
- Reduced incidence of pelvic infection.
- Acne and hirsutism may be improved with Dianette.
- Reduced risk of endometrial and ovarian cancer.
- Can be used in women over 35. Ideally a 20 μg pill can be used in slim, non-smoking women with no other contraindications.

Progestogen-only contraception

The progestogen-only pill (POP or mini-pill) is only used by about 5% of women. It is a useful alternative when the COCP is contraindicated because of oestrogenic effects. Precise explanations must be given to a woman commencing the POP. It must be taken at the same time each day, and taken continuously. If a pill is missed by more than 3 hours, a barrier method should be used for 7 days. If unprotected intercourse occurs after a missed pill, emergency contraception should be considered.

Mode of action

The POP acts to thicken cervical mucus and prevents sperm penetration. In 56–60% of women, ovulation may be inhibited and, in a small proportion, all follicular development may be suppressed, giving amenorrhoea.

Indications

- During breastfeeding.
- Women at risk of cardiovascular disease: diabetic women, smokers over 35, women with hypertension, women with hyperlipidaemia (not all).
- Migraine sufferers.
- Women at increased risk of thromboembolism.
- Side-effects from COCPs.

Contraindications

- Previous ectopic pregnancy.
- Ovarian cysts.

Side-effects

Erratic bleeding is common and around 20% of women will cease use because of this. The POP has a relatively short half-life and a slightly increased failure rate. However, the POP does not appear to be associated with any serious long-term risks.

Injectable contraceptives

There are two long-term injectable contraceptive progestogens—depot medroxyprogesterone acetate (DMPA, Depo-Provera, 150 mg intramuscularly (IM) every 12 weeks) and norethisterone oenanthate (NET-EN, 200 mgs IM every 8 weeks).

DMPA is widely used world-wide (9 million women). There do not appear to be any increased risks of cancer and there appears to be a powerful protective effect against endometrial cancer. Injections need to be given every 12 weeks, with the first injection during the first 5 days of menstruation. It is inexpensive, safe, and effective. It can be used for breastfeeding mothers and particularly for women with poor compliance on other methods. Dysmenorrhoea, menorrhagia, pelvic inflammatory disease (PID), and PMT may all be reduced.

However, weight gain and acne can be problems in the early stages of treatment. Amenorrhoea is common (over 50%). The return to fertility may be delayed after the normal 12-week duration of the injection.

Contraceptive implants

The first licensed contraceptive implant in the UK was Norplant. This consisted of six silastic rods containing levonorgestrel, inserted subdermally on the inner aspect of the upper arm. Local anaesthetic is needed for insertion and removal of the implants. The mode of action is similar to other progestogen-only methods and fertility returns swiftly after removal of the rods. This product is not now prescribed since the licensing of the newer product Implanon, but there are still patients who need removal of the Norplant rods. Implanon is a single silastic rod containing 3-keto-desogestrel, lasting for 3 years. Frequent and prolonged bleeds remain a problem, affecting 17% of women. Removal and insertion times are much reduced with the single rod.

Intrauterine contraceptive devices (IUCDs)

The IUCD is a longlasting and highly effective method of contraception. It causes local inflammatory response in the endometrium, interfering with sperm and egg function and inhibiting implantation. The IUCD consists of copper wire wound on an inert frame. This can be inserted with no anaesthetic, or with a local block, but is easier in women who have had a previous vaginal delivery. The newer GyneFix is frameless, the copper being attached around a nylon thread that is fixed to the fundus of the uterus. IUDs last 5–8 years.

risks of IUCDs include explusion, perforation, and pelvic infection. When fitting IUCDs, swabs should be taken to establish that the woman has no pelvic infection or prophylactic antibiotics should be prescribed at the time of insertion. If the IUCD user becomes pregnant, there is a higher likelihood that the pregnancy will be ectopic. Menorrhagia and dysmenorrhoea are common side-effects, related to increased local production of prostaglandins. These side-effects can be treated with nonsteroidal anti-inflammatory drugs (NSAIDs), but the side-effects limit the usefulness of IUCDs.

Intrauterine system (Mirena IUS)

The Mirena IUS is a levonorgestrel-releasing system similar to the copper coil in its insertion and removal. The hormone is contained in a reservoir on the stem of the device and lasts for 5 years. It releases approximately 20 µg of hormone daily locally to the endometrium, with only a small amount being absorbed into the circulation. This reduces the chance of progestogenic side-effects. The contraceptive efficacy is extremely good whilst blood loss is substantially reduced (80–95% in women with heavy periods).

Emergency contraception

Either hormonal contraception or a copper-containing IUCD can be used for emergency contraception. The Mirena IUS cannot be used in these circumstances.

Levonelle (750 µg levonorgestrel given immediately and repeated 12 hours later) is a more effective emergency contraceptive than the previously marketed PC4 (ethinyl oestradiol and progestogen). The failure rate is 0.4% if treatment is within 24 hours. Every 12-hour delay increases the failure rate by 50%. This may result in the treatment being available without prescription in the near future. There are fewer side-effects with the newer regimen (vomiting < 6%).

Absolute contraindications are:
   Existing pregnancy.
   Known acute porphyria.
   Current warfarin treatment (may alter anticoagulation and monitoring is
   necessary).

Chapter 76

Female sterilization

Sterilization is the method of contraception used by 26% of all couples and 50% of those over the age of 40.

Assessment

- Ask about the reasons for requesting sterilization, current contraception, menstrual history, and previous gynaecological or abdominal surgery.
- Women under the age of 25, those without children, or those who have had a recent relationship loss are more likely to regret sterilization. Try to assess whether the woman is making the decision of her own free will or being coerced by family or social or health-care professionals.

- Note any major medical problems, current medication, and allergies.
- Note the date and result of the last smear.
- On examination note especially the body mass index (BMI) and any abdominal scars and pelvic masses. Obese patients and those with a history of previous abdominal surgery are at increased risk of laparoscopic problems and may need to have an elective open rather than laparoscopic procedure.

Counselling

The following points should be covered.
- The *alternative methods* of long-term contraception should be discussed. Sterilization may be wrongly perceived as the only other solution to contraceptive needs in women who have problems with the contraceptive pill or barrier methods.
    —Injectables and the levonorgestrol intrauterine system have failure rates comparable to those of female sterilization.
    —The advantages and disadvantages of vasectomy should be discussed with couples. Vasectomy can be performed more readily under local anaesthetic and has a lower failure rate of one in 2000 (after two azoospermic samples 2–4 weeks apart).
- *The permanence of the operation.* Sterilization should only be undertaken by patients who are certain that their family is complete. Even so, 5–10% of patients will ask for reversal later. Additional care also needs to be taken when counselling women taking the decision during pregnancy. Funding for reversal operations is limited and success rates vary according to the method of sterilization used.
- *The procedure has a failure rate.* There is a one in 200 lifetime risk of failure. Pregnancies may occur several years after the operation. Early failures may occur if the procedure was incorrectly performed or if conception had already occurred when the sterilization was carried out in the second half of the cycle (luteal phase pregnancy). Later failures may be due to recanalization of the tubes. There is an increased risk of ectopic pregnancy (10%) if sterilization does fail. Patients should be warned to make sure they are not pregnant if they miss or have unusually light periods.

76 Female sterilization

- *The nature of the sterilization operation and its risks should be explained.* The nature of the operation, including the proposed method of access and the proposed method of tubal occlusion, should be explained. There is a risk associated with laparoscopy of bowel and vessel injury. A laparotomy may be required to repair injury and the hospital stay may be prolonged. A mini-laparotomy may also be required if the sterilization can not be completed laparoscopically.
  —Sterilization will not affect weight, menstruation, or the time of menopause. However, patients who are currently using contraception that might affect menstruation such as the combined contraceptive pill (COCP) may notice a change in their period pattern when these are stopped.

- *The need for adequate contraception prior to sterilization.* Effective contraception should be used until the first period following the procedure. An intrauterine contraceptive device (IUCD) *in situ* can be removed at the time of operation only if this is carried out in the first half of the menstrual cycle. Otherwise it should be left and removed at the time of the next period.

Patients should be offered printed information including the above points to take away and read prior to the operation. A record in the notes should be made that the patient has been told about the irreversibility, failure rate (and ectopic pregnancy risk), and the potential complications of the operation.

The operation

Prior to surgery check the date of the last menstrual period and current contraception. Separate consent forms are no longer usually used for sterilization. It is not necessary to obtain the partner's consent for sterilization but where there is doubt over mental capacity to consent prior sanction by a high court judge should be obtained.

The operation itself is usually carried out under general anaesthetic as a day case procedure. It can be done at any time of the menstrual cycle but a pregnancy test must be arranged for any woman whose period is late or who thinks she may be pregnant.

- The perineum and abdomen are cleaned, a pelvic examination performed, and the bladder emptied.
- The cervix is held with a valsellum or other forceps and the uterus instrumented to allow manipulation.
- A Veres needle (a large-bore needle with a retractable sharp tip) is inserted through a small incision usually made below the umbilicus and 2 to 3 L of carbon dioxide instilled into the peritoneal cavity. This displaces the anterior abdominal wall away from the abdominal contents so that a larger trochar can be introduced through the same incision. The pelvic organs are visualized through this portal using a laparoscope.
- A second incision is made in the lower abdomen for a second port through which the instrument used to perform the sterilization is inserted.
  —Sterilization is most commonly performed by applying occlusive clips or rings across the tubal isthmus 1–2 cm from the uterus.
  —Diathermy of the tubes is a suitable alternative if there is technical difficulty in applying rings or clips.
  —Partial or complete salpingectomy is more commonly done when sterilization is carried out at the time of Caesarean section or when there is pre-existing tubal disease.
  —The position of the clips or rings must be confirmed by positive identification of the fimbrial ends of the tubes and by ensuring that adjacent structures such as the round ligaments have not been incorporated into the clip.
- Local anaesthetic injection into the tube may be used to provide additional postoperative pain relief.
- The gas is released from the abdomen and the abdominal incision closed with a semi-absorbable suture.
- Routine curettage of the uterus to prevent luteal phase pregnancy is not recommended.

Postoperative care

- Inform the patient of the final method used for the sterilization and if any complications occurred.
- Check pulse and blood pressure.
- Inspect the wounds for any signs of bleeding. The abdomen should be soft.
- Patients should have been able to tolerate fluids and passed urine prior to discharge.
- She will need to take 3–7 days off work and may notice some abdominal discomfort for 2–3 weeks. Warn her that she may have some shoulder tip pain because of diaphragmatic irritation from the CO_2.
- Warn the patient to seek medical advice if her pain is not controlled by simple analgesia or if there is increasing pain or vomiting.
- Remember that fewer than 50% of bowel injuries occurring at laparoscopy are diagnosed at the time of surgery and signs of peritonitis may not be apparent for up to 72 hours.

647

Sterilization at the time of pregnancy

- Where possible, sterilization procedures after pregnancy should be performed as an interval procedure 3–6 months later. This is because sterilization performed at the time of pregnancy has a higher failure rate and may be associated with an increased risk of maternal complications such as thromboembolism. If carried out at the same time as termination there is likely to be an increased regret rate for both procedures. These drawbacks have to be balanced against the reliability of contraception during the interval period and in some cases will be outweighed by the risk of further unplanned pregnancy.
- Sterilization at the time of Caesarean section has the additional advantage of avoiding the need for a second operation. It is usually done by partial salpingectomy or by the use of clips after the uterus has been closed. Consent should have been obtained after counselling at least a week prior to the delivery.
- Sterilization at the time of pregnancy termination is normally carried out laparoscopically.

Urinary stress incontinence

649

Urinary stress incontinence is the involuntary loss of urine through an increase in intraabdominal pressure (coughing, sneezing, laughing, etc.). Occasionally this may be provoked by a detrusor contraction. However, genuine stress incontinence excludes this detrusor instability by defining it as 'involuntary' urethral loss of urine when the intravesical pressure exceeds the maximum urethral pressure in the absence of detrusor activity. Stress incontinence is usually due to urethral sphincter incompetence. However, because this loss of urine is so common, some judgement needs to be made as to whether this is a social or hygienic problem to the patient.

Aetiology

Stress incontinence occurs when the intravesical pressure exceeds the closing pressure on the urethra. Childbirth is the most common causative factor leading to denervation of the pelvic floor, usually during the trauma of delivery. Occasionally there can be congenital weakness of the bladder neck or trauma from other causes. Oestrogen deficiency at the time of the menopause leads to weakening of the pelvic supports and thinning of the urothelium. After pelvic surgery or radiotherapy, there may be fibrosis of the urethra precluding efficient closure.

Symptoms and signs

- *Symptoms*. Typically a woman will complain of leakage of urine when she coughs, sneezes, runs, jumps, carries heavy loads, etc. Patients are typically multiparous and the problem is more common in older than in younger patients. There may be associated frequency or urgency, but these symptoms can be due to detrusor instability.
- *Signs*. It may be helpful to demonstrate stress incontinence by asking the patient to cough with a fairly full bladder. The presence of a leak indicates incontinence, usually stress incontinence. Prolapse of the urethra and anterior vaginal wall may be present in 50% of women.

Investigations

Because the bladder is not a reliable witness, further investigations need to be performed.
- A midstream urine (MSU) sample should be taken to exclude infection or glycosuria.
- *Uroflowmetry* is a simple non-invasive test that will exclude voiding difficulties. The patient simply urinates into a toilet with a flow-measuring device in the pan. The normal flow rate is above 15 mL/second. Bladder outflow obstruction is rare in women, but much more common in men (enlarged prostate).

77 Urinary stress incontinence

- *Cystometry* and *videocystourethrography* are used to assess leakage and exclude detrusor instability. The bladder is filled with radio-opaque fluid via a urethral catheter. Fine pressure catheters in the bladder and rectum measure pressure rises. By subtracting the rectal pressure from the bladder pressure, detrusor pressure can be estimated. Leakage on coughing, estimated either by eye or by X-ray, should be assessed. If this occurs in the absence of a detrusor contraction then genuine stress incontinence is confirmed. Detrusor pressure can be estimated during the voiding phase.
- If there is still doubt about the extent of leakage, a 'pad test' can be performed. A dry pad is weighed, and the patient asked to wear this for an hour whilst exercising normally. The pad is re-weighed and the change in weight relates to the amount of urine lost. Whilst this gives an estimate of the loss, it does not indicate the cause of loss.

Treatment

Treatment can be either conservative or surgical. Almost all patients with genuine stress incontinence will undergo a course of conservative treatment before considering surgery.

Conservative treatment

Conservative treatment is carried out by either physiotherapists or continence nurses. General measures include the following.

- Treatment of obesity.
- Treatment of chronic cough.
- Treatment of chronic constipation.
- Treatment of urogenital oestrogen deficiency.

Specific training

Pelvic floor muscle exercise training can be taught to most patients. Patients need to understand why and how the training takes place. Feedback machines can be very helpful in this respect giving patients an idea of their progress (which will often precede symptomatic improvement). Electrical stimulation is helpful in women who have a denervated pelvic floor. Vaginal cones are a useful method of actively and passively exercising the pelvic floor. The patient starts by keeping an unweighted cone in the vagina, whilst walking round for 15 minutes. Once this is achieved, increasing weights can be added. Pelvic floor tone increases.

On average over 50% of patients will see objective benefit from pelvic floor muscle exercises. Hospital-based treatment is superior to home treatment. The success rate appears to depend very much on the enthusiasm of the patient and continence advisor. Patients with milder symptoms seem more likely to achieve a cure than those with severe stress incontinence.

Surgical treatment

There are many operations to cure genuine stress incontinence, but none are universally successful or without side-effects. The choice of operation depends on the type of incontinence, associated features (such as prolapse), and the personal experience of the operator. Patients will usually be offered a choice of operation because of the different success rates, complication rates, and recovery time.

- *Anterior colporrhaphy.* Vaginal repair with anterior colporrhaphy and suburethral buttressing can be useful in women with combined stress incontinence and vaginal prolapse. It has a lower success rate for curing stress incontinence than suprapubic operations, but is less likely to be associated with complications such as detrusor instability.
- *Endoscopic bladder neck suspension.* Techniques such as the Stamey or Ras have been used. In these techniques a needle is used to insert a suture on either side of the bladder neck, anchoring it with a buffer for sutures in the pubocervical fascia and tying the upper end of each suture to the rectus sheath. The principle is that a cough or strain of the intraabdominal muscles will pull up on the suture and 'tighten' the bladder neck. Whilst the short-term success may be useful, the long-term success is disappointing. However, this operation may be useful in elderly patients or in selected cases.

- *Tension-free vaginal tape.* This is a relatively new operation, usually performed under local or spinal anaesthetic. A proline mesh is inserted on either side of the urethra, with two needles, the needles emerging through the abdominal wall. The mesh is tensioned with the patient being asked to cough and adjusted until there is only a minimal leak. Care must be taken not to overtension the tape, which would lead to voiding difficulties. The tape remains in place permanently and sits suburethrally. The short-term success rate appears good (85%) with a low complication rate, but the long-term results are as yet uncertain.

- *Burch colposuspension.* The approach to the bladder neck is through a transverse abdominal incision. Dissection is made in the retropubic space and the bladder neck identified. Two or three sutures are placed in the vaginal tissue and fascia on either side of the bladder neck and tied to the iliopectineal ligament. When tightened, these create a shelf on the bladder neck. The success rate is again about 85%, but with well proven long-term success. The procedure can cure anterior vaginal wall proplapse at the same time. Complications include urinary retention, voiding difficulties, and the occurrence of detrusor instability. Posterior vaginal wall prolapse or enterocele may occur as a late complication.

653

- *Marshall–Marchetti–Krantz.* This operation is a widely used suprapubic procedure. As in the Burch procedure, retropubic space is dissected. The sutures are inserted between periurethral tissues along the proximal half of the urethra, which are then attached to the periosteum or perichondrium of the symphysis pubis. One major complication is that of osteitis pubis (up to 5% of cases). Unlike the colposuspension, this operation is unlikely to cure a cystocele.

- *Sling procedures.* There are many different types of sling using either organic or inorganic materials. Commonly, patient's rectus fascia is used, but tissues such as porcine dermis can also be used. Inorganic materials such as meshes are stronger, but if they get infected can be very difficult to remove. Cure rates for stress incontinence are again around 80–90%. Complications include voiding difficulties, detrusor instability, and sling erosion.

- *Periurethral injections.* Injections of substances such as collagen or Macroplastique are made either transurethrally or periurethrally. These form a cushion of tissue that reduces the calibre of the bladder neck and thus the chance of urinary incontinence. The injections are expensive, but have the advantage of being simple to insert with small risk of complications. However, some patients do go into retention. The success rate of periurethral injections is less good than that of other types of surgery (approximately 50% continence rate). The injection can be repeated with a small improvement in continence rate.

Failed continence surgery

For those patients with failed surgery, second or third operations may be successful. However, the success rate appears to be about 10% less than for a primary operation. The risk of developing problems such as bladder instability is greater for each subsequent operation. As a last resort, an artificial sphincter can be inserted, but there is a significant risk of infection or mechanical failure. For women, who are unfit for surgery, long-term catheterization may be an option.

Chapter 78

Frequency and urgency

655

Frequency of micturition is common and has many causes. Normally women would not empty their bladder more than 7 times a day or once at night. Voiding in excess of this is defined as frequency or nocturia. Urgency is the strong and sudden desire to void urine and may often be followed by urge incontinence. It tends to be due to an involuntary detrusor contraction, but some women may be unaware of this.

Causes

- *Gynaecological*. Pregnancy or pelvic mass can press on the bladder giving symptoms. A prolapse, particularly a cystocele, will often cause these symptoms as will postmenopausal urogenital atrophy.
- *Urological*. A urinary tract infection typically gives such symptoms. Detrusor instability will commonly present with multiple symptoms including urgency and frequency. Bladder pathology such as interstitial cystitis, bladder calculus, mucosal lesions, or urethral problems may all present in such a way.
- *Medical problems*. Treatment with diuretics causes frequency, mainly limited to the few hours following treatment.
- *Endocrine*. Diabetes mellitus, diabetes insipidus, and hypothyroidism can all cause frequency and urgency.
- *Psychological*. Some patients habitually have frequency, often in an attempt to prevent leakage of urine. Excessive fluid intake must be looked for also.

Investigation

The aetiology may be obvious from the history, but usually is not.
- The history should include information about the length of time for which the patient has had symptoms, fluid intake, associated diseases, previous surgery, and a history of childhood enuresis. Many women will have associated problems during sexual intercourse and may not complain of these unless asked directly.
- Investigations should include urine culture and an intake/output fluid volume chart.
- Urodynamic investigations may be helpful including uroflowmetry, and urodynamic assessment by cystometrogram. These will help identify an unstable bladder (one shown objectively to contract, spontaneously or on provocation, during the filling phase while the patient is attempting to inhibit micturition). Ambulatory urodynamics have not yet been validated adequately to recommend their widespread use although they can be helpful in difficult cases.
- Cystoscopy may be useful if intravesical pathology is suspected.

Treatment

Treatment depends on the cause. Excessive fluid intake can be curbed, and infections treated. It is helpful for a patient to avoid bladder stimulants such as tea, coffee, and alcohol. Ideally, they should limit their fluid intake to 1–1.5 L/day. Diuretic therapy may be changed or stopped.

- *Medication.* In postmenopausal women, local oestrogen treatment to the vagina can be helpful, particularly in those with sensory symptoms. A glass of cranberry juice each day appears to help some women's symptoms. Musculotropic relaxants such as oxybutynin or tolterodine will help the unstable bladder, although side-effects (dry mouth, blurred vision) limit their effectiveness. Tricyclic antidepressants can be useful, particularly for the treatment of nocturia and nocturnal enuresis.

- *Behavioural therapy.* In bladder drill, the patient is instructed to void by the clock commencing initially at one and a half hour intervals and then gradually increasing the time span. Concurrent treatment with musculotropic relaxants can increase the success rate but relapse is common. Biofeedback techniques can be helpful as can hypnotherapy. Electrical stimulation may also inhibit spontaneous detrusor contractions and can be performed by specialist nurses.

- Very rarely is *surgery* indicated but the 'clam' enterocystoplasty has been used with some success in severe cases. Conventional bladder neck surgery is not useful in the treatment of detrusor instability.

657

Uterovaginal prolapse

659

Prolapse is the protrusion of an organ or structure beyond the normal anatomical confines. Approximately 20% of all gynaecological operations are for prolapse repair.[1]

- *Normal pelvic anatomy*. The uterus, bladder, and rectum are supported by the pelvic floor, which includes the levator ani, the coccygeal, internal obturator, and piriformis muscles, along with the two transverse perineal muscles and pelvic fascia. Within the pelvis, the transverse cervical ligaments (cardinal ligaments), uterosacral ligaments, and pubocervical and pubourethral ligaments support the uterus. The round ligaments and broad ligaments do not contribute significantly to the support of the uterus.
- *Vaginal prolapse* is classified according to its contents.
  —*Urethrocele* involves the lower part of the anterior vaginal wall containing the urethra.
  —*Cystocele* is prolapse of the upper anterior wall and bladder.
  —*Rectocele* describes prolapse of the middle part of the posterior vaginal wall containing the rectum.
  —*Enterocele* involves the upper part of the posterior wall and may contain loops of small bowel from the pouch of Douglas.
  —After hysterectomy, the vaginal vault may prolapse and usually contains small bowel as well as omentum (vault prolapse).
  —Several types of prolapse may occur in the same patient.
- *Uterine prolapse* is divided into:
  —First-degree uterine prolapse when the uterus is within the vagina.
  —Second-degree prolapse when the cervix protrudes through the introitus.
  —Third-degree prolapse (procidentia) when the entire uterus has come outside the vagina.

Aetiology

Congenital weakness of pelvic floor ligaments and fascia may be found with spina bifida or bladder exstrophy, and congenital shortness of the vagina and deep uterovesical or uterorectal peritoneal pouches. Far more common are acquired causes of pelvic floor damage such as pregnancy, prolonged or difficult labour, bearing down before full dilatation, and multiparity. These cause denervation of the pelvic floor muscles. A gradual increase in denervation of the striated muscle of pelvic floor with age and oestrogen deficiency at the menopause can also occur in nulliparous women.[2] Prolapse may also be a sign of increased intraabdominal pressure due to pulmonary disease, heavy lifting, chronic straining (constipation), ascites, or a pelvic mass. Prolapse may occur after surgery such as hysterectomy or Burch colposuspension.

Symptoms

- Minor degrees may be asymptomatic.
- Patients with significant uterovaginal prolapse complain of a feeling of 'something coming down'.
- Cystocele and cysto-urethrocele lead to dragging discomfort and the sensation of a lump in the vagina. There may be associated urinary symptoms of incontinence and recurrent urinary tract infections. Voiding difficulties can occur if a large cystocele is present and the bladder neck is anchored normally. This can lead to overflow incontinence or incomplete emptying.
- Uterine descent may cause low backache, which is relieved by lying flat or temporarily using a pessary to support the prolapse.
- A patient with procidentia may present with protrusion of cervix and a blood-stained, sometimes purulent vaginal discharge due to decubitus ulceration of the vaginal skin.
- Rectocele may cause difficulty with defecation or a sensation of incomplete defecation, which is relieved by digital reduction of the prolapse.[1]

661

Diagnosis

Predisposing factors such as chronic cough or constipation may be present but the diagnosis is usually made by clinical examination.

- A speculum examination in the left lateral position is required to diagnose the type of vaginal prolapse.
- A bimanual pelvic examination should be performed to exclude any pelvic mass.
- When urinary symptoms are present stress incontinence may be demonstrated by asking the patient to cough with a full bladder.
- A midstream specimen of urine must be sent for culture and sensitivity testing.
- Cystometry and uroflowmetry may be necessary to differentiate detrusor instability from genuine stress incontinence.
- Renal function should be checked in patients with third-degree uterine prolapse.

Management

Prolapse carries no risk to life unless causing urinary obstruction. Asymptomatic patients do not require any treatment. Obese patients should be referred to a dietitian for dietary control and advised to reduce weight. Chronic cough and constipation should be corrected.

Prevention
- Minimize pelvic floor trauma during childbirth by decreasing parity and by avoiding prolonged pushing or difficult instrumental deliveries.
- Encourage the use of postnatal pelvic floor exercises.[2]
- Ensure adequate support of the vaginal vault at hysterectomy by securing the vault to the uterosacral ligaments.
- Use of hormone replacement therapy (HRT) may reduce the rate of denervation of the pelvic floor after the menopause.

Medical management

Minor degrees of prolapse should be treated conservatively.[3]

Physiotherapy
Pelvic floor exercises and electrical stimulation of the pelvic floor muscles may lessen the prolapse.

Hormone replacement therapy
HRT increases vaginal blood supply and collagen turnover.

Ring pessaries
Surgery is the treatment of choice for significant symptomatic prolapse but ring pessaries are indicated:
- During and after pregnancy if further pregnancies are planned.
- As a therapeutic test to confirm that surgery might help.
- When the patient is medically unfit for surgery.
- Patient's request.
- For relief of symptoms while the patient is awaiting surgery.

The ring is inserted between the posterior fornix and the pubic bone. Use the smallest diameter that keeps the prolapse reduced and does not fall out. Insertion is easier if the ring is softened in warm water first and lubricated with topical oestrogen cream.

The main complication of ring pessaries is vaginal ulceration leading to vaginal discharge and bleeding. Ulceration of the cervix may be managed by reducing the uterine prolapse and applying oestrogen cream. Shelf pessaries may be helpful in cases of failure of ring pessary and when there is no pelvic support.

Surgical management

Surgical management is carried out to correct prolapse, to maintain continence, and to preserve coital function. Sexual activity should be taken into account before surgical procedure to avoid overdoing the repair, which may lead to narrowing of the vagina and dyspareunia.

- *Urethrocele/cystocele.* Anterior repair (anterior colporrhaphy) is the operation of choice. A longitudinal incision is made on the anterior vaginal wall and the vaginal skin separated by dissection from the vesical fascia. One or more deep (buttressing) sutures are placed on either side of the vagina to support the bladder neck. The redundant vaginal skin is excised and the skin is closed. Approximately 50% of patients will suffer postoperative urinary retention following an anterior repair.[1] Colposuspension may be necessary to correct stress incontinence associated with cystocele.

663

- *Uterine prolapse.* Vaginal hysterectomy can be combined with an anterior or posterior colporrhaphy and correction of enterocele by coaptation of the uterosacral ligaments. The ovaries are inspected and, if there is ovarian pathology or the woman is over 50 years of age, vaginal oophorectomy can be accomplished at the same time. Uterine prolapse can also be treated by amputation of the cervix and suturing the cardinal (transverse cervical) ligaments in front of the shortened cervix (Manchester repair).

- *Enterocele.* The technique is similar to that used for hernia repair. The vaginal skin is incised and mobilized and the peritoneum opened. The neck of the sac of the prolapse is identified and closed with a purse-string suture.

- *Vault repair.* This may be done vaginally or abdominally depending on the patient's general condition and whether or not she wishes to continue intercourse. The vaginal route is simpler and provides a relatively pain-free postoperative recovery.
  - —*Sacrospinous fixation* is the most common operation done vaginally although it carries a risk of damage to the pudendal vessels and nerves. There is a significant risk of cystocele and stress incontinence.
  - —The abdominal approach includes the *sacrocolpopexy* where the vault is attached to the sacrum using a non-absorbable mesh. This procedure can be very vascular. Laparoscopic sacrocolpopexy has been undertaken in a number of centres.

- *Rectocele.* Posterior colporrhaphy is the operation for rectocele. Care must be taken when removing the redundant vaginal skin as vaginal narrowing can result in severe dyspareunia. A double plication of the vesicovaginal and rectovaginal tissues may prevent the recurrence of prolapse.[4]

References

1 Stanton, S.L. (1998). Vaginal prolapse. In *Gynaecology* (ed. R.W. Shaw, W.P. Soutter, and S.L. Stanton), pp. 759–70. Churchill Livingstone, Edinburgh.

2 Smith, A.R.B., Hosker, G.L., Smith, A.T.B., and Warrel, D.W. (1989). The role of partial denervation of the pelvic floor in the aetiology of genitourinary prolapse and stress incontinence of urine: a neurophysiological study. *British Journal of Obstetrics and Gynaecology* **96**, 24–8.

3 Jackson, S. and Smith, P. (1997). Fortnightly review: diagnosing and managing genitourinary prolapse. *British Medical Journal* **314**, 875–80.

4 Porges, R.F. and Smiler, J.W. (1994). Long-term analysis of the surgical management of pelvic support defects. *American Journal of Obstetrics and Gynecology* **171**, 1518–26.

Menopause

665

The menopause is defined as the last menstrual period when the cessation of menstruation occurs as a result of the loss of ovarian follicular activity and a reduction of oestradiol. The average age of menopause is 51–52 years. With an increasingly ageing population, most women in Western countries will expect to live 30 years postmenopause. This constitutes more than one-third of their life.

The climacteric is the time around the menopause when the menopausal transition takes place and symptoms begin. This is due to declining oestrogen and progesterone production from the failing ovary. The menopause transition starts on average 4 years before the menopause, although menstruation can cease abruptly. Bleeding more than 12 months after the last menstrual period is considered abnormal.

Causes

The menopause occurs when the store of oocytes is exhausted. Follicle-stimulating hormone (FSH) levels rise (FSH greater than 30 IU/L) but the ovary fails to respond adequately. Once oestradiol production falls below a certain threshold, endometrial stimulation does not occur and bleeding ceases. FSH and luteinizing hormone (LH) levels then remain permanently elevated.

Other causes for the menopause include surgery (bilateral oophorectomy), radiation, or chemotherapy used to treat malignancies such as Hodgkin's disease. A premature menopause is defined as menopause at less than 40 years of age, although, for practical clinical reasons, 45 years may be a more appropriate definition.

Short-term effects

Symptoms begin during the climacteric, before the last menstrual period.
- *Menstrual symptoms.* As the ovaries fail to respond, ovulation may not occur despite some oestradiol production. The ensuing anovulatory cycles may be erratic and heavy—initially more frequent and then becoming less frequent.
- *Vasomotor symptoms.* Hot flushes and sweats are the most common symptoms occurring in up to 80% of peri-menopausal women. The frequency can vary from many episodes each hour to only a few episodes during the week. The underlying pathophysiology is uncertain. Flushes are often associated with shivering, tachycardia, and sweating. They are associated with frequent wakening at night. These symptoms do not seem to occur in young women with hypo-oestrogenaemia, and priming with oestrogen before the eventual hypo-oestrogenism appears to be an important factor.
- *Urogenital ageing.* The vagina and the trigone of the bladder share a common embryological origin. Both are sensitive to changes in oestradiol levels. In the vagina, hypo-oestrogenism causes atrophy with thinning of the vaginal epithelium, loss of rugae, and dryness. The Gram-positive Doderlein's bacilli are lost with a resultant fall in lactic-acid production. The pH of the vaginal secretions rises and this gives decreased resistance to infections with bacteria and yeast. There is a loss of elasticity in the underlying tissues and this, associated with the dryness, may cause dyspareunia. The overall size of the vagina decreases with it becoming shorter and narrower.

- *Urinary tract effects.* Because the trigone and urethra are oestrogen-sensitive, atrophic changes may lead to the urethral syndrome—urinary frequency, urgency, and dysuria in the absence of infection.
  - —Stress incontinence is more common in older women, particularly around the time of the menopause. However, the association between low oestradiol levels and stress incontinence is much weaker than that with the urethral syndrome.
- *Psychological problems.* Although there may be an increase in psychological problems around the time of the menopause, the association between these and low plasma oestradiol levels is weak. However, psychological problems may well occur secondarily to other effects of the menopause (poor sleep, urogenital problems, sexual problems, poor concentration, etc.). Libido certainly appears to be reduced. There are cultural differences between attitudes to the menopause and these may have a strong underlying influence. Japanese women have far fewer complaints about menopausal symptoms than women from the USA.
- *Sexual problems.* Sexual problems are common complaints during the climacteric and postmenopause. About a third of women will complain of a loss of libido. However, there is a complex relationship between sexuality and the menopause.

Long-term effects

Cardiovascular disease

Coronary heart disease is a leading cause of death in women and the incidence increases with age. Compared to that in men, the onset of cardiovascular disease tends to be later and women have a relative protection premenopausally. After the menopause, there is a two–threefold increase in risk. There is uncertainty as to the relative influence of low oestradiol levels and ageing, and various mechanisms have been postulated for this increase in risk. These include adverse changes to lipids and lipoproteins, insulin resistance, and changes in clotting. There are also direct effects of oestrogen on the cardiovascular system and oestrogen receptors have been found throughout the cardiovascular system. A typical oestrogenic effect is a relaxation in arterial tone and a decrease in resistance.

Osteoporosis

This is a systemic skeletal disease leading to increased fragility and more susceptibility to fracture. Bone mass in women rises during childhood and reaches a peak during the third decade. This remains relatively stable until the menopausal transition when loss of bone density occurs. There is an accelerated rate of bone loss following the menopause and the rate of bone loss gradually slows into old age. Table 80.1 lists the risk factors for developing osteoporosis.

- *Prevalence of osteoporosis.* The World Health Organisation (WHO) has defined osteoporosis as a bone mineral density more than 2.5 standard deviations below the young adult mean (T-score). A reduction of 1.0–2.5 standard deviations represents osteopenia. Densitometry-defined osteoporosis associated with fragility fractures is called severe or established osteoporosis. The prevalence of osteoporosis increases with age with less than 1% of young women having osteoporosis but 70% of women aged over 80 being affected.
- Typical osteoporotic fractures occur in the femoral neck, vertebral body, or distal forearm (Colles' fracture). Many vertebral fractures go unnoticed. Hip fractures carry a much greater risk to significant morbidity with up to 50% of patients losing their independence following a hip fracture.
- DEXA (dual-energy X-ray absorptiometry) bone density scanning is the 'gold standard' for estimating bone density and risk of fracture. X-ray radiography is too imprecise to be useful. Quantitated CT scanning is accurate but involves a high radiation dose per scan. Biochemical markers will give a measure of bone turnover but not of overall bone density.

Alzheimer's disease

Like osteoporosis, the increasing age of the female population is leading to an increase in dementia. Alzheimer's disease is more common in women than men and there are observational data to suggest that oestrogen deficiency plays a role. The condition is more common in those with previous hip fracture, infarction, or low body mass index (BMI). Alzheimer's disease tends to occur later in women who take oestrogen.

Treatment for the consequences of the menopause is dealt with in Chapter 81.

Table 80.1 Risk factors for developing osteoporosis

Modifiable risk factors

Oestrogen deficiency (menopause, premature menopause, prolonged amenorrhoea)

Low body mass index (BMI)

Prolonged immobility

Smoking

Alcohol abuse

Nutritional factors

Susceptibility to falls

Secondary causes, e.g. coeliac disease

Non-modifiable risk factors

Age

Race

Positive family history

Prior fragile fracture

Chapter 81

Hormone replacement therapy

Hormone replacement therapy (HRT) constitutes treatment with oestrogen or oestrogen and progestogen to treat or prevent symptoms associated with the menopause. The aim of treatment is to increase circulating oestrogens to a level similar to that of the premenopause. Current evidence suggests that in hysterectomized women oestrogen-only treatment is needed, whereas in women with an intact uterus progesterone needs to be given cyclically or continuously.

Regimens

- *Oestrogen-only treatment.* For hysterectomized women oestrogen-only treatment is satisfactory. Treatment is given continuously (rather than cyclically as with the combined oral contraceptive (COC)).
- *Combined sequential (standard) HRT.* This is the standard regimen of HRT—continuous oestrogen with progestogen given cyclically for 10–14 days each cycle.
- *Continuous-combined (period-free) HRT.* In older women, where cyclical bleeding may be less acceptable, the continuous combined regimen can be used. Oestrogen and progestogen are given continuously in an attempt to induce an atrophic endometrium and 'no bleeding'. This regimen can only be used in women who are at least 1–2 years postmenopausal when the chance of endogenous oestrogen production has reduced.
- *Long-cycle HRT.* This regimen is used to give a 3-monthly withdrawal bleed, rather than the standard monthly bleed. Oestrogen is given continuously for 3 months with a higher dose of progestogen for the last 14 days of the 3-month cycle. This is followed by 1 week without treatment and then the cycle re-starts. This regimen can be used in a woman who is virtually or actually postmenopausal. If it is used too soon, breakthrough bleeding is common.

Drugs

- *Oestrogens.* Conjugated equine oestrogens (Premarin) have been used for over 50 years to treat menopausal symptoms. Once absorbed and metabolized, the major circulating product is oestrone. Many different oestrogens have been identified from the preparation and it has a proven 'track record'.
- *Oestradiol.* The ovary produces predominantly 17-beta oestradiol. Treatment can be given as 17-beta oestradiol but this is best given non-orally. Oestradiol valerate and micronized oestradiol are also used. All appear to be similarly effective in symptom relief and prevention.
- *Progestogens.* Synthetic progestogens are more potent than natural progesterone and can therefore be given in smaller quantities. The 19-nor-testosterone derivatives (norethisterone, norgestrel) and the C21 derivatives (medroxyprogesterone acetate, dydrogesterone) are effective in endometrial protection. Natural progesterone can be used but is poorly absorbed orally or transdermally. However, it is available as pessaries or vaginal gels.

Routes of administration

For most women there are no definite advantages of one route of administration over another and therefore it is often left to the patient to decide which route suits her best.

- Oral administration of oestrogens and progestogens has been used the longest and is simple to use. Most oestrogen tends to be absorbed and metabolized to oestrone even if administered as oestradiol. However, this is equally effective in symptom relief.
- Transdermal patches are highly effective and suit most women although a proportion can get skin irritation. The new generation matrix patches are easier to use than the older reservoir patches.
- Oestradiol can be given as a subdermal hormone implant, lasting 6–12 months. Testosterone implants can be useful in hysterectomized women who have poor libido, and these can be inserted at the same time.
- 17-Beta oestradiol can be given as a percutaneous gel, although progesterone creams, while widely advertised as useful for menopausal symptoms, are actually very poorly absorbed. Progesterone creams are unlikely to provide adequate endometrial protection.
- Progesterone can be given as pessaries or vaginal gel or by using a levonorgestrel intrauterine device and these will adequately protect the endometrium.
- Oestrogen can be given locally to the vagina and lower urogenital tract by creams, pessaries, or as an oestrogen-impregnated soft vaginal ring pessary that lasts 3 months.

673

Dosages

The dosage necessary for symptom relief tends to vary with the individual. In general, younger women require higher doses for symptom relief than older women. The bone-sparing doses shown in Table 81.1 are useful starting dosages, although a high dose may be given in young patients. In women more than 10 years past the menopause, lower dosages may be adequate—and starting at half the dosages in the table is also adequate.

Dosage should be altered after 3 months, according to symptoms or side-effects.

Table 81.1 The bone-sparing dosages of HRT

Drug	Dose
Oral oestradiol	1–2 mg daily
Transdermal oestradiol	50 mg daily
Oral conjugated equine oestrogens	0.625 mg daily
Oestradiol implants	50 mg implant 6- to 12-monthly

Indications and contraindications

There is still controversy as to the indications for HRT. Some enthusiasts advocate widespread use in almost every woman whilst others urge caution in view of side-effects. The generally agreed *indications* for treatment are the following.

- *The symptomatic patient.* In the absence of any contraindications, there is very little reason not to treat a woman if symptoms are affecting her quality of life.
- *Premature menopause.* In a woman who has a menopause, either natural or iatrogenic, before 45 years, there is abundant evidence that treatment with HRT is beneficial. Treatment for such women is considered virtually mandatory.
- *Treatment of prevention of osteoporosis.* HRT is still the 'gold standard' treatment for osteoporosis in postmenopausal women. However, in the older age group it can be difficult to get women on to HRT without side-effects.
- *Prevention of cardiovascular disease.* Although previous observational studies had suggested a protective effect against heart disease, the results of the largest prospective controlled study have in fact shown an increase in the incidence of heart attacks on combined HRT. HRT is no longer indicated for the prevention of cardiovascular disease.

Contraindications are as follows.
- HRT should not be given to women with an oestrogen-dependent malignant tumour.
- Postmenopausal bleeding or abnormal perimenopausal bleeding should be investigated before starting HRT.
- A history of recent or active thrombosis contraindicates HRT.

Precautions

- In view of the increased risk of thrombosis (see below) any woman with a past history of thrombosis or strong family history should have a thrombophilia screen before starting HRT.
- Fibroids are likely to grow under the influence of HRT and, if present, patients should be warned that this may be the case. However, they will normally regress once HRT is stopped.
- With all HRT there is an increased risk of gallstones and endometriosis may be re-activated by combined sequential HRT.
- The risk of breast cancer is discussed below.

These risks should be discussed and documented prior to starting HRT. It is wise to check blood pressure prior to starting HRT as a small proportion (possibly 1%) may get an increase in blood pressure with oestrogens. However, the majority will notice a small decrease in blood pressure. If there is hypertension, this is best treated before starting HRT.

Benefits and risks

Benefits

- There is abundant evidence to show good symptom relief with HRT. As a general rule, if symptom relief does not occur, it is either because the dosage is too low, absorption poor, or because the symptom is not due to oestrogen deficiency.
- The risk of osteoporotic fracture is roughly halved for women taking HRT.
- Women with a premature menopause have a much reduced risk of osteoporosis, or symptoms in later life.
- It is uncertain how much protection women get from Alzheimer's disease but recent studies suggest that the incidence is reduced by approximately a third in women taking HRT.
- There is a reduction in risk of colon cancer (relative risk 0.58 among HRT users compared to non-users) but no difference in rectal cancer.

Risks

675

- *Thromboembolism*. Oral HRT confers an increased risk of 1–2 in 5000 of venous thrombosis in HRT users. The increased risk of thrombosis mainly occurs in the first year of treatment. The risk appears to be smaller in non-oral oestrogen preparations (patches, gels, or implants).
- *Breast cancer*. The main concern for women is the risk of breast cancer. The biggest recent study by the Collaborative Group on Hormonal Factors in Breast Cancer reported an analysis of 51 studies comprising 52 705 breast cancer patients and 108 411 control women. For each year of use, the risk of breast cancer increased by 1.023, a similar relative risk for non-users for each extra year before the menopause (1.028). This translates into an increased risk of 2 per 1000 cases of breast cancer for 5 years of treatment and 7 per 1000 for 10 years treatment. However, breast cancers in women on HRT appear to be at an earlier stage and at a better grade than those in women not on HRT. The prognosis for women on HRT at the time of diagnosis is better, and it appears that HRT does not cause any increase in mortality from breast cancer.
- *Vascular disease*. The relative risk of heart attacks and stroke are increased (1.29 and 1.41 respectively)[1] in women taking combined HRT for 5 years. It is not clear whether this is related to the type of progestogen used.

Each individual woman must weigh up the risks and benefits for her of taking HRT. The most common indication for use is still symptom relief.

References
1 Womens Health Initiative Study. (2002). *Journal of American Medical Association* **288**, 321–33.

Benign neoplasms of the genital tract

The genital tract can be the seat of various benign tumours that can be clinically significant and require intervention but can often be asymptomatic. Benign neoplastic lesions arising from different parts of the genital tract are described below.

Vulva

Clinically significant diseases of the vulva are rare in gynaecological practice. Inflammatory disorders (vulvitis) are far more common than benign neoplasms and are described in Chapter 40. Benign neoplasms can be categorized as solid lesions and cystic lesions.

Solid lesions

- *Lipoma/fibroma.* Fibrofatty and muscular tissues of the labia and mons pubis or ischiorectal fascia may give rise to benign fibromas, lipomas, and leiomyomas. These tumours are relatively infrequent and histologically may contain a mixture of both elements. Clinically, they may cause discomfort or interfere with sexual intercourse. These growths should be excised.
- *Granular myoblastoma* is a benign lesion arising from the nerve sheath. Myoblastoma is not a well localized tumour and may locally recur. Treatment is local resection of the lesion.
- *Haemangiomas.* Different varieties of these can occur. Pyogenic granuloma is a type of haemangioma characterized by the proliferation of capillaries of labia. It usually occurs during pregnancy. These lesions are the largest and most symptomatic of adult vulvar haemangiomas. Bleeding and infection are common and can often give rise to purulent discharge. Treatment is by deep excision.
- *Endometrioma.* Ectopic endometrium may arise by metaplasia or by implantation of viable endometrium at the time of surgery or delivery in a genetically susceptible individual. A history of cyclical enlargement of nodule and pain with menses is highly suggestive. Local excision is diagnostic and curative.
- *Hidradenoma.* This tumour usually occurs in the vulva of sexually active Caucasian women. It arises from the sweat gland. These tumours are rare and excisional biopsies are both diagnostic and curative.

Cystic lesions

- *Inclusion cysts* are also known as epidermal cysts. They are lined by a smooth layer of keratinizing squamous epithelium and the contents of the cysts are largely keratin and cellular debris. They have a sebaceous appearance and odour. Acutely inflamed cysts should be treated with a warm pack and incision and drainage. Excision may become necessary to prevent recurrence.
- *Bartholin's cyst.* Dilatation of the Bartholin's duct is the most common cystic swelling of the vulva. Most of these cysts occur because of a purely mechanical problem, i.e. a blockage of outflow of the mucus. Rapid enlargement and pain can be secondary to abscess formation. Marsupialization is the treatment of choice, i.e. the inner cyst wall is folded back and stitched to the skin. Gonococcal infection should be excluded. Persistent episodes of abscess formation may require excision of the gland.
- *Hydrocele of the canal of Nuck.* Cysts of the canal of Nuck are not true hernia, but are analogous to hydrocele in men. Treatment is often not indicated unless cysts become symptomatic at which point excision is indicated.

Vagina

Neoplasms of vagina can present with a sensation of fullness in the vagina. Benign neoplasms can be either solid or cystic.

- *Inclusion cysts* arise from inclusion of the vaginal skin underneath the surface resulting from perineal lacerations or from imperfect surgical repair of the perineum. Treatment is surgical removal and is only indicated when the cysts cause symptoms such as discomfort or dyspareunia or infection.
- *Gartner duct cyst.* This arises from vestigial remnants of the Wolffian or mesonephric system. Gartner duct cysts are generally located on the anterolateral aspect of the vagina and are usually small. Occasionally, they may be large and bulge from the introitus. No treatment is necessary if the cysts are small and not symptomatic but surgical excision may be required if the cysts are large and obstruct the outlet.
- *Condyloma acuminatum* is a viral disease caused by human papillomavirus. It is multifocal in character and is associated with vulvar and cervical lesions. It is mostly benign but specific subtypes may give rise to cervical or vaginal cancers. This disease is considered to be sexually transmitted. Rarely, lesions are passed to the offspring of infected mothers and may be found in the mucous membrane of the newborn as well as in the larynx. Lesions have a flowery appearance classically known as wart. Biopsies are recommended to rule out verrucous carcinoma. Laser vaporization or cryotherapy may be used to treat the lesions. Medical treatment with 5-fluorouracil or podophyllin is also effective. Lesions in pregnant women can hypertrophy and proliferate and may develop to the degree that they obstruct the outlet of the vagina, necessitating Caesarean section. However this is extremely rare.
- *Endometriosis.* Endometriotic implants in the vagina are rare. They are usually seen on the top of the vagina. They usually respond to medical therapy.
- *Leiomyoma* is very rarely seen in the vagina. It may be locally excised.
- *Adenosis vaginae* is found in female offspring of women who were exposed to diethylstilboestrol during pregnancy. Adenosis is a benign lesion and requires no treatment. However, it should be carefully observed for malignant transformation.

Cervix

- *Cervical polyps* are the most common benign growth of the cervix. They are usually pedunculated arising from the endocervical mucosa but they occasionally arise from the external or vaginal surface of the cervix. Clinically, they present as small bright-red growths that protrude from the cervical canal. They may be inflammatory in origin and range up to few centimetres in diameter. Polyps can be asymptomatic and are discovered as an incidental finding during routine smear test. They can produce intermenstrual spotting or contact bleeding after coitus. When polyps are identified removal is indicated because of the low risk of malignancy (said to be 1:6000). Sometime (e.g. in the presence of irregular bleeding) this may need to be combined with hysteroscopy and curettage of the endometrial cavity to rule out any polyps in the uterus. Recurrence is not uncommon.
- *Nabothian cysts* are mucus-retention cysts caused by blockage of the openings of the endocervical mucous glands. They are usually seen on the surface of the cervix and may be associated with chronic cervicitis and chronic infection of the endocervical canal. Normally no treatment is required unless they are infected, at which point cryotherapy or cautery to the cervix may be indicated.

82 Benign neoplasms of the genital tract

Uterus

Leiomyomas are the most common benign tumour of the uterus, occurring in an estimated 25–30% of women of reproductive age. They arise from the smooth muscle cells of the myometrium (hence the name) but, perhaps because they are firm or for some illogical reason, they are more often referred to as fibroids. They have not been reported before menarche and rarely develop after menopause. Genetic influences are involved, because these tumours are considerably more frequent in AfroCaribbean than in other ethnic groups. Oestrogens probably stimulate their growth. Conversely, they shrink in size after menopause. Leiomyomas can be single but are usually multiple. They can be entirely asymptomatic and be discovered only on routine pelvic examination or postmortem. The most frequent manifestation when present is menorrhagia with or without intermenstrual bleeding. Large masses may present with lower abdominal swelling, dragging sensation, or urinary symptoms. Whether these benign tumours ever become transformed into sarcomas is highly questionable, and indeed this may never occur.

681

Leiomyomas are classified by their location in the myometrium and their proximity to endometrial and serosal surfaces. Submucous, intramural, and subserous are the three most common types.

Treatment

Leiomyomas can be treated conservatively or with surgery. Radiation therapy was used in the past for patients considered poor surgical risks and those with excessive bleeding to induce menopause, but this management is now rare. Shrinkage of fibroids by embolization of feeding vessel may be possible but is still under research.

Conservative treatment

Leiomyomas discovered during routine pelvic examination in a patient without any symptoms usually require no active treatment but pelvic examinations should be done to monitor the growth perhaps at 6–12-monthly intervals unless there are indications of rapid growth and symptoms are reported.

Surgical treatment

Surgical treatment is usually indicated in patients with large leiomyomas and for those associated with heavy periods or other symptoms. Occasionally the position of the tumour within the uterine cavity may be the cause of repeated miscarriages, or even subfertility.

- *Myomectomy* can be used to remove single or multiple leiomyomas. It is indicated when fertility is a concern and if the patient does not wish to part with her uterus for social or religious reasons. Excessive bleeding during operation is a significant risk factor and may even necessitate a hysterectomy and patients should be appropriately counselled.
- *Hysterectomy* is indicated when there are large leiomyomas and the possibility of preserving the uterus by myomectomy is minimal or nonexistent. The risk of recurrence is high so hysterectomy is the treatment of choice for those patients who do not intend further childbearing. In younger patients the ovaries are conserved.

Endometrial polyps

Endometrial polyps are the result of focal overgrowth of endometrial glands and stroma. Recent cytogenetic studies confirm that most endometrial polyps are monoclonal and stromal cells are the neoplastic component. Although endometrial polyps may occur at any age, they develop more commonly at the time of menopause. Their clinical significance lies in the production of abnormal uterine bleeding and, more importantly, the risk of giving rise to cancer. Approximately 1% of endometrial polyps are malignant.

Ovary

Neoplasms of the ovary make up an amazing diversity of pathological entities. This is due to the presence of three cell types in the normal ovary: the multipotential surface (coelomic) epithelium; the totipotential germ cells; and the sex cord stromal cells. Each of these cell types can give rise to a variety of tumours.

- Cystadenoma (serous or mucinous).
- Brenner tumour (rarely malignant).
- Neoplastic tumours arising from germ cells.
- Dermoid (benign cystic teratoma).
- Neoplasms arising from ovarian stroma.
- Fibroma.
- Adenofibroma.
- Thecoma.
- Physiological cysts.
- Follicular cysts.
- Luteal cysts.

Overall, 90% of ovarian tumours are benign although they are more likely to be malignant in the older women. The most common solid tumour in younger women is the cystic teratoma, also commonly known as a dermoid. Among older women, epithelial cell tumours are more common. Benign ovarian tumours are often asymptomatic, but they can present with pain, abdominal swelling, pressure effects, menstrual disturbances, or hormonal effects. Pain may be due to torsion or bleeding inside the cyst. Masses that are 12 cm or more in diameter may be palpable abdominally above the symphysis pubis. Bimanual examination usually reveals a mass in the pelvis and it may be possible to assess the mobility, consistency, and tenderness of the mass and the presence of nodules in the pouch of Douglas. The presence of ascites and a hard irregular fixed mass suggests malignancy.

Pelvic ultrasound, computerized tomography (CT) scan, and measurement of tumour markers (CA125) are useful adjuncts for diagnostic evaluation of ovarian cysts.

Treatment

- Even when asymptomatic, older women gain little from conservative treatment. As the risk of malignancy is high, detailed evaluation of the cysts and removal is usually indicated. Often this involves hysterectomy and bilateral salpingo-oophorectomy.
- Women under 35 are less likely to have malignancy and may also wish to have children. Ovarian cysts more than 10 cm in diameter are unlikely to be physiological or to resolve spontaneously. Smaller cysts can be followed up with ultrasound. If the cyst does not regress or becomes symptomatic, laparoscopy or laparotomy is indicated. Ovarian cystectomy or oophorectomy is usually carried out provided the clinical appearance of the cyst is entirely benign. Frozen section (histology report intra-operatively) should be arranged where possible to guide therapy.
- Ovarian cysts detected during pregnancy are mostly benign. The conservative approach of monitoring cyst size with ultrasound is often adequate. In the presence of acute symptoms or if the cyst is large or is growing rapidly, laparotomy may well be required regardless of gestation.

Chapter 83

Cancer screening in gynaecology

Screening

Screening is the process of identifying those asymptomatic individuals in the population who are at sufficiently increased risk of a condition to justify referral for further investigation and treatment. As such, a screening test does not necessarily diagnose the condition. The ultimate aim of screening programmes in cancer is to reduce deaths and morbidity from the disease.

Conditions suitable for screening should ideally satisfy a number of criteria.
- The condition should represent an important public health problem.
- The natural history of the condition should be known.
- There should be a recognizable early stage of the condition.
- An effective intervention should be available.
- There should be a suitable screening test available.
- The benefits should be greater than the harm caused by screening.

A suitable screening test should:
- Have a high sensitivity and specificity.
- Be acceptable to patients.
- Be cost-effective.
- Be reproducible.

Here are some useful definitions.
- *Sensitivity* is the proportion of subjects tested who have the disease who have a positive screening test.
- *Specificity* is the proportion of people who do not have the disease and who have a negative test.
- The *positive predictive value* of a test is the chance that, given a positive result, you will have the condition and the *negative predictive value* is the probability that you do not have the disease if the test is negative.
- The *odds ratio* of a test is the number of individuals with a positive screening result for each person with confirmed disease.

Although, clearly, a test must have sufficient sensitivity to be able to detect cases of the disease, it is the specificity of the test that is most important in screening. This is especially true when an invasive and potentially dangerous procedure is required to confirm the diagnosis, as would be the case for example in ovarian cancer (laparoscopy, laparotomy). In these circumstances a screening test with an odds ratio of greater than 10 to 1 is unlikely to be acceptable. In order to have an odds ratio of 10 a screening test for ovarian cancer in women over the age of 40 needs to have a specificity of 99.6%.

687

Cervical carcinoma

Rationale

Invasive disease is preceded by cervical intraepithelial neoplasia (CIN). Effective treatment of CIN prevents progression. Women at risk of having CIN can be identified by exfoliative cytology.

Methods

Papanicolau smear

Screening is by cervical cytology (Papanicolaou smear). In England and Wales this is carried out every 3 to 5 years from the age of 20 to 65. A national call and recall system sends reminders to patients. Three-yearly testing identifies more than 95% of abnormalities detected by annual screening and so is more cost-effective. Interpretation of smears in postmenopausal women may be difficult and cervical neoplasia is unlikely if smears prior to this have been normal.

- A pelvic examination is performed using a speculum. A suitable spatula inserted into the external cervical os is rotated through 360°, smeared evenly over a glass slide, and fixed immediately with an acetic acid/alcohol mixture.
- After staining, the slide is examined by a technician or pathologist for the presence of epithelial cells with neoplastic changes (increased nuclear to cytoplasmic ratio, mitotic figures). The presence of cells from the endocervix is used as an indication that the sample has been taken across the squamocolumnar junction and has included the transformation zone.

Smears are reported as: normal; unsatisfactory; inflammatory; borderline; mild, moderate, or severe dyskaryosis; suspicious of malignancy; or showing abnormal glandular cells.

- *Unsatisfactory smears* occur in 10–15% of cases and can be due to insufficient cells, inflammatory cells, or red blood cells obscuring the epithelial cells. A repeat after 3 months is recommended and, if a second repeat is unsatisfactory, referral for colposcopy.
- Patients with *borderline nuclear abnormalities* (BNA) and *mild dyskaryosis* should have a repeat smear after 6 months and are referred if successive smears are abnormal.
- All other women are referred for colposcopy.

Note that the diagnosis of CIN itself requires a tissue sample from biopsy and the correlation between the degree of abnormality on cytology and histology is poor. False-negative results (i.e. women with CIN who are reported as having a normal smear) occur in up to 20% of cases. Reasons include errors in sampling technique, distortion of the cervix from previous surgery, and laboratory error. Of women, 10–15% will have an abnormal smear and 5–10% will be referred for colposcopy. Premalignant changes in the endocervical epithelium (cervical glandular intraepithelial neoplasia (CGIN)) cannot be reliably detected by cervical screening. The introduction of cervical screening has been associated with a 40% fall in deaths from cervical cancer in the UK over the last 20 years. Regular cervical screening reduces (but does not eliminate) the risk of death from cervical carcinoma by 75%.

Other methods of screening

Cervical carcinoma is the second most common cause of female cancer-related deaths worldwide. Using cervical smears for screening requires a sophisticated infrastructure, laboratories, and trained staff. These are expensive and therefore not available in many developed countries where mortality rates from cervical carcinoma are higher. Other alternative approaches to screening are visual inspection of the cervix by trained non-medical health workers looking for early stage disease and photographing the cervix after staining with acetic acid (cervicography).

Testing for the human papillomavirus (HPV)

Infection with the HPV is common in sexually active women. However certain serotypes (16, 18, 31, and 33) are more commonly found in the presence of invasive disease. Routine testing for a limited range of HPV types using samples taken from the cervix at the time of cervical smear testing identifies a higher proportion of women with CIN than conventional cytology. HPV testing may also be of value in predicting whether or not low-grade changes will progress. However, the routine use of HPV testing in addition to conventional cytology would significantly increase the cost per case detected. The role of HPV testing is currently under evaluation. Possible strategies might include:

- Using HPV testing to determine whether patients with low-grade CIN or borderline changes require treatment or referral for colposcopy.
- Only screening women who are positive for certain HPV types by cytology.
- Referring women with high-risk HPV disease for colposcopy.

Ovarian carcinoma

Rationale

75% of cases present with advanced disease. The prognosis for early-stage disease is better than that for advanced disease. If the disease could be diagnosed earlier in asymptomatic women, overall survival might be improved.

Methods

- Ultrasound examination to look for ovarian cysts. As many cysts in premenopausal women are functional (follicular or corpus luteum), more than one measurement may be required. Suspicious features are; increasing size, internal septa, solid areas within the cyst, and increased blood flow (Doppler). False-positive results may be due to benign ovarian tumours (which might need to be removed in any case), endometriosis, and inflammatory masses. Screening needs to be done centrally and requires some operator expertise. There have been significant improvements in odds ratio for both ovarian malignancy (7:1) and all abnormalities (2:1).

- CA125 is a glycoprotein shed by 85% of epithelial tumours. Cut-off levels of between 30 and 65 IU/L have been used for screening. CA125 lacks sufficient specificity if used alone but can be used as a primary screen to identify candidates for ultrasound. It does not require specialist expertise or equipment at point of collection. False-positives occur in other malignancies (liver, pancreas), endometriosis, pelvic inflammatory disease (PID), and early pregnancy. Sensitivity can be improved by looking at serial measurements in women with borderline values. Up to 50% of stage 1 tumours will have a value of less than 35 IU/L.

The current situation

Early disease can be identified by current screening tests. Ultrasound, either used alone or in combination with CA125, now appears to have sufficient sensitivity and specificity but most studies to date have not compared long-term death rates in screened and unscreened populations. Large multicentre studies randomizing women into screened and unscreened controls are in progress but at the moment the value of screening the general population remains unproven. Women with hereditary disease should be offered testing where possible to see if they are carriers of an abnormal *BRCA* gene. Carriers may be offered annual screening with ultrasound sonography and CA125 and prophylactic oophorectomy when their family is complete. Even in these groups the value of such an approach in increased survival is unproven.

Endometrial carcinoma

There is no screening programme for endometrial carcinoma. Possible methods of screening would be the use of ultrasound to detect increases in endometrial thickness in postmenopausal women or the routine use of endometrial sampling. The value of doing this even in high-risk groups is unproven.

Chapter 84

Pathology and management of cervical intraepithelial neoplasia (CIN) lesions of the cervix

The cervical canal is lined by endocervical glandular epithelium. The vaginal portion of the cervix is covered by squamous epithelium. The junction between these two epithelia is called the squamo-columnar junction (SCJ). From late fetal life to the menopause the position of this junction changes. When columnar epithelium is exposed to the acid vaginal pH, transformation occurs. Whilst in most cases physiological squamous metaplasia occurs, the transformation zone (TZ) is where cervical intraepithelial neoplasia (CIN) develops.

Early intercourse, multiple sexual partners, smoking, human papillomavirus (HPV) infection, and immunocompromise are associated with an increased risk of CIN.

Pathology

CIN is a single continuous disease process with disordered growth and development of the epithelial lining of the TZ of the cervix, with varying degrees of nuclear enlargement and pleomorphism. CIN1 is defined as disordered growth of the lower one-third of the epithelial lining. In CIN2 there is failure of the cells to mature in the lower one- to two-thirds of the epithelium with a greater degree of nuclear atypia. In CIN3 undifferentiated cells extend into the upper third of the epithelium. Cytologically, the dyskaryotic cell is characterized by anaplasia, increased nuclear/cytoplasmic ratio (the nucleus is larger), hyperchromatism with changes in nuclear chromatin, multinucleation, and abnormalities in differentiation. CIN is a precursor of squamous cell carcinoma. Possibly only 30% of untreated CIN3 cases will progress to invasive squamous cell carcinoma within 20 years with spontaneous regression in one-third of cases.

Screening for CIN

The National Health Service (NHS) Cervical Screening Programme recommends that all women aged 20–64 should be screened by cervical cytology at least once every 5 years. The following patients should be referred for colposcopy.
- Suspected carcinoma of the cervix.
- One smear showing moderate or severe dyskaryosis.
- Two successive smears showing mild dyskaryosis.
- Persistent smears showing borderline nuclear abnormalities or being unsatisfactory for reporting.
- Glandular changes.

84 Pathology and management of CIN lesions

Colposcopy

At colposcopy the cervix is examined under low power (6–20 ×) binocular magnification and an intense light source. Abnormalities in the appearance of the epithelium and its capillary blood supply are not visible to the naked eye but can be identified at colposcopy. After application of 3–5% acetic acid to the cervix a transient coagulation of the protein of the superficial cells occurs and atypical areas stand out from normal epithelium. The major abnormal patterns at colposcopy are acetowhite epithelium, punctation, mosaicism, and atypical vessels. Acetowhite epithelium is related to the abnormal nuclear/cytoplasmic ratio that occurs in dysplastic or neoplastic cells. After application of acetic acid the application of Schiller's or Lugol's iodine (a weak aqueous solution) may enhance the definition of the outer limit of the TZ and enable detection of any abnormal areas of vaginal epithelium. The Schiller test is based on the principle that normal squamous epithelium of the cervix contains glycogen, which combines with iodine to produce a deep mahogany-brown colour. Non-staining indicates abnormal squamous (or columnar) epithelium. The test is not specific for dysplasia but merely reveals non-glycogen-containing epithelium. Immature metaplasia may be non-staining.

At colposcopy one must assess:
- Whether the SCJ can completely be seen.
- The area of acetowhite epithelium and any atypical vessel patterns.
- The outer limit of the TZ including any evidence of extension on to the vaginal wall.

A diagnostic biopsy for histological assessment must be taken from abnormal areas if treatment by a local ablation technique is contemplated.

Treatment

It is customary to recommend treatment for all patients with higher-grade (CIN2 and CIN3) lesions.

The following therapies are used for the treatment of CIN.
- *Local ablation methods*: cryocautery, coldcoagulator, electrodiathermy, and carbon dioxide laser vapourization.
- *Excision methods*: large loop excision of the transformation zone (LLETZ), knife cone biopsy, laser cut cone (CO_2), hysterectomy.

Local ablation should only be used when:
- The SCJ can be seen completely.
- There is no cytological, histological, or colposcopic suggestion of microinvasive or frankly invasive disease.
- There is no suggestion of glandular abnormality.
- The patient is considered reliable and will attend for regular follow-up.

If the SCJ is not completely seen or the patient has previously been treated, local ablation is contraindicated. Excision of the abnormal epithelium enabling histological assessment of the total abnormal area should be undertaken.

Knife cone biopsy and hysterectomy will usually be performed under general anaesthetic but most other treatments are suitable for out-patient management. Hysterectomy is rarely required for the management of CIN. It may, however, be indicated in those who have completed their childbearing and have coexisting gynaecological problems, or in postmenopausal women where cone biopsy may be technically difficult. Where the lesion involves the upper vagina a combination of local ablative or excisional treatment with laser vapourization of the vaginal part of the lesion may be appropriate.

Management of minor changes (CIN1) is controversial. Low-grade changes can be treated immediately or kept under surveillance by a combination of cytology and colposcopy. It is likely that a significant proportion may regress. Unfortunately, we are as yet unable to identify those patients whose CIN is likely to progress. It is possible that HPV testing may identify those patients in whom progression of CIN might be more likely to occur, and hence identify those to treat rather than observe. Prospective randomized trials are required to validate this possibility.

Follow-up

All patients treated for CIN require follow-up. Routinely, all patients should have two cervical smears within the first year and then annual smears for at least 5 years. Thereafter 3-yearly smears may be appropriate. It is recommended that patients treated by hysterectomy without vaginal extension of their intraepithelial neoplasia should have a vaginal vault smear at 6 and 12 months. They may then discontinue follow-up. If the histological report of the removed cervical tissue suggests incomplete excision or that there has been a wide lesion extending beyond the cervix, follow-up by colposcopy and smears is indicated.

Special situations

Pregnancy. Abnormal cervical smears in pregnancy may be assessed by colposcopy to rule out an invasive lesion. Although the gravid cervix is more vascular, directed biopsies can be performed. If CIN is confirmed serial colposcopic examinations can be performed and treatment undertaken postpartum. Pregnancy does not appear to cause abnormal progression.

Immunosuppression. Women who are immunosuppressed such as those on immunosuppressive agents following organ transplant or those with autoimmune diseases have an increased incidence of lower genital tract dysplasia. An annual cervical smear with colposcopic surveillance if the smear is abnormal is recommended.

Cervical glandular intraepithelial neoplasia (CGIN)

There is probably a continuum of glandular change ranging from normality to adenocarcinoma *in situ* (AIS). Histological diagnosis of AIS is based on changes suggesting malignancy without evidence of penetration of the basement membrane. It is recognized in the mucin-secreting columnar epithelium by: stratification of the epithelial cells; loss of nuclear polarity; loss of mucin-secreting capacity; an increase in the nucleocytoplasmic ratios; cellular pleomorphism and nuclear hyperchromatism; and the presence of numerous, sometimes atypical mitoses. Because of the difficulties of distinguishing glandular abnormalities it has been suggested that the spectrum is divided into two grades, low- and high-grade CGIN or glandular atypia and AIS.

Colposcopy should be undertaken in all cases of glandular anomalies noted on cervical smear. A squamous lesion may be identified in the absence of other anomaly.

 If the smear shows high-grade anomalies a cone biopsy with uterine curettage should be performed.
  —AIS may be multifocal. Even if the surgical margins of the cone biopsy are clear of abnormal epithelium, follow-up with careful sampling with an endocervical brush is essential.

Chapter 85

Malignant disease of the cervix

Carcinoma of the cervix is the second most common female cancer worldwid In England and Wales it constitutes around 4% of female malignancies. In th UK the annual incidence is 9.5/100 000. The overall incidence of the cervic cancer and death rate (approximately 3.1/100 000 per annum) from it hav declined recently due to aggressive screening programmes.

Aetiology

Sexual activity has been correlated with the disease, especially age at first inter course and number of sexual partners. Cancer of the cervix is four times a frequent in prostitutes as in other women. A strong link between smoking an cervical cancer has been noted. Smoking reduces the number of Langerhan cells, which are involved in local immune surveillance. Human papillomaviru (HPV) types 16, 18, and 33 are associated with invasive tumours. HPV 16 and 1 produce E6 and E7 proteins, which alter normal cell function by forming com plexes with cell proteins involved in cell cycle regulation. Other factors associ ated with the disease include immunocompromised host, oral contraceptiv use, and a high-risk male sexual partner.

Pathogenesis

The columnar epithelium of the uterine cervix meets the stratified squamou epithelium of the vagina and cervix at the squamo-columnar junction (trans formation zone). Most of the cases of pre-invasive and invasive disease occur a this site. Most of the cervical cancers probably begin as dysplastic changes wit gradual progression over a period of several years. Cervical cancers sprea mainly by direct local invasion and by the lymphatics and blood vessels in ver advanced cases. Lymphatic spread occurs via parametrial lymphatics to th internal and external iliac nodes and from there to lymph plexuses surroundin aorta and vena cava. Blood-borne spread to distant organs is noted in advance cases. The age distribution of the tumour shows a bimodal type with peaks a 35–44 years and 75–85 years.

Pathology

Most of the cervical tumours are squamous (70%), and adenocarcinoma an adenosquamous carcinoma, in roughly equal proportions, form about 25% The rest involves rarer types such as small cell, transitional cell, lymphomas, an sarcomas.

FIGO[1] has dropped the term 'early stromal invasion' and uses the term microinvasive and invasive carcinoma of cervix (detailed in Table 85.1).

Table 85.1 Staging of cervical carcinoma[1]

Stage	Features
0	Pre-invasive carcinoma (carcinoma *in situ*, CIN).
I	Carcinoma confined to cervix (extension to the corpus should be disregarded)
Ia	Invasive cancer identified only microscopically. All gross lesions even with superficial invasion are stage Ib cancers. Measured stromal depth should not be more than 5 mm and no wider than 7 mm*
Ia1	Measured invasion no greater than 3 mm in depth and no wider than 7 mm
Ia2	Measured depth of invasion greater than 3 mm and no greater than 5 mm and no wider than 7 mm
Ib	Clinical lesions confined to cervix or preclincal leisons greater than Ia
Ib1	Clinical lesions < 4 cm in diameter
Ib2	Clinical lesions > 4 cm in diameter
II	Carcinoma extending beyond the cervix but not on to the pelvic wall. The carcinoma involves the vagina but not as far as the lower third
IIa	No obvious parametrial involvement
IIb	Obvious parametrial involvement
III	The carcinoma has extended on to the pelvic wall. On rectal examination there is no cancer-free space between the tumour and the pelvic wall. The tumour involves the lower third of vagina. All cases with hydronephrosis or non-functioning kidney should be included unless they are known to be due to another cause
IIIa	No extension to pelvic wall but involvement of lower third of vagina
IIIb	Extension to the pelvic wall or hydronephrosis or non-functioning kidney
IV	The carcinoma has extended beyond the true pelvis or has clinically involved the mucosa of the bladder or rectum
IVa	Spread of the growth to adjacent organs
IVb	Spread to distant organs

*The depth of invasion should not be more than 5 mm from the base of the epithelium, either surface or glandular, from which it originates. Vascular space involvement, either venous or lymphatic, should not alter the staging.

Clinical features

- The common presenting features are postcoital bleeding, foul-smelling blood-stained discharge, postmenopausal bleeding, and irregular vaginal bleeding. In abnormal bleeding in pregnancy cervical pathology needs to be ruled out.
- In very early cases the disease may be asymptomatic and detected by abnormal cervical cytology.
- Late cases present with pelvic/leg pain, backache, haematuria, oedema of the lower legs, malaise, and weight loss.
- Invasion of the parametrium may involve the ureters leading to ureteric obstruction and renal failure.
- Bone and nerve involvement causes severe pain. Involvement of the lymphatics causes intractable oedema of the legs.
- Involvement of the bladder causes dysuria, frequency, and haematuria.
- Involvement of the bowels causes tenesmus, diarrhoea, and rectal bleeding.
- Fistula formation may occur between the bladder or bowel and the vagina.
- Death occurs from uraemia following ureteric obstruction or from haemorrhage and sepsis.

Examinations and investigations

Physical examination includes checking the supraclavicular glands, inguinal glands, and palpation of the abdomen to detect any organomegaly (liver/kidney). In early cases colposcopic examination is required to visualize suspicious features such as atypical vessels, intense acetowhiteness, and/or raised/ulcerated surfaces. Diagnosis is based on histology. Sufficient material for histological assessment should be obtained by cone/wedge biopsy. Bimanual examination may reveal a hard, irregular, friable cervix. The cervix becomes fixed as tumour invades the parametrium. Per rectal examination has to be done to assess parametrial and posterior spread. The tumour may grow within the endocervix producing barrel-shaped, cylindrical enlargement of the cervix.

Routine examination includes full blood count (FBC), urea and electrolytes (U&Es), liver function tests, chest X-ray, and intravenous urogram.

Examination under anaesthesia including per rectal examination should be done for proper staging. Cystoscopy and proctoscopy/sigmoidoscopy should be done in cases that are suspected to have locally advanced. In selected cases lymphangiography may be needed. In all cases diagnosis is established histologically by biopsy of the tumour.

703

Treatment

Microinvasive disease

For stage Ia1 diseases local excisions by cone biopsy may be done, especially in young women who want to preserve fertility. In older women who have completed their family a total hysterectomy is performed. Treatment of stage Ia2 with marked lymphatic space involvement includes radical hysterectomy or hysterectomy with lympadenectomy or hysterectomy with radiotherapy.

Invasive disease

Treatment of invasive disease involves surgery or radiotherapy or a combination of both. Surgery is preferred in younger patients with stage Ib with low volume tumours as it allows conservation of ovaries, fewer bowel and bladder problems than with radiotherapy, and preservation of a more normal vagina. Radiotherapy is used for bulky stage Ib, IIa, and advanced cases and also in older and surgically unfit patients.

- *Surgery.* Radical hysterectomy and pelvic node dissection (Wertheim's hysterectomy) include removal of the uterus, upper third of the vagina, and internal and external iliac and obturator lymph nodes. In older women, bilateral salpingo-oophorectomy is done, but the ovaries may be conserved and may be placed outside the field of radiotherapy should it be needed. Complications include haemorrhage, infection, damage to urinary or intestinal tracts, and, postoperatively, pulmonary embolism, atonic bladder, and fistula of the urinary tract.

- *Radiotherapy* is given by intracavity and external beam irradiation. Intracavity irradiation gives effective treatment to the cervix and surrounding tissues and external beam irradiation is used to control spread within the pelvis especially to lymph nodes. Complications of radiotherapy include diarrhoea, colicky abdominal pain, and urinary symptoms. Late complications include subacute obstruction, diarrhoea due to radiation colitis, haematuria due to radiation cystitis, and, rarely, vesicovaginal fistula.

- *Chemotherapy* as single-agent (cisplatin, bleomycin, methotrexate) and combination regimens with either radiotherapy or surgery has been used. The use of neoadjuvant chemotherapy and radiotherapy has not resulted in improved survival.

- *Combination of surgery and radiotherapy.* Postoperative radiotherapy is considered if multiple lymph nodes are involved or the resection margin was inadequate or in cases of large tumour volume. This reduces the incidence of pelvic recurrence. Preoperative intracavity radiotherapy followed by surgery has not shown improved survival.

85 Malignant disease of the cervix

Special cases

The management of cancer of cervix in pregnancy depends on the stage of the disease, gestational age, and the patient's wishes. Before 24 weeks, treatment is the same as that for non-pregnant women and after that treatment may be delayed to allow fetal maturity. Treatment of carcinoma of the cervix after simple hysterectomy depends on the stage. Usually pelvic irradiation followed by vault irradiation is given. Alternatively, the parametrium, upper vagina, and pelvic lymph nodes are removed surgically.

Treatment of cancer of cervix in cervical stump is by radiotherapy. Recurrent cervical cancer following surgery is managed by radiotherapy. In postradiation failures or in local recurrence involving bladder or rectum, pelvic exenteration is offered to suitable surgical candidates.

New procedures such as radical trachylectomy (removing cervix and paracervical tissue) after a meticulous lymph node dissection are being evaluated. This procedure is for women with early ectocervical disease so that they have a chance to have children.

Results of treatment

The overall 5-year survival rate in stage Ib following surgery is around 82%. In good radiotherapy centres the figures are stage I (80%), stage II (61%), stage III (32%), and stage IV (15%).

Follow-up

All patients need follow-up for reassurance, symptomatic relief, psychosexual counselling, hormone replacement therapy in younger patients, evaluation of treatment, and early detection of recurrence.

Reference

FIGO (International Federation of Gynecology and Obstetrics) (1994). *FIGO annual report on the results of treatment in gynecologic cancer*, Vol. 24. FIGO, London.

Ovarian cancer

There is an incidence of 18.7 per 100 000 women or 6000 new cases per year ▮ England and Wales. There is a 1.3% risk of developing the disease by the age ▮ 74. Ovarian carcinoma is the fifth most common cause of cancer in women in ▮ UK but the fourth most common cause of death from cancer. It is rare under ▮ age of 30. The incidence increases with age but reaches a plateau of 60 per 100 ◖ women per year after the age of 65. About 6% of all ovarian cysts are maligna▮

Aetiology

Of cases of ovarian cancer, 1% occur in women with a family history of two ▮ more affected first-degree relatives (mother or sister). In most of these famil▮ a predisposition to breast and ovarian cancer is inherited in an autosomal do▮ inant manner by an abnormal tumour suppressor gene (*BRCA1*) located ▮ chromosome 17. Carriers of the abnormal gene have up to a 70% risk of dev▮ oping cancer. Other family members can be tested once the site of the def▮ has been determined. Women with a single affected relative have a 2–3-f▮ increased risk. The majority of cases are sporadic and the cause unknown. T▮ relative risk of epithelial tumours is increased in nulliparous women, infertil▮ late menopause, and early menarche. There may be an increased risk after tre▮ ment for infertility using drugs to induce ovulation if pregnancy does not occ▮ The risk is reduced by use of the combined oral contraceptive pill (up to 60%▮ and having children (up to 40%). Abnormal ovarian development, such as t▮ streak gonads seen in Turner's syndrome, is associated with an increased risk▮ dysgerminomas.

Pathology

Epithelial tumours

Epithelial ovarian cancer (EOC) accounts for 85% of all ovarian cancers. T▮ tumours may be undifferentiated or lined by epithelium that resembles th▮ seen elsewhere in the female genitourinary tract. The most common types a▮ the following.

- *Serous cystadenocarcinomas* (40%) are usually unilocular cysts containing serous fluid lined by ciliated columnar epithelium in papillary fronds, wit▮ solid areas. They are bilateral in 30% of cases.
- *Mucinous cystadenocarciomas* (10%) are more often multilocular, mucin-fille▮ and lined by columnar glandular cells. They are associated with tumours of the appendix and gall bladder. Rupture of a mucinous cyst may disseminate mucin-secreting cells leading to a build up of mucinous fluid in the abdome▮ (pseudomyxoma peritonei) requiring interval laparotomy to clear.
- *Endometrioid cystadenocarcinomas* (20%) resemble endometrial adenocarcinoma (associated in 15% of cases).
- *Clear cell* (*mesonephroid*) *cystadenocarcinomas* (5%) are thin-walled, unilocular tumours with cells characterized by clear cytoplasm. These are the most common tumours found in association with endometriosis.
- *Borderline tumours or tumours of low malignant potential* comprise 10% of EOC and can occur in any of the above epithelial types, although mucinou▮ borderline tumours are the most common. They are characterized by cellular atypia with increased mitosis and multilayering without invasion. The prognosis is much better than that for invasive carcinomas although late recurrence (> 10 years) may occur.

ther tumours

Sex-cord stromal tumours (6%) are usually of low-grade malignancy.
—They include granulosa cell tumours, the most common oestrogen-
producing tumours (menstrual problems, postmenopausal bleeding,
precocious puberty), and Sertoli–Leydig cell tumours, the most common
androgen-producing lesions (amenorrhoea, hirsutism, virilization).

Fibromas are solid fibrous tissue tumours that may be associated with
pleural effusions (Meig's syndrome) and ascites but are benign.

Germ cell tumours (2–3%). Teratomas contain multiple tissue types
including hair, teeth, and skin. Mature cystic teratomas or dermoid cysts
are more common and benign. Teratomas may be hormonally active
(human chorionic gonadotrophin (hCG), α-fetoprotein (AFP), thyroxine).
Immature teratomas are solid, malignant, unilateral, and heterogeneous.
The, prognosis depends on the amount of embryonal tissue present and
degrees of atypia. Other malignant tumours are rare and include:
dysgerminomas, solid, nodular tumours similar to seminomas of the testis;
ectodermal sinus tumours (yolk sac tumours), which may produce AFP;
and non-gestational choriocarcinomas, which secrete hCG. They usually
occur in women under 30.

Secondary tumours comprise 6% of presentations. The most common
primary sites are breast, stomach (Krukenberg), and colon.

Presentation

Ovarian carcinoma commonly remains asymptomatic until late in the course of the disease and is detected as a mass on pelvic examination. Where symptoms do occur these are due to distension, torsion or bleeding (causing pain), pressure effects on adjacent structures, and hormone effects (postmenopausal bleeding, virilization). The staging of ovarian cancer is given in Table 86.1.

Screening and diagnosis

Pelvic examination is of no proven value as a method of screening for ovarian carcinoma. Transvaginal ultrasound with or without tumour marker measurement (CA 125) can be used to detect early-stage asymptomatic disease. However, the value of routine screening in reducing mortality from ovarian carcinoma remains unproven.

Diagnosis is on the basis of the clinical findings of a solid or cystic mass arising from the pelvis. The uterus is felt separately. There may be associated ascites. Arrange an ultrasound to exclude other causes of pelvic mass such as fibroids and to look for suspicious features such as solid areas within the cyst or free fluid. A chest X-ray should be done to look for pleural effusions. Computerized tomography (CT) or magnetic resonance imaging (MRI) scans may give an indication of spread but will not usually alter management. Ovarian carcinoma is associated with increased serum levels of a number of oncofetal proteins of which CA125 is the most important. However, 15% of epithelial ovarian cancer (EOC) will have normal levels. Blood should be taken for tumour markers, full blood count, liver function tests, and electrolytes.

Table 86.1 Staging of ovarian cancer

Stage	Description
	Disease confined to the ovaries (25% of presentations)
Ia	Involving only one ovary
Ib	Involving both ovaries
Ic	Positive cytology or ascites or breaching the capsule of either ovary
I	Confined to pelvis (5–10% presentations)
II	Confined to peritoneal cavity (45% presentations)
IIIa	Micronodular disease outside the pelvis
IIIb	Macroscopic tumour deposits < 2 cm
IIIc	Tumour > 2 cm or retroperitoneal node involvement
IV	Distant metastases (20% of presentations)

Management

Patients with suspected ovarian cancer should be managed where possible in specialist gynaecolgical cancer centre.

- *Surgery* is the primary method of treatment as well as the method of obtaining histological confirmation of the diagnosis and staging the disease. A laparotomy is performed through a midline incision with careful inspection of the liver and peritoneal surfaces. Washings from the peritoneal cavity or any ascites are sent for cytology. Where possible a total abdominal hysterectomy and bilateral salpingo-oophorectomy and infracolic omentectomy are performed. The aim is to remove all macroscopic disease if possible, as this outcome is associated with a better prognosis. If this is not possible the aim should be to remove as much tumour more than 2 cm in size, as possible. The retroperitoneal lymph nodes are biopsied in women with clinically less than stage IIIc disease. This is controversial, but is performed because up to 20% of clinically 'stage I + II' disease will have positive nodes.

- *Chemotherapy* is given to all patients after surgery including now those with stage I tumours. The overall response rate is 70–80%. Chemotherapy has improved median survival but has had minimal effect on overall mortality rates from the disease. Platinum-based drugs (cisplatin/carboplatin; 50–100 mg/m^2) give the highest response rates. Addition of other agents in primary chemotherapy does not appear to give better results although it does increase morbidity. Treatment is given at 3–4 weekly intervals for 6 months (but stop if no response after 3 months). Side-effects are nausea, bone marrow suppression, neurotoxicity, renal toxicity (with cisplatin to reduce risks, prehydrate), and neuropathy. Carboplatin is less toxic and is less likely to require hospital admission. Leucopenia and thrombocytopenia are the dose-limiting side-effects. Further details can be found in Chapter 90.

- Radiotherapy is used in some centres (more outside of the UK).

Follow-up/recurrence

The routine use of second look operations does not improve survival. Follow up is usually for 5 years at 3–12-monthly intervals. A rising serum CA 125 has high predictive value for recurrence with a 3–6 month lead-time over clinical signs. CT/ultrasound scanning is of value in assessing response to treatment and identifying localized recurrence. The prognosis for recurrent disease is poor although it is more likely to respond to further chemotherapy if it occurs more than 3 years after original diagnosis or if previous treatment didn't use platinum. Better response rates in recurrent disease may be obtained with other drugs such as paclitaxel. Surgery may be palliative for obstruction or isolated recurrences.

Prognosis

Prognosis depends on stage, differentiation, residual tumour bulk, and chemosensitivity. The 5-year survival for EOC is 30–35% overall with 67% for stage I disease, 51% for stage IIa, 20% for stage III, and 5% for stage IV. The overall survival for germ cell tumours is 77%.

Endometrial cancer

Endometrial cancer, or cancer of the body of the uterus, is the second most common gynaecological cancer in the UK (14.3/100 000 cases pa). The incidence of endometrial cancer worldwide is on the increase, which reflects the impact of the age structure of the Western population being 4–5 times more common in Western industrialized countries compared to developing countries of Southeast Asia. Furthermore, the reduction in the incidence of cervical cancer has also contributed to the prominence of endometrial cancer. Endometrial cancer is predominantly a disease of postmenopausal women, most cases occurring in the sixth and seventh decades, with less than 5% of cases in women under 40 years of age. The lifetime risk of developing endometrial cancer is 1.1%, while the lifetime risk of dying of endometrial cancer is 0.4%, reflecting the good prognosis of the condition with early diagnosis.

Risk factors

- *Age.* This is principally a disease of postmenopausal women with peak incidence in the age group 65–75 years, with less than 5% of cases occurring in women under 40 years of age.
- *Excessive endogenous oestrogens.* This is the common pathway shared by most of the common risk factors such as early menarche (before age 12), late menopause (after age 52), obesity, nulliparity, and/or continuous anovulation associated with polycystic ovarian disease.
  —An important source of extraovarian oestrogens in postmenopausal women is the aromatization of adrenal androgens in fat tissue. Thus it is not surprising that endometrial cancer is more common in obese postmenopausal women.
  —A rare sex cord stromal tumour of the ovary, a granulosa-theca cell tumour, also produces endogenous oestrogens and is associated with endometrial hyperplasia and endometrial carcinoma in 10% of cases.
  —There may also be an increased risk in women with cirrhosis of the liver due to decreased degradation of oestrogens.
  —Endometrial hyperplasia, excessive proliferation of the endometrial glands and to a lesser extent of the endometrial stroma, is thought to be due to excessive endometrial oestrogen stimulation. The severity of endometrial hyperplasia is divided into simple, complex, or atypical and may progress to well differentiated endometrial carcinoma. The risks associated with simple and complex hyperplasia are in the region of 1–3%, while hyperplasia with cytological and architectural atypia is associated with a 23% risk of endometrial carcinoma over 10 years.
- *Unopposed oestrogen therapy* in postmenopausal women increases the risk of endometrial carcinoma 6–8-fold as observed in the 1970s in the USA. The addition of 10–14 days of progestogens significantly reduced this risk.
- *Tamoxifen* is an anti-oestrogen widely used in the treatment of postmenopausal breast cancer but it also has weak oestrogenic action on the genital tract. It is associated with a twofold increase in the risk of endometrial cancer when used for 5 years or more. It is also associated with increased risks of developing other benign endometrial changes such as hyperplasia and polyps.
- *Miscellaneous.* There appears to be a higher risk of endometrial cancer in women with breast, ovarian (endometrium type), and colorectal cancers.

Presentation

- The most common presenting symptom of endometrial cancer is postmenopausal bleeding.
- Endometrial cancer may also present with postmenopausal vaginal discharge or pyometra.
- Endometrial cancer should also be excluded in peri- or premenopausal women with persistent intermenstrual bleeding or polymenorrhoea especially if the latter fails to respond to hormonal treatments.
- It is also important to consider endometrial carcinoma as part of the differential diagnosis of asymptomatic women with glandular abnormalities on routine cervical cytology.
- Over 90% of women with endometrial cancer will present with vaginal bleeding, and 7–10% of women with postmenopausal bleeding may turn out to have the disease.
- Advanced disease may present with symptoms attributable to local and distant metastases or paraneoplastic syndromes.

Pathology

Endometrial carcinomas are predominantly (80–85%) endometrioid adenocarcinomas, which at the well-differentiated end of the spectrum may be difficult to distinguish from complex endometrial hyperplasia. Within adenocarcinomas there may be foci of squamous metaplasia, which, where benign, are known as adenoacanthomas and, where malignant, are referred to as adenosquamous carcinoma.

Approximately 10% of endometrial carcinomas are papillary serous type, and 4% are clear cell carcinomas. Both these subtypes are associated with more aggressive tumours and poorer prognosis and, despite their relative infrequency, account for 50% of treatment failures. They are both similar to tumours found in the ovaries and Fallopian tubes and tend to spread in a fashion akin to that of ovarian cancer.

Spread

Endometrial cancer spreads directly through the endometrial cavity to the cervix and through the Fallopian tubes to the ovaries and peritoneal cavity. The tumour invades and infiltrates the myometrium reaching the serosal surface and parametria. Very rarely, there may be direct invasion of the pubic bones.

Lymphatic spread is to pelvic and para-aortic nodes, the former being more common and, although para-aortic node involvement may occur in the absence of pelvic node involvement, pelvic node involvement when para-aortic nodes are involved is the more likely finding. Inguinal node involvement is a rare finding.

Haematogenous spread is rare, but may occur to the lungs.

Prognostic factors

- *Stage.* The overall survival is affected by stage at diagnosis. Stage I disease is associated with a 72% overall survival dropping to 56%, 32%, and 11% moving up from stages II, III, and IV, respectively. Table 87.1 gives the staging of endometrial cancer.
- *Depth of myometrium invasion.* The depth of myometrial involvement is reflected in the subclassification of stage I disease (see Table 87.1). The depth of myometrial invasion correlates well with pelvic and para-aortic lymph node involvement in early disease. There is also a close correlation between tumour grade and depth of myometrial invasion.
- *Tumour grade.* As tumour grade increases (the tumour becoming less differentiated), the risk of associated myometrial invasion and lymph node involvement increases. Thus, 90% of grade 1 tumours will be limited to the endometrium or inner half of the myometrium, while almost half of the grade 3 tumours will be found invading the outer half of the myometrium. Tumours are graded as follows:
  - —Grade 1. Well differentiated tumours have less than 5% squamous solid growth pattern.
  - —Grade 2. Moderately differentiated tumours have 6–50% solid squamous growth pattern.
  - —Grade 3. Poorly differentiated tumours have > 50% solid squamous growth pattern.

  The presence of nuclear atypia in addition to the growth pattern, raises grade 1 and 2 tumours to the next grade.
- *Histological type.* Endometrioid adenocarcinomas have the best prognosis while clear cell and papillary cell tumours are associated with a poorer prognosis. Over 70% of endometrial cancers are positive for oestrogen and progesterone receptors. Absence of receptors is associated with a poorer prognosis.
- *Lymphovascular space involvement* appears to be an important prognostic factor in terms of survival and disease recurrence for stage I disease.

Investigations

All women with symptoms and signs suggestive of or suspicious of endometrial carcinoma should be investigated. In the past the 'gold standard' was a dilatation and curettage (D&C) to obtain an endometrial sample for histopathological assessment. This has the shortfall that it is performed 'blindly' and therefore randomly samples a proportion of the uterine cavity, potentially missing isolated foci of disease.

- The current gold standard is a combination of visualization of the cavity by hysteroscopy combined with targeted endometrial biopsy either as an out-patient/local anaesthetic procedure or under a general anaesthetic.
- Alternatives to hysteroscopy and directed biopsy include a combination of out-patient endometrial sampling with a pipelle (randomly samples a small proportion of the cavity) in combination with assessment of the uterine cavity by means of a transvaginal ultrasound to assess endometrial thickness, homogeneity, and the presence of fluid or polyps within the cavity as well as presence of ovarian masses. A transvaginal ultrasound indicating a thin midline homogeneous endometrium less than 5 mm in thickness has a high negative predictive value.

- Ultrasound also has a role in assessing the depth of endometrial invasion in cases of confirmed endometrial cancer, but magnetic resonance imaging (MRI) is superior in this respect, as it assesses cervical involvement and metastases to pelvic and paraortic nodes.
- In confirmed cases of endometrial cancer a chest radiograph is essential to exclude pulmonary spread.

Table 87.1 Staging of endometrial cancer

Stage	Description
I	Disease confined to the body of the uterus
Ia	Carcinoma confined to the endometrium
Ib	Myometrial invasion < 50%
Ic	Myometrial invasion > 50%
II	Cervix involved
IIa	Endocervical gland involvement only
IIb	Cervical stromal invasion but does not extend beyond the uterus
III	Spread to serosa of uterus, peritoneal cavity, or lymph nodes
IIIa	Carcinoma involving serosa of uterus or adnexae, positive ascites, or positive peritoneal washings
IIIb	Vaginal involvement either direct or metastatic
IIIc	Para-aortic or pelvic node involvement
IV	Local or distant metastases
IVa	Carcinoma involving the mucosa of the bladder or rectum
IVb	Distant metastases and involvement of other abdominal or inguinal lymph nodes

Treatment

Surgery
The treatment of choice for patients with early (stages I and II) disease is a total abdominal hysterectomy and bilateral salpingo-oophorectomy (TAH + BSO). The exceptions to this are patients who are medically unfit or a very high surgical risk, in whom radical radiotherapy may be the chosen mode of treatment accepting that the surgery with or without radiotherapy offers a better prognosis than radiotherapy alone. For patients with clinical stage III or IV disease radical radiotherapy with or without hormonal manipulation and/or chemotherapy is the standard mode of therapy. Patients with stage III disease may sometimes be suitable for radical surgery and therefore treatment should be individualized aiming to perform TAH + BSO and maximally debulk the disease followed by radiotherapy.

Routine lymphadenectomy is not performed at the time of TAH + BSO in the UK. This is due to a number of reasons including the fact that the extent of optimum lymph node dissection remains unclear, along with the increase in morbidity that this entails in a generally unfit group of patients. The UK Medical Research Council (MRC) ASTEC trial is currently assessing the morbidity and effectiveness of complete pelvic lymphadenectomy.

Radiotherapy
In practice most patients with early disease get a combination of surgery and radiotherapy after review of any adverse features of the operative and histopathological findings. Patients who are treated by surgery alone are limited to those where the carcinoma is of endometrioid type, confined to less than 50% of the myometrial thickness, and is grade 1 or 2 (well or moderately differentiated). The widely used radiotherapy regime involves a combination of high-dose intracavitary brachytherapy to reduce risk of vault recurrence and 25 fractions of low-dose external beam radiotherapy to reduce the risk of pelvic recurrence. Radiotherapy may also be used in the palliative setting with advanced disease to control vaginal bleeding and bone pain.

Hormone therapy
Progestogens are the most commonly used form of hormonal therapy in endometrial cancer. They have no role in the prevention of recurrence but their main contribution is to the management of recurrent disease with a response rate of up to 30% (higher in oestrogen and progesterone receptor positive tumours) reported using medroxyprogesterone acetate (MPA) in doses of 200–400 mg daily. Other hormonal agents that have been reported to have limited roles in achieving a response include gonadotrophin-releasing hormone (GnRH) analogues and tamoxifen.

Chemotherapy
The use of chemotherapy in endometrial cancer is uncommon but should be considered in fit patients with systemic disease. Drugs with response rates of 25–30% include epirubicin and doxorubicin (anthracyclines) and cisplatin or carboplatin (platinum drugs) either alone or in combination, but their responses are partial and short-lived and their use may be limited by a patient's advanced age and poor performance status.

Prognosis

The 5-year survival rates for endometrial cancer by stage are:

- Stage I, 75%.
- Stage II, 58%.
- Stage III, 30%.
- Stage IV, 10%.

The overall 5-year survival for the disease is around 70% reflecting the fact that the majority of endometrial cancers present early due to abnormal vaginal bleeding.

Chapter 88

Premalignant and malignant diseases of the vulva

Premalignant disease

Premalignant lesions (vulval intraepithelial neoplasia (VIN)) of the vulva are seen more commonly recently. Though also seen in postmenopausal women, about 41% of cases are seen in premenopausal women. It is not clear whether increased detection represents greater awareness of the problem. The vulval skin is part of the anogenital epithelium that extends from the perianal skin and perineum to the cervix. Multiple foci of dysplasia are seen when there are neoplastic changes of the vulval skin. Viral aetiological factors such as human papillomavirus (HPV) are thought to be involved but their role is uncertain at present.

Pathology
The International Society for the Study of Vulvar Diseases have standardized the reporting of vulval dysplastic lesions as VIN1, 2, or 3 depending on the degree of loss of cellular maturation. This has replaced older and more confusing terminology such as Bowen's disease, Bowenoid papulosis, and erythroplasia of Queyrat. Dysplasia of the vulva is multicentric. Vulval dysplasia is usually squamous VIN though very rarely adenocarcinoma *in situ* (Paget's disease) occurs on the vulva. The histological features and terminology of VIN are the same as those of cervical intraepithelial neoplasia (CIN) and the histology of Paget's disease is similar to that of the lesions seen in the breast.

Presenting features
The most common presenting symptom is pruritus. However, VIN may be asymptomatic and detected only during treatment of the pre-invasive/invasive lesions of the cervix/lower genital tract. The lesions may be raised or flat, single or multiple, and diffuse or discrete. They may form papules. The colour is variable, white in cases of hyperkeratinization and red due to thinness of the epithelium or dark brown due to increased melanin deposition in epithelial cells.

Diagnosis
Careful inspection of the local area is needed to identify the full extent of the disease. This is helped by application of 5% acetic acid. The changes may be seen by naked eye but it becomes easier if the colposcope is used. VIN lesions turn white and mosaicism or punctation may be visible. An abnormal vascular pattern is associated with a severe degree of VIN/invasive disease. Toluidine blue is sometimes used as a nuclear stain. As mentioned earlier, due to VIN's developmental origin, a thorough colposcopic evaluation of cervix and upper vagina needs to be done. Frequently, condyloma of the genital tract is associated with these lesions.

Adequate biopsies must be taken from abnormal areas to rule out invasive disease. This can usually be done in an out-patient clinic with Keyes or a 4 mm Stiefel punch biopsy. Microscopic appearances are characterized by cellular disorganization and loss of stratification depending on the grade of the lesion. Cellular changes involve size variability, multinucleated and giant cells, numerous mitotic figures, and hyperchromatinism.

Treatment

The treatment of VIN poses a few problems such as the multifocal nature of the disease and the discomfort and the mutilation from the therapy especially in young patients. However, it must be remembered that VIN 3 may progress to vulvar cancer if not treated. The incidence of unifocal lesions is higher in older women whereas multifocal lesions are commoner in younger women.

- Excision of a small lesion may be diagnostic and therapeutic.
- Multifocal lesions and lesions covering wide areas may need skinning vulvectomy with or without skin grafting or simple vulvectomy.
- Carbon dioxide laser treatment is an alternative to surgical excision but careful control of the depth of destruction is essential for a good cosmetic result. The depth of treatment required in VIN is not clear and hair follicle involvement makes this treatment unsuitable. In some cases treatment of whole vulva to such a depth will cause third-degree burns. Laser treatment is not very popular in the UK.
- The purpose of medical treatment is to relieve the symptoms. If invasion has been excluded, topical fluorodinated steroids are used but not for more than 6 months.
  —Topical 5-fluorouracil (5-FU) therapy is painful and hyperkeratotic lesions do not respond.
  —Topical alpha-interferon therapy has also been tried.

VIN is becoming more common in younger women. Careful observation and treatment should be tailored to suit individual cases.

Follow-up

Recurrence has been noted in both surgical and laser-treated cases and thus follow-up is needed. Regular follow-ups with colposcopy every 6 months are needed until the patient is disease-free for 2 years.

Vulval cancer

Carcinoma of the vulva is a relatively uncommon gynaecological cancer. Its annual incidence is around 3/100 000 women per year. It is common in the elderly with a peak incidence at around 65 and one-third of all patients are more than 70 years old. Of this cancer, 85–90% is squamous and less common lesions are melanoma, basal cell carcinoma, carcinoma of the Bartholin gland, Paget's disease, sarcoma, and metastatic carcinoma.

Not much is known about its aetiology but viral factors have been suggested (HPV 16/18 and herpes simplex virus 2 (HSV2)). However, this cancer has been associated with smoking, immunosuppression, and a history of cervical neoplasia.

Clinical presentation

The most common symptom is longstanding vulval pruritus. Vulval pain, discharge, and bleeding are less frequently reported. Most commonly (66%), the tumour involves the labia majora and in the rest of the cases it involves the clitoris, labia minora, posterior fourchette, and perineum. The lesions may be exophytic, ulcerated, or flat. The incidence of complicating medical disease (diabetes, obesity, hypertension) is greater in the older age group. Younger patients have more chance of having multicentric disease. Frequently, patients delay reporting the symptoms or any abnormality they have seen. Sometimes physicians delay in referring cases. Doing a vulval biopsy in suspected lesions is important for appropriate management.

Route of spread

The tumour spreads by the lymphatic to the regional lymph nodes and locally to involve the adjoining organs (vagina, urethra, anal canal, clitoris, etc.). Blood spread occurs if the tumour involves blood vessels. The lymph drains from the vulva to the superficial inguinal nodes initially and then to the inguinofemoral chain and on to the pelvic nodes. In general, central vulvar structures drain bilaterally whereas lateral structures drain to nodes on the same side. Deep pelvic nodes may be involved from the clitoris and central vulvar structures but involvement of the deep glands in the absence of inguinal node disease is very rare.

Differential diagnosis

Ulcerative lesions on the vulva may be due to sexually transmitted diseases, benign or malignant tumours, or viral infections. Tumours of the vulva are diagnosed by biopsy and excision. The groin nodes may require fine-needle aspiration biopsy or preferably excision biopsy to establish a histological diagnosis. Usually this is done after establishing the diagnosis of the primary lesion.

Assessment and staging

As this tumour is multicentric in nature, a thorough inspection of the cervix, vagina, and adjoining organs should be done. Cervical cytology and chest X-ray are required and at times intravenous pyelography, lymphangiography , ultrasonography (including Doppler studies), and magnetic resonance imaging (MRI) may be used. Examination under anaesthesia including the groin nodes and a full thickness generous biopsy of the primary lesion are the most important diagnostic measures. Cystoscopy and barium-enema may be needed in some cases. Apart from review by an anaesthetist, examination by an internal medicine specialist is required if there are concomitant medical problems. The International Federation of Gynaecologists and Obstetricians (FIGO) staging of vulval cancer is given in Table 88.1.

Table 88.1 FIGO staging of vulval cancer

Stage	Description
0	Carcinoma *in situ*, intraepithelial cancers
I	Tumour confined to vulva or perineum or both. 2 cm or less in greatest diameter (no nodal metastasis)
Ia	Stromal invasion no greater than 1.0 mm
Ib	Stromal invasion greater than 1.0 mm
II	Tumour confined to vulva or perineum or both. More than 2 cm in greatest diameter (no nodal metastasis)
III	Tumour of any size with one or both of the following: (1) adjacent spread to the lower urethra, the vagina, and the anus; (2) unilateral regional lymph node metastasis
IVa	Tumour invading any of the upper urethra, bladder mucosa, rectal mucosa, or pelvic bones or bilateral regional node metastasis
IVb	Any distant metastasis including pelvis lymph nodes

Vulval cancer (*continued*)

Prognostic factors

The main prognostic factor is the condition of the inguinofemoral nodes. Five-year survival declines with positive nodes (from 90% in node-negative to 58% in node-positive cases). Other factors include depth of invasion, tumour diameter, tumour differentiation, lymph–vascular space involvement, margin status, and the number of nodes involved.

Treatment

- *Surgery* is the primary treatment of cancer of vulva. The principle is wide excision (healthy margin) of the tumour and extirpation of the potential route of spread (radical vulvectomy and regional lymphadenectomy). This involves a large area of skin. Modifications to this include doing simple vulvectomy and vertical groin incision to reduce morbidity rather than butterfly incisions where lymph-bearing tissues and vulva are removed in continuity.
  —Regional lymphadenectomy involves bilateral superficial and deep inguinal lymph nodes.
  —Ipsilateral lymphadenectomy may be considered in a relatively small lesion in the midportion of the labia and when all nodes examined are negative.
  —If superficial lymphadenectomy of inguinal nodes is negative by thorough sampling, deep inguinal lymphadenectomy may be avoided to reduce the morbidity of the operation.
  —However, cases must be selected very thoroughly whenever modifications to radical vulvectomy and regional lymphadenectomy are made as reports of recurrence with devastating results have been noted.
- *Radiotherapy.* Improvements in radiotherapy technique with the use of megavoltage external beam therapy and the judicious use of electrons and brachytherapy have now resulted in its use in vulval cancer. Radiotherapy has been used preoperatively when the tumour is large and in advanced cases where the tumour involves or is very close to the vagina, urethra, or anus. Postoperatively, it is used for groin node diseases after inguinofemoral lymphadenectomy and to prevent vulval local recurrence in cases with insufficient tumour-free margin.
- *Chemotherapy.* 5-FU and mitomycin-C have produced encouraging results. They are used as radio-sensitizers.

Morbidities

The most frequent complication of radical surgical treatment is wound breakdown (50%). Other complications include lymphoedema of the lower extremities, lymphocyst formation in the groin, development of rectocele and cystocele due to lack of support, and loss of body image and impaired sexual functions.

Recurrent disease

The outcome of recurrent disease is poor. Treatment is usually palliative in the form of radiotherapy or combined with chemotherapy. In selected cases surgical excision of the recurrence can be done. Single-agent as well as combined therapy has also been used.

Follow-up

All patients need follow-up though prognosis depends on the adverse prognostic factors present in the case. A 5-year survival of 75% should be expected after surgical treatment of invasive squamous cancer. Five-year survival rates are as follows: stage I, 97%; stage II, 85%; stage III, 74%; and stage IV, 30%.

Paget's disease of the vulva

Paget's disease of the vulva is of apocrine origin and is confined to the epithelium in most cases. Invasive disease is present in 15–25% of cases either as underlying apocrine gland adenocarcinoma or breach of the basement membrane. It is not a common tumour. Pruritus is the presenting complaint. Velvety-red discoloration with development of eczemoid changes and white plaques is usually seen. Diagnosis is made by biopsy and histology shows large pale cells, often in nests, infiltrating upward in the hyperkeratotic epithelium. It occurs with other malignancies (15–25%) and the most common organs involved are breast, genitalia, and underlying adnexa. Treatment involves wide local excision in intraepithelial cases, but in invasive cases radical surgery like that for squamous cell carcinoma is needed.

Other tumours of the vulva

The other vulval tumours include melanoma, basal cell carcinoma, Bartholin gland carcinoma, verrucous carcinoma, Merkel cell cancer, and, very rarely, sarcoma and metastatic tumours. The mainstay of the treatment is wide local excision and lymphadenectomy depending on the type of the cancer. Bartholin gland tumours are radiosensitive. Sarcomas are treated by vulvectomy and groin node dissection.

Conclusion

Vulval cancers are more common in elderly people. Surgery is the cornerstone of the treatment and efforts are made to reduce the morbidity from surgery and to improve the modalities of chemo/radiotherapy.

Chapter 89

Vulval pain and pruritus

The moist hair-bearing and delicate skin of the vulva is vulnerable to many non-specific microbe-induced inflammations and dermatological disorders. The vulva has a rich somatic nerve supply and responds to acute stimuli, which are well perceived with exquisite sensitivity. The sensations experienced vary from the pain of trauma to the itching and irritation due to inflammatory or infective causes. The majority of women presenting with vulval symptoms will complain of pruritus but a significant number will complain of burning pain of the vulva or rawness. Often no obvious cause is demonstrated and this can be a perplexing problem for both the patient and clinician.

Causes of vulval pain

- Infection.
- Dermatoses (discussed below under the heading 'Causes of pruritus').
- Vulvodynia.
- Urinary tract disorders.
- Malignant disease.

Infections
Herpes simplex virus
The primary attack usually presents with an extremely painful vulval ulceration together with generalized malaise, fever, and often inguinal lymphadenopathy. Intact vesicles may be visible. Recurrences are not uncommon and can be of variable severity. Sometimes the patient only complains of mild vulval itching and soreness that is dismissed and treated as thrush, particularly if the primary attack was missed. An acute attack should be treated with oral and topical acyclovir (oral dose of 200 mg 5 times daily for 5 days). Acyclovir may be used on a long-term basis to prevent recurrences.

Other causes
Other causes such as candidiasis, syphillis, gonococcal vulvovaginitis, tropical infections such as lymphogranuloma venereum caused by certain subtypes of *Chlamydia trachomatis*, and chancroid caused by *Haemophilus ducreyi* can all give rise to vulval ulceration and pain (see Chapter 64).

Vulvodynia
Vulvodynia is a syndrome of unexplained vulval pain often coupled with sexual dysfunction and psychological disability. The pain is often described by the patient as a burning, stinging irritation and/or rawness. The pain characteristically occurs in response to stretching or pressure. The following types or subsets of vulvodynia can occur alone, simultaneously, or sequentially.

Cyclic vulvodynia
Vulval symptoms that recur in association with menstruation or coitus may be due to changes in vaginal pH. This creates an environment susceptible to infection, e.g. candidosis, bacterial vaginosis, or genital herpes. The clinical features are vulval itching and soreness that is sometimes cyclical, being worse in the luteal phase. Sexual intercourse may be uncomfortable at this time or may be associated with pain on the following day. Diagnosis is confirmed by the finding of fungal hyphae. Treatment is usually local clotrimazole or econazole pessary and/or topical application of 2% clotrimazole cream.

Vestibular papillomatosis

Vulvar squamous papillomatosis describes the appearance of multiple tiny filamentous papillae occurring on the vulva in women of all ages. They are usually found in the vestibule and posterior aspect of the introitus but sometimes cover the entire surface of the labia minora. This is now considered to be a variation of the normal and of uncertain clinical significance. Most of the women with vulval papillae are asymptomatic. Symptomatic women may require colposcopy to exclude other lesions. They do not themselves require treatment and, in fact, treatment with laser or 5-fluorouracil has sometimes led to a new set of painful symptoms.

Vulvar vestibulitis

The criteria for diagnosis are:
- Pain on entry or touch.
- Vestibular erythema.
- Tenderness on pressure.

This triad of dyspareunia, erythema, and tenderness to touch restricted to the vestibule distinguishes vulvar vestibulitis from vulvitis. Dyspareunia can be a minor nuisance or completely prevent sexual intercourse. The pain experienced by the patient is described as severe burning, whereas itching is not usually present.

The aetiology of vulvar vestibulitis remains uncertain. Postulated causes or triggering events include infection (*Candida* in particular), bacterial vaginosis, chlamydial infection, excess urinary oxalate, human papillomavirus (HPV) infection, hypersensitivity reactions, and psychosexual problems. Vulvar vestibulitis is uncommon in the Afro-Caribbean population and is mostly found in Caucasian women aged 30–60 years.

733

Management depends to some extent upon its severity as many minor cases clear up spontaneously.
- Acute vestibulitis causing sufficient symptoms may be treated medically with the removal of allergen or irritant, the treatment of infection, and local corticosteroid application.
- The chronic condition is more difficult to resolve. Treatment with a topical steroid preparation containing antifungals and antibacterials (Trimovate) may relieve symptoms.
- Dyspareunia may respond to the use of a local anaesthetic gel, e.g 5% lignocaine applied 15–30 minutes before intercourse. Surgical excision of the vestibule should be considered as the last resort for patients with significant dyspareunia. However, the results of vestibulectomy are variable and it is not without complications.

Causes of vulval pain (*continued*)

Essential vulvodynia

This is characterized by a constant diffuse, unremitting burning that may extend into the thigh or buttock. Patients are usually peri- or postmenopausal and have no consistent history of previous trauma or infection. There is no cyclical pattern to the pain and both dyspareunia and point tenderness are less marked than with vulvar vestibulitis. Essential vulvodynia is of unknown aetiology; but is believed to be an altered perception of cutaneous pain rather like postherpetic neuralgia. There are no physical findings as the problem is essentially neural. Treatment is with tricyclic antidepressants such as amitryptyline 10 mg at night increasing to 50 mg.

Idiopathic vulvodynia

There will be some patients who do not fulfil any of the diagnostic criteria discussed. There may be underlying psychological problems and psychiatric assessment will provide patients with appropriate support and insight. Even reassurance about the normality of the anatomy can be therapeutic to some women.

Urinary tract disorders

Urological disorders, such as urethral mucosa prolapse; urethral syndrome, urethral caruncle, and urogenital sinus syndrome, can give rise to vulval pain. Close cooperation between the referring doctor, the gynaecologist, and the urologist is required to treat these conditions.

Malignant diseases

Carcinoma of the vulva represents about 3% of all genital tract cancers in women, occurring especially in women over the age of 60. Approximately 90% of these tumours are squamous cell carcinomas. The remainder are adenocarcinomas, melanomas, or basal cell carcinomas. HPV infection may be an aetiological factor. Non-neoplastic epithelial changes, especially lichen sclerosus, can often precede invasive carcinoma of vulva.

Miscellaneous

Musculoskeletal causes of referred pain to the vulva are uncommon. Levator ani myalgia can cause vulval pain and usually responds to nonsteroidal anti-inflammatory drugs (NSAIDs). Nerve entrapment or neuroma may result after an episiotomy or the repair of tears sustained during childbirth. It can present with superficial dyspareunia and vulval pain. Pain may be relieved by injection of 0.5% bupivacaine. Pudendal nerve neuralgia may follow an injury by certain activities such as riding or herplex simplex infection.

Causes of vulval pruritus

Dermatoses

The dermatoses are classified as non-neoplastic epithelial disorders (vulval dystrophies) of the skin and mucosa.

Eczema

Eczema can be considered as synonymous with dermatitis and therefore can have different causes. It may occur elsewhere in the body. Allergic responses to substances such as washing powders, deodorant, or perfume can result in an acutely swollen, well defined area that can be extremely itchy with a burning sensation. Secondary infection can occur giving rise to offensive discharge. Acute moniliasis is the common differential diagnosis. Referral to a dermatologist is advised for patch-testing. Treatment is by removal of the offending agent(s) and symptom control may be achieved by using soothing applications, emollients, or local corticosteroids.

Lichen sclerosus

Lichen sclerosus is one of the skin conditions of the vulva that causes intense itching and inflammation with secondary excoriation. Characteristically the skin is white, thin, and wrinkled and the condition may involve the whole vulva, perineum, and perianal region. Atrophy of the labia minora occurs often associated with labial fusion, clitoral oedema, and introital narrowing. Microscopially the epithelium is thin with disappearance of rete pegs. This is accompanied by superficial hyperkeratosis and dermal fibrosis with scant perivascular, mononuclear infiltrate. It occurs in all age groups, but is most common in postmenopausal women. The pathogenesis is uncertain but autoimmune reaction is suspected. About 1–4% of cases undergo malignant change, so regular follow-up with particular attention to the periclitoral area is essential. Diagnosis is made on the basis of the patient's history, physical signs, and, finally, by biopsy. The treatment is with potent topical steroids initially, reducing to a maintenance regimen with moderately potent steroids.

735

Squamous cell hyperplasia

Previously called hyperplastic dystrophy, this disorder is marked by epithelial thickening and significant surface hyperkeratosis. It presents with itching or vulval pain and appears clinically as an area of leucoplakia. The hyperplastic epithelial changes show no atypia. No increased predisposition to cancer is generally held to be the case but, suspiciously, squamous hyperplasia is often present at the margins of established cancer of the vulva. Treatment is by local application of fluorinated corticosteroids for 4–6 weeks or until symptoms resolve.

Chapter 90

Chemotherapy in gynaecological cancer

Most chemotherapy is given every 3 weeks but some types may be given more or less frequently depending upon the nature of the drugs being used. Side effects are common and potentially serious, but may be prevented by a variety of measures.

Side-effects

- *Leucopenia* and *thrombocytopenia* are common for most regimens and treatment should not be given unless the white cell count is 3.0×10^9/L or more, the absolute neutrophil count is 1.5×10^9/L or more, and the platelet count is 100×10^9/L or more. The nadir count is normally 7–14 days after giving treatment and it is essential to be aware of the possibility of neutropenic sepsis at this time as this is potentially fatal unless treated very rapidly with intravenous (IV) antibiotics. Granulocyte colony-stimulating factor (GCSF) may prevent leucopenia but it is expensive.
- *Nausea and vomiting* are largely things of the past with the use of modern antiemetics, such as ondansetron and granisetron, coupled with high-dose dexamethasone and other more conventional oral antiemetics.
- *Hair loss* is common with many drugs and a wig must be provided for the patient before she loses her hair, which is usually 3 weeks after the start of treatment. Hair grows back in again after 6 months and usually grows back in curly, but may revert to normal after 6 months. Hair loss may be prevented for some drugs by the use of scalp cooling, but this is not effective for doxorubicin and taxol. Cisplatin and carboplatin do not normally give rise to hair loss.
- *Anaemia.* Platinum compounds frequently give rise to anaemia after three or four courses and, if symptomatic, the patient can be transfused. Erythropoietin may be used instead of a blood transfusion but it is expensive.
- *Renal toxicity* is a potential problem with cisplatin but may be minimized by before and during therapy hydration and by ensuring an adequate urine flow of at least 100 mL/hour whilst having treatment and for a minimum of 4 hours afterwards. Mannitol may be used to produce this diuresis. Extreme caution should be used if frusemide is thought necessary. Methotrexate is excreted unchanged in accordance with renal function and the dose must be reduced in patients with poor renal function.
- *Neurotoxicity* is exhibited by those receiving cisplatin and the taxanes, with taxol giving rise to 18% grade 2 or 3 neurotoxicity lasting for up to 2 years. The main effect is peripheral neuropathy, which gives tingling initially in some cases, loss of sensation, and difficulty in walking. Vincristine can also give rise to neurotoxicity and the total dose of vincristine should not exceed 12 mg (1–2 mg/week).
- *Doxorubicin* and to a lesser extent epirubicin can give rise to cardiomyopathy in a high cumulative dose. A total dose of 500 mg/m^2 should not be exceeded. Concurrent use of cyclophosphamide potentiates the cardiomyopathic effect of doxorubicin and in this case a total dose of 450 mg/m^2 of doxorubicin should not be exceeded.
- *Palmar–plantar erythrodysaesthesia* is a side-effect of Caelyx® (pegylated liposomal doxorubicin) and further treatment should not be given until all evidence of this side-effect has gone. Patients should be advised to wear loose clothing to minimize this problem.

Cyclophosphamide and *ifosfamide* can give rise to cystitis due to the breakdown products. In the case of cyclophosphamide this may be prevented by adequate daily fluid intake, but for ifosfamide routine use of mesna is required.

Methotrexate is bound to albumin and only the unbound drug is available for cytotoxic action. Drugs such as sulfonamides and aspirin can increase the dissociation of methotrexate from its bound form and hence increase its toxicity. Methotrexate also accumulates in ascites and pleural effusions and caution is required in such patients as the effusions and ascites can act as a reservoir for methotrexate giving rise to prolonged exposure. Folinic acid is an effective 'antidote' to methotrexate.

Bleomycin can give rise to lung fibrosis and lung function tests are required in patients receiving this drug. Bleomycin also accumulates in skin and will produce excess sensitivity to sunlight within approximately 30 minutes of being given. More commonly, it will give rise to dark skin markings at pressure areas such as elbows and knuckles and may give rise to permanent black marks where there has been local trauma, e.g. scratching.

Ovarian cancer

Germ cell tumours

Intensive treatment with bleomycin, etoposide, and cisplatin with monitoring
markers in such patients is curative in more than 95% of patients.

Tumours of stromal origin

This very rare subvariant of anaplastic granulosa cell tumour can be cured
approximately two-thirds of patients with the same combination of bleomycin
etoposide, and cisplatin.

Tumours of epithelial origin

Stage I disease

Until recently, there was no evidence that adjuvant chemotherapy was of an
value in these patients after complete removal of all evidence of tumour, but th
International Collaborative Ovarian Neoplasm (ICON) 1 and ACTION tria
have now ceased recruitment and results show a 9% increase in survival with th
use of adjuvant chemotherapy. All such patients should be offered six courses
single-agent carboplatin given at 4-weekly intervals.

Stages II, III, and IV

A combination of doxorubicin, cyclophosphamide, and cisplatin has for mar
years been regarded as standard treatment for these patients, giving six course
at 3-weekly intervals assuming that the patient has adequate renal function wit
a glomerular filtration rate (GFR) of more than 60 mL/minute.

- The ICON 2 trial showed that carboplatin at an AUC (area under the
  curve) of 5 given every 3 weeks is equally effective and is much better
  tolerated particularly by the elderly. Nausea and vomiting are relatively
  easily controlled with carboplatin. Leucopenia and thrombocytopenia can
  be a problem but neutropenic sepsis is rare. Hair loss does not occur, but
  anaemia is common after three or four courses.
- The combination of doxorubicin, cyclophosphamide, and cisplatin
  produces nausea and vomiting which is more difficult to control. Hair loss
  is inevitable and some loss of renal function may occur even with adequate
  hydration. Neutropenic sepsis is much more common than with
  carboplatin.
- With both regimens combined complete and partial response of 70–80% is
  to be expected with approximately 2 years median survival and 25% of
  patients still alive at 5 years.
- The taxanes (taxol and taxotere) are also effective in epithelial ovarian
  cancer and many, particularly in the USA, believe they should be the
  treatment of choice. This is still debatable, but the ICON 3 trial with over
  2000 patients in it has shown no survival advantage for a combination of
  taxol and carboplatin compared with carboplatin alone, this trial being the
  largest ever undertaken in the history of ovarian cancer. Median survival
  was approximately 3 years.

Second-line treatment

The longer the treatment-free interval before recurrence, the more likely it
that the patient will respond to further platinum-based chemotherapy. After
long treatment-free interval responses can be almost as high as with first-lin
treatment. New drugs such as topotecan, gemcitabine, and liposomal doxoru
bicin are all currently being investigated as second-line treatments. The resul
of the recently published ICON 4 trial suggest some improvement in survival a
2 years in women treated with a combination of taxol and platinum.

Other gynaecological cancers

Fallopian tube
This responds to the same treatment as that for epithelial ovarian cancer.

Uterine sarcoma
A recent meta-analysis has shown that patients with poor prognosis sarcoma should receive adjuvant chemotherapy based on doxorubicin, as this will markedly improve their chances of survival. A combination of doxorubicin and ifosfamide is the most commonly used combination.

Carcinoma of the endometrium
Cytotoxic chemotherapy is not commonly used in the UK for this condition, but is more commonly used in other countries. Chemotherapy should only be used in patients with advanced disease that is not amenable to other forms of treatment such as surgery, radiotherapy, and hormonal manipulation. A combination of cyclophosphamide, doxorubicin, and cisplatin can be effective in up to 60% of patients. Carboplatin has also been used and, more recently, taxol is being investigated.

Carcinoma of the cervix
Any chemotherapy should be based on cisplatin and common regimens involve combining one or more of the following drugs with cisplatin: 5-fluorouracil (5-FU), ifosfamide, bleomycin, vindesine, mitomycin-c, vinblastine, methotrexate. In the UK it is common to use a combination of cisplatin and methotrexate with folinic acid rescue given every 2 weeks with studies looking into giving such treatment more frequently. It would seem that, the more frequently the chemotherapy is given in carcinoma of the cervix, the more likely it is to be effective in view of the very rapid turnover of the cells in this condition.

- *Adjuvant chemotherapy* is not established in the management of cervical cancer, but is being investigated in trials at present.
- *Neo-adjuvant chemotherapy* has been used in many trials and a meta-analysis is currently being undertaken by the Medical Research Council (MRC) in the UK looking into all such trials to determine whether this treatment is effective.
- *Concurrent chemotherapy*. Five recent papers in the *New England Journal of Medicine* have indicated that cisplatin-based chemotherapy given at the same time as radiotherapy can markedly increase the cure rate of the radiotherapy and such treatment has become the norm in the past year. There is increased toxicity as a result of giving such treatment concurrently and ideal methods of giving this treatment have yet to be devised.
- *Palliative chemotherapy*. At present chemotherapy is mainly reserved for those with advanced disease that is not amenable to radiotherapy or surgery and where palliation is required.

Carcinoma of the vagina
The chemotherapy regimens used for carcinoma of the cervix can be effective in this situation.

Carcinoma of the vulva

The use of chemotherapy in this elderly population remains controversial. Combinations of CCNU (lomustine), methotrexate, and bleomycin given in small doses over 6 weeks have been shown to shrink tumours sufficiently to make them operable and hence potentially curable, and other drugs such as the taxanes and 5-FU are currently being investigated in this disease. The concurrent use of chemotherapy and radiotherapy for those not amenable to surgery is currently being investigated in trials and such treatment may be used for palliative purposes.

743

Radiotherapy in gynaecological cancer

Radical radiotherapy is given daily 5 days a week lasting a few minutes per day. Once a course of treatment is started, there should not be any breaks at all. Before the patient undergoes treatment she has to go through the planning process which involves measuring her body contour, noting the fields that have to be treated, making appropriate marks on the patient for later setting up, and feeding all of this information into a computer to determine the dose distribution within the treatment volume and adjustment of the various beams to ensure an even distribution of no more than 5% variation throughout the treatment volume. Most patients receiving gynaecological external beam radiotherapy are treated with a 10 MV or higher energy linear accelerator using three or four fields to the pelvis. Standard fields cover from the L5/S1 junction down to the bottom of the obturator fossa and are out laterally to 1 cm outside the pelvic sidewall. Posteriorly, they cover the cervix and part of the adjacent rectum and anteriorly halfway through the pubic bone. Most pelvic gynaecological treatments are within the range 44–50 Gy in 4–5 weeks with or without brachytherapy and/or para-aortic irradiation where the dose does not usually exceed 40 Gy.

Brachytherapy

Brachytherapy in gynaecological cancer involves the placing of applicators either in the vagina or in the uterus or both which allows radioactive sources (usually caesium) to be placed inside these applicators by a remote technique, hence avoiding irradiation to anyone other than the patient. Such treatment is commonly given by a Selectron machine. If intrauterine treatment is required the patient will be anaesthetized in theatre. If vaginal treatment alone is required an anaesthetic is not usually necessary. Various dose schedules exist, but commonly the patient has a single application of brachytherapy which involves staying in hospital for 1, 2, or even 3 nights depending on the dose rate for the particular machine. High dose rate brachytherapy machines are available where the dose is given over a very short period of time and may be repeated on a weekly basis with up to four insertions, depending upon dose schedule. The total dose of irradiation is reduced in patients treated with high dose rate brachytherapy but with the intention that they receive a dose that is radiobiologically equivalent.

Side-effects

These are common to all forms of pelvic radiotherapy. The short-term side-effects normally subside by 6 weeks after completion of radiotherapy. Late side-effects are possible. Lethargy is common to all patients.
- Diarrhoea may occur during the last 7–10 days of treatment, but is easily dealt with using simple medication, such as codeine phosphate.
- Frequency of micturition may also occur in the last 7–10 days and urinary tract infection should be excluded as a cause of this. If it is due to radiation it is not as easy to alleviate this symptom in the short-term.
- Vaginal stenosis will be common to all patients unless they are sexually active, but a suitable stent that should be used for 1 year after completion of treatment eliminates this problem.
- Fistulae in the bladder, rectum, or small bowel are all very rare.
- Skin changes with modern high-energy radiotherapy are very uncommon.

Radiotherapy in ovarian cancer and uterine sarcomas

- There is little place for the use of radiotherapy in ovarian cancer although it was common practice as an adjuvant treatment 20 years ago. The current use of radiotherapy is mainly for palliative treatment of solitary metastases, either in the abdominal wall or in the vaginal vault, with such lesions not responding to chemotherapy and giving rise to symptoms sufficient to warrant radiotherapy.
- There is no evidence to support the routine use of adjuvant radiotherapy after complete surgical removal of uterine sarcoma. Large trials are in progress to assess whether adjuvant radiotherapy has any part to play.

Carcinoma of the endometrium

Adjuvant radiotherapy

In patients with stage I disease such treatment has frequently been used in the past when the patient had disease with a poor prognosis (penetration more than halfway through the myometrium, poorly differentiated tumour, or vascular invasion) but there is no evidence that such treatment is of value. The UK Medical Research Council (MRC) is currently conducting a trial to determine whether such adjuvant radiotherapy is of value in these poor prognosis patients. The trial is also assessing the value or otherwise of pelvic lymphadenectomy in this situation.

If the patient has more than stage I disease but all evidence of tumour has been removed then adjuvant pelvic radiotherapy is conventionally given.

Vaginal vault brachytherapy is widely used in stage I patients with poor prognosis disease to prevent vaginal vault recurrence. Such patients have an approximately 16% chance of vaginal vault recurrence and brachytherapy may reduce this down to 2%, but such treatment has *no* effect on survival.

Primary treatment

Radiotherapy is inferior to surgery in the treatment of stage I endometrial cancer with a cure rate on average of 20% less. Such treatment should therefore only be used when the risks of surgery are very high.

Carcinoma of the cervix

Adjuvant radiotherapy

In patients who have had surgery with radical hysterectomy and node dissection and where the nodes have been found to be involved with tumour, it is standard practice to give adjuvant radiotherapy to the pelvis, but there is no good evidence that such treatment is of value with regard to survival. It is also common practice to use vaginal vault brachytherapy in addition to the external beam therapy.

Primary treatment

Stage I

Treatment with radiotherapy involving external beam radiotherapy and brachytherapy is equally as effective as radical hysterectomy and node dissection in stage I disease. With modern anaesthetics and surgical techniques the tendency is to do more in the way of surgery and reserve radiotherapy for those patients with involved nodes or inadequate excision margins. Patients with poor general health will be treated by radiotherapy alone.

Stage II/III

For those with more advanced disease radiotherapy is the treatment of choice using the doses given above together with intrauterine and intravaginal brachytherapy usually giving a dose of 20 Gy to point A, which is a point 2 cm superior and lateral to the cervix.

Advanced disease

In patients in whom cure is not possible, palliative radiotherapy involving the whole of the pelvis, usually by a two-field anterior and posterior technique giving 30 Gy in a 2-week period, can be very effective in relieving the symptoms of disease such as bleeding. Pain from bone metastases can also be relieved by a single exposure of 8 Gy to the affected area.

Chemo-radiation

Cisplatin-based chemotherapy concurrent with radiotherapy would produce a higher cure rate but more side-effects in patients with carcinoma of the cervix. Trials are currently being devised to determine the ideal combination of these two modalities of treatment.

Carcinoma of the vagina

Treatment is principally by external beam radiotherapy but the fields will come down much lower in the pelvis to ensure that all disease is covered. This may give rise to radiation covering the vulva, which is very sensitive and becomes very sore. Treatment may then be followed by vaginal caesium using an appropriate applicator. In some patients with very localized disease such brachytherapy may be used alone.

Carcinoma of the vulva

Although surgery remains the mainstay of treatment in this condition, many will give adjuvant radiotherapy to the nodal areas if they were involved, although such treatment is still debatable. Studies are currently being devised to look at the place of chemo-radiation as an adjuvant in such patients.

749

For patients with advanced disease radiotherapy can be effective in shrinking the tumour down prior to definitive surgery and long-term survival has been obtained by this method. A short course of radiotherapy can also be effective palliation in patients with recurrent disease.

Palliative care

Palliative care describes a range of care and support provided to meet the needs of patients with progressive illness and their carers. It can be usefully subdivided into general palliative care and specialist palliative care.

- *General palliative care*. This is integral to all areas of clinical practice and aims to promote physical and psychosocial well-being whatever the stage of the disease. Its key principles comprise:
  —Focus on quality of life that includes good symptom control.
  —Whole person approach taking into account the person's past life experiences and current situation.
  —Care that encompasses both the person with the life-threatening disease and those who matter to that person.
  —Respect for patient autonomy and choice (e.g. over place of care, treatment options).
- *Specialist palliative care*. This is provided by a multiprofessional team who have undergone recognized specialist palliative care training. It addresses a level of complexity of problems that cannot be managed solely by health-care professionals providing general palliative care. It may be appropriate at various stages of a patient's illness and in a variety of settings.

Principles of symptom management

Symptoms associated with gynaecological malignancy may be due to:
- The effects of treatment.
- Locally progressive disease.
- Specific metastatic disease.
- General effects of advanced malignancy, e.g. weakness.

The severity of symptoms perceived by patients, particularly those with advancing disease, may also be affected by psychosocial and spiritual issues, e.g. fear, anxiety, or depression may exacerbate pain.

Successful symptom management depends upon a number of key principles:
- Defining the underlying cause of the symptom.
- Consideration of any psychosocial and spiritual issues.

- Explanation of the cause of the symptom to the patient (and family where appropriate).
- Treatment of reversible causes of symptoms, e.g. anaemia, hypercalcaemia.
- Consideration of any appropriate disease-orientated treatment, e.g. chemotherapy in ovarian cancer; localized radiotherapy for pain from bone metastases from endometrial cancer.
- Specific drug treatments to relieve symptoms, e.g. analgesia.
- Consideration of non-drug measures.
- The use of regular medication for persistent symptoms rather than 'p.r.n.' (*pro re nata*, whenever needed).
- Discussion of treatment options.
- The burden of treatment should not outweigh the benefits.
- Emphasis on open and sensitive communication that extends to patients, informal carers, and professional colleagues.
- Provision of information (including written).
- Review of the response to the treatment.
- Review of treatment options if present treatment is ineffective or incompletely effective.

The detailed assessment of the patient is an essential part of managing difficult symptoms. This may include the use of investigations but for patients with far advanced disease the trauma of having even simple investigations such as an X-ray may outweigh the possible benefit. The patient's view on this is therefore extremely important.

Many symptoms can be managed in a general setting using the guidelines in the following sections. However, for complex problems and for patients who do not seem to be responding as expected, referral to a specialist in palliative medicine is advised.

Pain

Pain is a common symptom in advanced gynaecological malignancy with over 40% of patients with advanced ovarian cancer suffering significant pain. Severe pain is also a major symptom for patients with recurrent carcinoma of the cervix.

It is estimated that cancer pain can generally be well controlled in around 80% of patients if the World Health Organization's (WHO) analgesic ladder guidelines are followed (Table 92.1). Patients are prescribed the weakest analgesic on a regular basis and, if the pain is not fully controlled on this, a stronger analgesic from the next 'rung of the ladder' is given and so on, until pain relief is adequate. It may be necessary to add other drugs to achieve satisfactory pain control (see later sections).

Morphine

Morphine remains the strong opioid of choice. It should be used when necessary to control severe pain regardless of the stage of a patient's illness. It should be given orally where possible and the dose titrated to achieve adequate pain relief. Initial titration is usually best achieved using a short-acting (4-hourly) preparation, e.g. morphine sulfate solution or tablets. Once the pain is under control change to a slow-release preparation is usually more convenient for the patient.

The starting dose of morphine will depend upon previous analgesics used, e.g. taking into account that 10 mg of codeine/dihydrocodeine is approximately equivalent to 1 mg of morphine. Dose increments for titration should be in the range 25–50% such that a typical titration of 4-hourly oral morphine doses may be

5 mg $\rightarrow$ 7.5 mg $\rightarrow$ 10 mg $\rightarrow$ 15 mg $\rightarrow$ 20 mg $\rightarrow$ 30 mg $\rightarrow$ 45 mg $\rightarrow$ 60 mg, etc.

For some patients, e.g. those whose pain is almost controlled on weaker opioids, the initial use of a long-acting morphine preparation together with p.r.n. doses of a short-acting morphine preparation for 'breakthrough' pain may be appropriate. It is recommended that the appropriate 'breakthrough' dose should be equivalent to one-sixth of the total daily dose, e.g. for a patient taking a 12-hourly slow-release morphine preparation 30 mg bd (twice daily), the appropriate breakthrough dose would be 10 mg 4-hourly p.r.n.

For patients who are unable to take oral morphine because of weakness, vomiting, etc., subcutaneous (SC) morphine or diamorphine can be given. Diamorphine is more soluble in water, and is therefore preferred as the volume of injection can be smaller. SC diamorphine can be given as 4-hourly bolus injections or as a continuous infusion using a battery-operated syringe driver. Approximate dose equivalents of oral and subcutaneous opioids are:
- 3 mg oral morphine = 1 mg SC diamorphine.
- 2 mg oral morphine = 1 mg SC morphine.

Side-effects of morphine

It is useful to discuss potential side-effects with patients when morphine is first prescribed. The most common are:

- *Constipation* is almost universal and dose-dependent. It can be a distressing symptom and it is important to try to prevent it by the prescription of a regular dose of oral laxative whenever morphine is commenced (unless the patient has diarrhoea), e.g. co-danthramer or co-danthrusate, which both soften the stool and stimulate bowel activity. Dose titration is important and will often avoid the need for rectal intervention. If faecal impaction develops, however, the use of enemas may be necessary, e.g. for faecal impaction with a hard faecal mass, arachis oil enema overnight followed by a phosphate enema.
- *Nausea and vomiting* occur in a minority of patients and seem to be largely related to changes in morphine dose. They therefore usually settle once a patient has been stabilized on a regular dose of morphine. It can be helped by haloperidol 1.5 mg nocte to bd orally.
- *Drowsiness/lightheadedness* is quite common, particularly in the initial stages of titration, but usually resolves when the patient is on the minimum appropriate dose to control the pain.
- *Confusion* may occur, particularly in the elderly, and may be helped by dose reduction followed by more gradual titration.

Respiratory depression is not usually encountered if oral morphine doses for pain are titrated according to the above guidelines. It is extremely important that, when an increase in morphine dose has been prescribed, the patient's response to this change is assessed. If the increased dose has not brought about an increase in pain relief then side-effects such as drowsiness and confusion may be encountered. The dose should therefore be reduced to the previous level and the cause of the pain reassessed.

Fears associated with morphine use

Patients and their families may be concerned that:
- The use of morphine means that the patient is about to die.
- The early use of morphine means that the pain will no longer respond when it becomes worse later on.
- The patient will become addicted to morphine.

755

Table 92.1 WHO analgesic ladder

Simple/non-opioid analgesic, e.g. paracetamol 1 g qds (4 times a day)
Weak opioid, e.g. codeine 30–60 mg 4-hourly
Strong opioid, e.g. morphine

Pain (*continued*)

The following discussion may therefore be helpful:

- Morphine is used earlier in patients' illnesses than it was in the past and its use is determined by the severity of pain rather than the stage of disease.
- Pain does not always become worse as the disease progresses but, if it does, further adjustment of morphine dose may help. Other methods of pain relief are also available for some types of pain.
- Psychological addiction is not usually encountered in patients taking morphine for cancer pain. Physical addiction does occur but, if the patient no longer needs opioid analgesia because the cause of the pain has resolved then the morphine dose can be reduced gradually and discontinued without withdrawal symptoms.

Other strong opioids

A number of other strong opioids are becoming available as alternatives to morphine. Their exact place in the management of cancer pain is yet to be established For some patients, however, who do not seem to be able to tolerate morphine because of side-effects, alternatives may be worth considering, e.g. transderma fentanyl.

Features of transdermal fentanyl:

- Applied as a skin patch that is changed every 3 days.
- Associated with less constipation and drowsiness than morphine.
- Useful when patients are unable to take oral morphine.
- More expensive than oral morphine.

Opioid responsiveness of pain

For those pains that do not respond fully to strong opioids other measures are necessary. It may often be appropriate to seek the advice of specialists in palliative medicine or pain clinics for these patients.

The causes of physical pains can be broadly classified in terms of their opioid responsiveness as follows:

1. Opioid-responsive, e.g. nociceptive pain from tumours.
2. Partially opioid-responsive, i.e. opioid titration seems to reach a ceiling above which an increased dose causes more side-effects but no improved pain relief, e.g. bone pain and nerve compression pain.
3. Opioid non-responsive, where opioids seem to have little effect on the pain, e.g. neuropathic pain due to nerve damage and pain from muscle spasm.

The detailed assessment of the physical cause of pain as described above is therefore essential in determining the best approach and likely responsiveness to the analgesic ladder. Where there are psychosocial issues that contribute to the severity of the pain perceived, then opioids may not be fully effective and other ways of addressing these issues need to be considered.

Thus, effective pain relief with minimized side-effects from inappropriate drug doses depends upon:

- An understanding of the opioid responsiveness of physical pains.
- Careful assessment of the cause of pain including psychosocial and spiritual issues.
- A review of the response of pain to opioids.

In advanced gynaecological malignancy pains may be complex in that there may be a number of physical components of different opioid responsiveness. For example, an expanding pelvic tumour mass may produce opioid-responsive pain but may also cause nerve compression or damage resulting in opioid non-responsive neuropathic pain. Para-aortic node involvement, e.g. in carcinoma of the cervix, may produce back pain and associated paravertebral muscle spasm that may also not respond to opioids.

Other drugs used in pain management

- Nonsteroidal anti-inflammatory drugs (NSAIDs) may be helpful in pain due to bone metastases or associated with inflammatory processes.
- Muscle relaxants, e.g. diazepam, may be helpful for muscular spasm pain.
- Tricyclic antidepressants, e.g. amitriptyline, and anticonvulsants, e.g. carbamazepine, may be helpful in neuropathic pain.
- Corticosteroids, e.g. dexamethasone, may be helpful in combination with opioids in a number of pains, e.g. hepatic capsular pain from liver metastases, perineal pain resulting from pelvic tumour, and pain associated with nerve compression. It is believed that the steroids work by reducing peritumour oedema and thereby relieving pressure.

Intestinal obstruction

Approximately 25% of patients with late-stage ovarian carcinoma develop intestinal obstruction with a median survival of 14 weeks. Surgical relief of the obstruction where possible offers approximately 2 months palliation but there is a significant risk of re-obstruction.

Symptoms include:
- Abdominal pain from:
  —distension.
  —colic.
  Nausea and vomiting.
- Constipation.

Where surgery is not appropriate the following medical management may relieve symptoms.

Medical management

In intestinal obstruction, oral medication is unlikely to be absorbed so the SC route is preferable and an SC infusion of drugs using a syringe driver can be extremely beneficial. Specific symptoms and their appropriate treatments include:
- *Pain.*
  —Pain from distension: opioids.
  —Pain from colic: anticholinergic drugs, e.g. hyoscine butylbromide.
- *Nausea and vomiting.*
  —If there is no colic, the first choice is metoclopramide, but if this is not successful change to cyclizine.
  —If there is colic, use hyoscine butylbromide and consider a trial of corticosteroids.
  —If there is residual nausea, cyclizine may be added and, if there are persistent large-volume vomits, SC octreotide may reduce these, or a nasogastric tube may be considered.
  —*NB.* In the presence of small intestinal obstruction with colic, metoclopramide and stimulant laxatives may exacerbate the colic and should therefore be avoided.
- *Constipation.* In some situations, e.g. recurrent subacute intestinal obstruction, a stool softener, e.g. docusate, may be helpful.
- *Hydration.* Depending upon the stage of disease and likelihood of reversing the obstruction, the issue of parenteral hydration should be considered, also taking into account the patient's wishes. In some situations SC fluids may help to relieve symptoms of dehydration.

Malignant ascites

Malignant ascites is common in advanced ovarian malignancy and may be associated with leg oedema, dyspnoea, reduced appetite, nausea and vomiting, and uncomfortable distension.

Treatment options include:
- Anticancer therapy.
- Paracentesis.
- Diuretic therapy, e.g. with spironolactone with or without frusemide (furosemide).
- Peritoneo-venous shunt: may be helpful in some situations where other therapies have failed.

Renal failure

Ureteric obstruction causing renal failure is a common feature of end-stage carcinoma of the cervix. Symptoms arising from progressive renal failure can be varied but at times distressing. These include:
- Drowsiness.
- Confusion and agitation.
- Nausea and vomiting.
- Myoclonic jerks.
- Itching.

It should also be remembered that renal failure may affect the metabolism of many drugs already being used, e.g. opioids, and the doses of these may need to be reduced.

Drug management of these symptoms includes:
- Confusion/agitation: haloperidol, methotrimeprazine.
- Nausea and vomiting: haloperidol, methotrimeprazine.
- Myoclonic jerks: diazepam (oral or rectal), midazolam (SC).

759

Fistulae, haemorrhage, vaginal discharge, and other symptoms

- *Fistulae.* In advanced gynaecological malignancy, particularly carcinoma of the cervix, a variety of fistulae may occur, especially between rectum and genitourinary tract or bladder and vagina. Surgical management, e.g. defunctioning colostomy for a rectovaginal fistula, may give the best symptom relief but may not be possible in far advanced disease. Under these circumstances simple measures such as using laxatives to keep the stool soft often reduces the flow through the fistula. A urinary catheter may help to reduce leakage from a vesicovaginal fistula.
- *Haemorrhage.* Rectal and vaginal bleeding may occur with local tumour invasion, particularly from carcinoma of the cervix, which may erode into the rectum. Palliative radiotherapy may be helpful and the use of antifibrinolytic drugs, such as tranexamic acid, may reduce bleeding.
- *Vaginal discharge.* Foul-smelling vaginal discharge may occur in patients with advanced carcinoma of the cervix. This is often due to anaerobic infection of fungating tumour. The smell can be reduced by using metronidazole either orally or vaginally.
- *Other symptoms.* Depending upon the site of metastatic disease numerous other symptoms may be encountered, e.g. dyspnoea from pleural effusions; anorexia and cachexia; lymphoedema; right hypochondrial pain from liver metastases; headache, nausea, and vomiting from cerebral metastases. Detailed discussion of the management of these is beyond the scope of this chapter.

Terminal care

In the last days of life it is important to continue to manage distressing symptoms. This may require the use of SC medication by bolus injection or SC infusion. Support of both the patient and family are particularly important at this stage and the explanation of symptoms such as Cheyne–Stokes breathing is helpful.

In general, unnecessary medication should be withdrawn but additional medication may be necessary for particular problems:
- *Retained bronchial secretions* can cause a rattling sound particularly distressing for those sitting by the bedside. Helpful measures include changing the patient's position, use of anticholinergics such as hyoscine butylbromide subcutaneously, and, occasionally, suction.
- *Terminal restlessness* may be caused by distended bladder or rectum, cerebral hypoxia, pain, dyspnoea, drugs, e.g. steroids, metabolic factors, anxiety, or fear. It is important to determine any reversible causes, e.g. distended bladder (in which case consider catheterization). In the absence of reversible causes, drug treatment by midazolam by SC infusion is helpful.

Recommended further reading

1 Twycross, R. (1997). *Symptom management in advanced cancer*, 2nd edn. Radcliffe Medical Press, Oxford.

2 NHS Executive (1996). *Policy framework for commissioning cancer services: palliative care services*, no. EL(96)85. NHS Executive, Leeds.

Chapter 93

Urinary tract injuries in obstetric and gynaecological practice

The close anatomical relationship between the urinary tract and the internal genital organs and lower genital tract predisposes the distal ureter and bladder to iatrogenic injury during pelvic and gynaecological surgery.

Incidence and risk factors

The incidence of ureteric injuries at the time of major gynaecological surgery has been reported to be 0.4–2.5%. The incidence of ureteric injury during hysterectomy for benign causes is reported at 1:500 cases, rising to 1% in cases of malignancy and even higher where preoperative radiotherapy has been used. Damage to the bladder occurs in 1:200 cases, being more common after previous Caesarean section. The risk of ureteric injury is higher during abdominal compared to vaginal hysterectomies especially when the former is associated with pelvic and para-aortic lymphadenectomy. Obstetric procedures such as repeat Caesarean sections and Caesarean and postpartum hysterectomies are also associated with increased risks of injury to the lower urinary tract.

Conditions that directly or indirectly distort, scar, or infiltrate pelvic tissues and thus predispose to injury of the lower urinary tract include the following.
- Large pelvic masses.
- Cervical fibroids.
- Widespread endometriosis.
- Oophorectomy after previous total abdominal hysterectomy (TAH).
- Chronic pelvic inflammatory disease (PID).
- Pelvic abscess/pelvic haematomas, lymphocyst.
- Gynaecological/lower gastrointestinal cancer.
- Prolapse—procidentia.
- Prior pelvic surgery/radiotherapy.
- Placenta accreta in the lower segment.
- Congenital abnormalities of the urinary tract.

Ureteral injury

The majority of ureteric injuries in gynaecological surgery occur in the lower third of the ureter. Thus the most common sites of such injury at the time of abdominal hysterectomy are:

- At the pelvic brim where the ureter lies beneath the infundibulopelvic ligament, overlying the bifurcation of the common iliac artey.
- Lateral to the cervix where the ureter crosses under the uterine artery.
- Lateral to the vaginal fornix as the ureter passes lateral to the cervix and upper vagina on its course to enter the bladder.

Ureteric damage in the form of 'kinking', perforation, or ligation may also occur during reperitonealization of the pelvis or during retropubic urethropexy procedures. In the obstetric setting, ureteral injury may occur as a result of extension of the uterine incision or during suturing of the uterine incision or an attempt to control haemorrhage within the broad ligament. The increased vascularity of the pelvis, distortion of anatomy, and total hysterectomy, when the cervix is not palpable due to effacement, all contribute to the increased risk of ureteric injuries during Caesarean and postpartum hysterectomies.

Bladder injury

Injury to the bladder may be an immediate result of sharp or blunt dissection during hysterectomy or repeat Caesarean section or a result of later avascular necrosis. The bladder may also be accidentally opened during entry into the peritoneal cavity at the time of hysterectomy or, more commonly, Caesarean section where the bladder is 'hitched up' from previous surgery.

765

Prevention of urological injuries

In selected cases, preoperative intravenous urogram (IVU) may assist in the detection of congenital abnormalities of the urinary tract as well as identify any distortion due to involvement by pelvic tumours, PID, endometriosis, or cancer. Perioperative insertion of ureteric catheters or stents may assist in identification and dissection of ureters but does not reduce the overall incidence of urological injuries as most cases occur in patients where there was no indication for use of such stents.

Intraoperatively, the basic principles of safety for all pelvic procedures should be adopted including adequate exposure of the surgical field, adequate light and assistance, restoration of normal anatomic relationships, traction and counter-traction to expose adjacent structures, and dissection along tissue planes. Furthermore, it is important to avoid mass ligation of tissues. Clamping, cutting, and suturing of tissues should take place under direct vision at all times. During complex pelvic surgery, the most effective way of preventing ureteral injury is to identify the ureters as they enter the pelvis over the bifurcation of the common iliac arteries and trace each ureter through their pelvic course in the retroperitoneal space preserving its pelvic peritoneal attachment and thus the blood supply within the adventitial sheath.

Detection of urological injuries

If, intraoperatively, there is a suspicion of urological injury this needs to be investigated to confirm or refute such a possibility. If a cystotomy is suspected, the bladder can be filled with methylene blue per urethra and leakage of dye will confirm inadvertent cystotomy. If injury to the ureter is suspected a number of options are available. Dissection of the ureter throughout its course in the retroperitoneal space and observing 'peristalsis' is the gold standard. Other options include intraoperative ureteral catheterization, intravenous dye injection to detect leakage of coloured urine, and intraoperative excretory urography.

Unrecognized ureteric or bladder injuries may present with symptoms and signs of intraperitoneal or retroperitoneal leakage of urine causing abdominal distension, ileus, and urinoma. There may also be symptoms of oliguria or anuria, fever, chills, and flank pain especially with ureteric obstruction. An abdominal ultrasound, excretory urography, or a cystogram may be required depending on the working diagnosis.

Repair of urological injuries

A cystotomy can usually be repaired at the time of initial injury. It is essential to identify the ureteric orifices if the cystotomy is proximal to the point of entry of the ureters to the bladder to avoid causing a ureteric obstruction as a result of the repair. If there is difficulty in identifying the ureteric orifices then intravenous frusemide will increase the urine output allowing easier identification of the ureteric orifices. The bladder should be repaired in 2 layers with a fine absorbable suture and its water tightness be tested postrepair by filling the bladder with methylene blue. Postoperatively the bladder should be drained for 7–10 days.

Ureteric injuries may take the form of angulation (kinking), crushing, ligation, transection (complete or partial), and devascularization. The general principles of successful ureteric repair include meticulous ureteric dissection with atraumatic instruments, while preserving the ureteric blood supply by maintaining the peritoneal attachment.

- A tension-free anastomosis needs to be performed using the minimum of absorbable suture to maintain a watertight anastomosis and surrounding it with retroperitoneal fat or omentum to help healing.
- Draining the site to prevent accumulation of urine, lymph, or blood is important. A proximal urinary diversion or urinary stenting may be required. Prophylactic antibiotics are recommended until all stents and drains are removed.
- Any significant angulation or kinking of the ureter should be released to prevent obstruction.
- Minor devascularization, crush injuries, or ligated ureters after release of the suture may require no other treatment but sometimes stenting the damaged ureter may help recovery.
- Lacerations of the ureter are dealt with using fine absorbable sutures to close the defect after insertion of stents.
- Where the ureter has been transected, repair depends on the nature and location of the injury and may include uretero-neocystostomy (ureteric reimplantation) with or without bladder flap, end-to-end ureteroureterostomy, ureteroureterostomy to contralateral ureter, and creation of a cutaneous ureterostomy to name just a few.

In general when a urological complication has occurred the assistance and advice of a urological surgeon should be sought, given that the best results are obtained when the complication is appropriately dealt with in the first instance.

Chapter 94

Communication/ record-keeping

History-taking

Start by introducing yourself and explaining who you are. Establish and maintain eye contact. Try to adopt an open and conducive posture and avoid sitting with a desk or other object between yourself and the patient. Indicate that you are interested in what the patient is saying by sitting forward, asking questions, and using non-verbal encouragement such as nodding. Avoid rustling through papers, looking at the time, or concentrating on writing in the notes or on to a computer. Try to ensure that you are not interrupted during the interview by telephone calls or other people entering the room. During the interview note the patient's appearance and manner.

- *Introduction.* Check the patient's name and whether she prefers to be addressed as Mrs. or Miss if you are unsure about her marital status. Ask about age and occupation. Occupation may be relevant both to the level of understanding that can be assumed and the impact of different gynaecolgical problems on the patient's life.
- *Presenting complaint.* Start with open questions and allow the patient to describe her own symptoms without interruption. Use more specific closed questions to fill in additional details if necessary. Establish the effect of the problem on the patient's life and family. Use the history-taking process to explore the patient's own concerns about her condition.
- *Previous gynaecological history.* Ask about any previous gynaecological problems and treatments. For all women of reproductive age ask about contraception if sexually active. Ask about the date and results of the last cervical smear for women over the age of 20. Unless it has already been covered in the presenting complaint ask about the date of the last menstrual period (LMP) and whether it was normal and occurred at the expected time. If the menstrual cycle varies note the minimum and maximum length.
- *Previous pregnancies.* Ask about the number of previous pregnancies and their outcome (miscarriage, ectopic, abortion, or delivery after 24 weeks). Ask about the mode of delivery and if there were any antenatal problems.
- *Previous medical history.* Ask about previous medical problems especially any endocrine disease and major cardiovascular/respiratory disease and venous thromboembolism. Ask about previous operations, especially abdominal surgery, and any anaesthetic problems. Ask about current medication, especially sex steroids and their antagonists and anticoagulants. Check for any allergies.
- *Social and family history.* A strong family history of ovarian cancer is associated with an increased risk of developing the disease. Ask about what support the patient has at home and work. This will have a bearing on the arrangements she will need to make to come into hospital and the support she will require after discharge. Ask about smoking and consumption of alcohol.

During an examination

Before any examination explain to the patient what is involved and why the examination needs to be performed and obtain her permission. Allow the patient to undress in privacy. Expose only those areas of the body that are needed at that time to carry out the examination. During the examination itself restrict you comments to an explanation of what is being done and relevant questions about any symptoms. Avoid unnecessary personal comments. After the examination explain your findings and encourage questions and discussion. Avoid giving advice or discussing management during the examination itself.

Presenting a history

Being able to accurately and concisely summarize the history and examination findings is essential when communicating with other health professionals.

Start the history by introducing the patient by name and giving a clear indication of the presenting complaint or the reason why the patient is in the ward or clinic. If there are several problems say so and deal with each in turn. If the history consists of a long narrative of events try to summarize these rather than recap each event in chronological sequence. Present the remainder of the history in a logical structured way, not skipping back and forward between items. Always include the date of the last menstrual period and cervical smear. Include details of the social history.

- Don't appear disorganized or waffle.
- Don't simply read back your notes.
- Don't reprise past history or systems review if not relevant.
- Don't use abbreviations or medical terms you can't define.

At the end of your history give a summary in no more than one or two sentences.

Giving patients information

This includes counselling about the results of tests or the implications of a particular diagnosis as well as counselling about a particular procedure.
- Use appropriate (simple) language and avoid medical jargon.
- Give information at an appropriate rate pausing where necessary. This may involve making an assessment of the patient's level of understanding and medical knowledge.
- Start with the most important items of information first.
- If giving advice make this specific and detailed.
- Use short sentences and use more than one way of giving information such as repetition, diagrams, or written summaries.
- Pausing to summarize can also be a useful way to check the patient's understanding of the information given.
- At the end of the interview try to summarize what has been said and give the patient enough time to ask any questions.
- Make an accurate record in the case notes of what has been said to the patient and/or her relatives.
- Provide appropriate information leaflets for the patient to take away or write to the patient after the interview.

Breaking bad news
- Ensure that adequate time is set aside free from interruptions for the interview.
- Read through the notes, especially the results of recent investigations, before speaking to the patient.
- Encourage the patient to have a friend or relative present during the discussion. They are more likely to remember information than a patient who is trying to come to terms with what she has been told.
- Avoid medical jargon and euphemisms for conditions such as cancer.
- Encourage the patient and/or her family to ask questions and check their understanding of what has been said.
- Make sure the patient knows what will happen next.
- Offer a further appointment or give a contact number for an appropriate team member (such as a nurse specialist) to follow up with further information.
- Make a record in the case notes of what has been said and, where possible, comment on the patient's and/or her relatives' reactions.

Dealing with an angry patient or relative
If the patient or her relatives become angry or abusive during the interview stay calm. Remain seated and invite the patient to sit down. Keep talking in a normal tone of voice whilst acknowledging the patient's anger and inviting her to talk about the reasons for her reaction. Try to convey an impression of remaining professional and in control without appearing dismissive of the patient's concerns.

Record keeping: essential elements

- Write legibly in black ink.
- Be clear and unambiguous.
- Be accurate in each entry, as to date and time. Use the same clock.
- Sign each entry: print name and grade on first entry.
- Should be contemporaneous. If written in retrospect, state this and add date and time the entry was made.
- Do not use abbreviations, meaningless phrases, or offensive subjective statements.
- Ensure that wrong entries are scored out with a single line and initialled.
- Record any warnings given to women about the risks of a particular treatment.
- Note any cardiotocograph (CTG) abnormality in the case notes and the action taken.
- Record all decisions made even if the decision is only to observe closely.
- If a woman refuses treatment, record anything said about the possible consequences of ignoring advice given. Patient should ideally countersign such an entry.
- Meconium. Record presence, thick or thin, and amount of liquor.
- CTG trace. Patient details, date and time of commencement, and maternal pulse rate should be recorded.
- Check that the fetal monitor clock displays/records the correct time.
- Record on CTG when the trace ends (it may be alleged that part is missing).

Chapter 95

Medico-legal issues in obstetrics and gynaecology

Throughout the Western world there has been a significant increase in medico-legal claims in obstetrics and gynaecology over the past decade. Few clinical practitioners in the speciality have not experienced allegations of medical negligence against them, and such claims cause considerable personal anxiety and stress. However, those receiving such claims should remember that the vast majority of allegations of medical negligence eventually are not proven and, furthermore, because of the high level of claims, the receipt of such a claim is not the medical disgrace that it may have been 50 years ago.

It is the nature of obstetrics and gynaecology, particularly the former, that things can go wrong quickly, sometimes without warning, and yet a perfect outcome is expected by everybody. Equally, because in gynaecology our patients are often very fit preoperatively, again a perfect outcome is expected. It is for this reason that the speciality of obstetrics and gynaecology was historically one of the first specialities to be hit by medical negligence claims, although other specialities are now equally affected. Because of the nature of our speciality, it is therefore difficult to avoid absolutely the risk of a claim. However, the fundamentals of good medical practice will go a long way to diminishing the risk. These are:

- Be courteous to patients and relatives at all times.
- Pay careful attention to the detail of the management of a case.
- Maintain a high standard of note-keeping in medical records.

What is negligence?

To a medical layman the expression 'negligence' carries the connotation of a wilful act on behalf of the individual practitioner. Apart from a very small number of notorious individuals, the concept of a wilful misdeed is horrific to most. However, the term negligence in law means that a duty of care owed by the practitioner (then becoming a defendant) to the patient (who has become the claimant) has been breached. Such a breach may be caused by omission rather than commission. In simple terms, the claimant alleges that the defendant has been careless. In determining the degree of carelessness, particularly in surgical procedures, recognition is made of the level of skill an individual practitioner may have. For example, if a consultant instructs a first-year specialist registrar to carry out a Wertheim's hysterectomy alone, and both ureters are damaged, this outcome may have been expected and the specialist registrar alone could not necessarily be held negligent in this respect. However, the consultant could be deemed to be negligent for inappropriate delegation of the task and, equally, the registrar could be deemed negligent for taking it on. This could also apply in other instances where a registrar undertook a difficult emergency case without discussing it with the consultant. In another example, where the rectal mucosa was breached by a suture during the repair of a second-degree tear after childbirth, whether it was caused by the senior house officer or consultant, both could equally be liable if they had not carried out a rectal examination at the completion of the procedure to check that this had not happened. In other words, this would be exercise of a skill that all levels of practitioners should possess.

At the present time, patients and politicians expect all non-consultant grade doctors to be supervised. Unfortunately, the term supervision means different things to different people. To most, supervision of a surgical procedure by a consultant means that he/she is scrubbed and taking part in the operation. However, it is possible to supervise an operation while standing in the theatre unscrubbed, by being in the theatre suite but not necessarily in the operating room, by being in the hospital, or even by not necessarily being in the hospital at all. In all situations, it would have to be demonstrated that the operating junior had been adequately trained, and was adequately experienced to operate on the patient at that level of supervision and, where the case had been specifically chosen by the consultant, that the case was matched to the surgeon's known level of skill and ability. Furthermore, if the consultant is not present in the hospital, then proper arrangements have to be made for assisting the operating practitioner in the event of unexpected difficulties.

If it can be demonstrated that the duty of care had been breached by the above means, a causal connection between such a breach and the alleged damage suffered by the patient has to be demonstrated. This process is called determination of causation. In a lot of cases this is straightforward, e.g. 'surgeon operates on wrong leg', or may be more difficult than the claimant's supporters may believe, e.g. 'failure to remove intrauterine contraceptive device (IUCD) at time of sterilization resulting in long-term pelvic pain'. Furthermore, how much of the damage resulting from such incidents is attributable to the negligence and how much is attributable to other causes needs to be determined.

Finally, a monetary value of such damage needs to be determined and the legal term for this is 'quantum'.

Civil Justice Reforms 1999

Until recently, the natural course of medico-legal claims resulted in many cases being dropped after a response from the defendant. In other cases claims were settled but approximately 5% resulted in a court case following the traditional adversarial pattern. The overall effect of this was that, in this small group of cases, the legal process often went on for many years and finally culminated in a very expensive time in court where the legal costs could be more than any settlement achieved by the plaintiff. It was with this background in mind that Lord Woolf carried out a review of the procedure for litigation (not only for medical cases but for others as well) and introduced what have now been called the Woolf Reforms. These introduced new rules for dealing with litigation cases and introduced plain-speaking language, e.g. replacing the term plaintiff with claimant. The Woolf Reforms have an overriding objective of 'enabling the court to deal with cases justly'. The court now manages the progress of a case and does not tolerate delays for any reason. It also strictly limits the number of experts that each side may employ to provide evidence. The court also may instruct the experts from each side to discuss the points of the case on which they can agree and demonstrate those on which they cannot agree. This process, of course, replaces the time-consuming and expensive process of cross-examination in court to arrive at the same end. The purpose of such a meeting would seem to be to avoid a court process altogether so that, once the points of agreement and disagreement can be arrived at, it is easier for the lawyers of both parties to debate a settlement if appropriate.

One further element that is new is the so-called part 36 offer (named after the number of its section in the new rules). For the first time a claimant will be given the right to make an offer to settle for a certain sum of money. Previously, this facility was only available to the defence and it does give a guidance to the thinking of the claimant and her advisers. Once a claimant has made a part 36 offer, however, there is strict timescale in which the defence is able to respond and general denial to stonewall the claim is no longer acceptable. There must be a response between 14 and 28 days after the offer and, where the defence thinks there may be liability, although limited, the defence will have to also put in a value. Some clinicians may see this as a considerable weakening of their case and resist this. However, if liability is subsequently found against the defence, and no realistic valuation of a settlement sum has been proposed, then the new rules allow the legal costs to be heaped upon the defence out of all proportion to the value of the settlement. It is therefore important that doctors who are unfortunately involved in this situation be pragmatic and strongly heed the advice of their legal advisers.

Consent for operative procedures

It is incumbent on anybody performing an operative procedure to ensure that adequate signed consent has been obtained from the patient beforehand. It is also important to check that the planned procedure matches that which is written on the consent form. There can be very little defence if tubes and ovaries are removed at the time of hysterectomy when the patient only consented to the hysterectomy itself. Similarly, if it has been agreed that something be done, e.g. removal of an IUCD at sterilization, and this is not carried out (and the patient not advised), again there is little defence.

There is currently a view being put forward that consent should only be taken from patients by practitioners who are capable of performing the operation, on the grounds that such a practitioner can adequately brief the patient on the procedure and any complications. Usually, this means that the consent should be taken by the surgeon concerned. However, in practice this may be difficult to achieve for all situations. Provided a practitioner is familiar with the procedure, whilst not necessarily being able to perform it, this could be considered as sufficient. This could mean that junior members of the team could readily take consent for hysteroscopy and perhaps even for straightforward hysterectomy. However, in more complex cases, such as minimal access surgery or radical oncology procedures, the consultant should ensure (and be capable of demonstrating by the medical record) that the patient has been adequately briefed on the procedure and complications at the very least even if he/she is not necessarily the signatory of the consent form.

Common obstetric problems

Most medico-legal problems in obstetrics revolve around very consistent themes even if the details of individual cases vary. Problems invariably arise due to failure to elucidate, disclose, or discuss information about a pregnancy with patients, failure to take or maintain adequate medical records about a case, and, in particular, failure to act appropriately in the presence of abnormalities.

All first-class obstetric units (and who would wish to be otherwise) should possess a manual of guidelines/protocol of action in the event of abnormal situations arising. If it can be demonstrated, preferably through the medical report, that these guidelines and protocols have been observed, an adequate defence may usually be achieved even in the event of an adverse outcome.

95 Medico-legal issues

Common causes of medico-legal problems in obstetrics are the following.

- *Antenatal period.*
  —Failure to explain investigations and results, scan findings, etc.
  —Failure to act on abnormal results.
  —Failure to keep good records.
  —Failure to obtain good antenatal CTG recordings or appropriately annotate them.
- *Intrapartum period.*
  —Failure to keep continuous, timed and signed, detailed records of progress.
  —Failure to achieve good quality CTG recordings, with event annotation.
  —Failure to act in the presence of abnormal physical signs, progress, or CTG recording.
  —Failure to make and record adequate observations on a patient in the postpartum period, particularly in the event of an operative delivery, or complications such as pre-eclampsia.
  —Failure to act on observations and thus avoid postoperative collapse or eclampsia, for example.
- *Complicated pregnancies* such as multiple, breech, or placenta praevia, all require the presence of a senior obstetrician, paediatrician, and anaesthetist at delivery.
- *Shoulder dystocia* is a major and often unexpected sudden complication of the second stage of labour, which can have serious long-term results for the baby particularly in the form of brachial plexus nerve palsy. For this reason each unit should have a distinct protocol for the management of such an emergency and the protocol should be rehearsed regularly.

Common medico-legal problems in gynaecology

The same principles as previously discussed apply. Failure to adequately counsel patients on their condition and any proposed surgical procedure is a common cause of litigation. Sterilization procedures and termination of pregnancy are frequent cases seen in gynaecology and, individually, they represent the highest risk of adverse outcome and litigation. It is therefore prudent to ensure that patients are adequately briefed and in some centres information leaflets are issued to patients prior to operation and patients are asked to sign that they have read and understood the contents. If these are not available, it is incumbent to record in the notes that the patients have been specifically counselled in the following areas in both topics.

- *Sterilization.* The following areas must be discussed.
  —The type of operative procedure and devices used.
  —The failure rate (now usually described as 1 in 200–500 cases)
  —Potential irreversibility of the procedure.
  —Laparoscopic risks involving bowel or vessel damage that may result in laparotomy.
  —Preoperatively—the importance of determining LMP and/or excluding pregnancy.
  —Failure to remove/discuss removal of IUCD if present.
- —*Termination of pregnancy*. It is important to counsel concerning/discuss the following:
  —Primary or secondary haemorrhage that may lead to hysterectomy.
  —Incomplete evacuation requiring a subsequent repeat procedure.
  —Infection subsequent to procedure.
  —Infertility subsequent to procedure.
  —Uterine perforation at procedure leading to laparoscopy/laparotomy/ hysterectomy.

The disclosure of operative risks

Minimal access gynaecological surgery carries particular risks. Because there is very little to show on the external body surface, patients tend to think they have had a small operation. Similarly, particularly in the early days, surgeons also tended to think that these were small procedures. In fact, many of them are not—they tend to be complex procedures involving high technology equipment. Despite this, some senior surgeons, who perhaps should have known better, went straight into performing these operations without any training on the equipment or the procedures. Some dreadful accidents ensued that, of course, were medico-legally indefensible. It is important, particularly in the current climate, that anyone undertaking new operative procedures, particularly when they are complex, can demonstrate they have been adequately trained in the procedure and the equipment to be used. Equally, it is very important that patients are counselled as to the expected outcomes and complications of these procedures. In particular, it must be explained that in endometrial ablative procedures there is a risk of perforation leading on to hysterectomy and that, in laparoscopic procedures, the very nature of the surgery makes damage tp collateral structures a higher risk than in open surgery even in the hands of the most experienced of laparoscopic surgeons.

In more traditional operations and those of lower medico-legal risks than sterilization and termination of pregnancy, there is a debate as to how much operative risk needs to be disclosed to the patient. For example, ureteric and bladder damage is a known risk of total abdominal hysterectomy. In North America, surgeons are advised to disclose such risks in detailed information sheets to patients. In Western Europe, such an extreme approach is considered (at least at present) to be unnecessary and perhaps counterproductive in that such details would alarm patients to the point of declining the surgery when offered, even in cases where there was an overwhelming medical reason for it. There is also a general impression amongst gynaecologists that risks only need to be disclosed to patients if they are higher than 1 in 1000 cases, 1 in 2000 cases, or so on. It is by no means certain that such specificity is the case despite efforts by certain medico-legal experts to make it so. For some operations, e.g. bowel/blood vessel damage at laparoscopy, an incidence of 1 in 2500 needs to be disclosed to a patient, whilst other experts maintain that an incidence of less than 1 in 1000 need not be disclosed at all. The simple reason for this disparity is because the courts decide what the 'ordinary skilled practitioner' would do in a given set of circumstances rather than there being any set rules. Furthermore, in the case of known complications such as ureteric/bladder damage at hysterectomy, contemporary cases would suggest that, if all due care and attention has been taken at the operation and this has been properly documented, in the case of complications such as significant pelvic haemorrhage during the procedure, this can be a mitigating and acceptable circumstance. However, if there is subsequently a delay at diagnosis of the resulting fistula, then this could be construed as negligent. Similarly, significant wound infection with abscess formation, which certainly has a significance of greater than 1 in 1000 cases, need not specifically be counselled for preoperatively and the occurrence of such a complication would not be construed as negligent. However, if it were managed inappropriately, it could be so construed.

Special types of hysterectomy, such as radical (Wertheim's) hysterectomy where the incidence of complications is higher, do need to have particular special attention applied to the preoperative counselling. Subtotal hysterectomy, which is now becoming more popular as an elective procedure, does have particular possible problems concerning outcome, e.g. continued regular menstruation and the need for continued regular cervical cytology. These make it important that patients are counselled about the details of this particular procedure preoperatively.

783

Recommended further reading

1 Chamberlain, G.V.P. (ed.) (1992). *How to avoid medico-legal problems in obstetrics and gynaecology*, 2nd edn. Royal College of Obstetricians and Gynaecologists, London.

Clinical risk management

Risk is a part of everyday life. We all seek to manage such risks, e.g. by wearing seat belts, locking houses, and insuring property. Clinical risk management is a mechanism for dealing with risk exposure in obstetric and midwifery practice. This process enables us to recognize those events that may result in unfortunate or damaging consequences for patients, their frequency and severity, and how the risks may be controlled.

The overall objective of clinical risk management is to improve the quality of patient care by reducing or eliminating accidental harm to patients whenever possible. A review of the literature suggests that many more patients are harmed or traumatized by clinical treatment than those who consider legal action.[1, 2] The scale and effects of injury to patients should therefore be the primary focus for risk management. Where quality is good litigation is likely to be low.

Clinical staff involved in adverse incidents are often seriously affected by such events. Genn[3] states that doctors involved in legal claims report great distress, worry, anger, and frustration. Loss of professional confidence and the adoption of defensive medical practice may result. Media interest in clinical negligence and professional competence issues would appear likely to increase staff stress and may also result in a loss of reputation for the National Health Service (NHS) Trust.

Costs of clinical negligence claims are currently around £200 million per year[4] with obstetric practice generally being regarded as 'high risk' for legal claims. In addition, obstetric claims may involve very large financial settlements, e.g. up to £3 million damages in cerebral palsy cases. Extra costs associated with increased hospital stay and further investigation and treatment must also be considered. Equally important are the costs to the injured patient—increased pain, disability, and disruption to relationships, work, and social life.

With the possibility of litigation and/or prosecution under the UK Health and Safety at Work legislation the NHS is becoming more aware of the consequences of a wide range of risks that occur by accident through mischance, mishap, or mistake.

The clinical governance initiative[5] places a strong emphasis on risk management, clinical audit, and professional competence. The main aims of this process are to improve standards of care and define best practice in order to improve quality. It is essential that health-care practitioners can demonstrate a commitment to clinical and cost effectiveness as for the first time NHS Trusts have a legal duty to provide *quality* health care. Controls assurance also requires Trusts to identify and prioritize risks.

- A proactive move towards managing clinical risk means anticipating any potential hazards that may cause harm to patients and taking steps to prevent or limit any harm that may occur.
- Reactive approaches include dealing appropriately with injured patients, learning from past mistakes, and effective claims management.
- Both approaches will require risk assessment and prioritization skills.

Risk identification

Risks to service users can be identified by a combination of methods:
- Incident reporting.
- Analysis of complaints/legal claims/user views.
- Confidential enquiries and audit.
- Risk assessments.

Incident reporting

All grades and disciplines of staff should be encouraged to report any situation where the individual considers that a threat to patient safety may exist. This includes incidents where actual harm is caused to a patient and 'near miss' events, i.e. where something has gone wrong but no actual harm has occurred to the patient. In order to achieve the compliance of clinical staff it is important that organizational culture is encouraged to move from one of blame to a culture of openess and honesty. Assurances need to be given at board level that disciplinary action will not result against employees who commit errors, unless serious professional misconduct or a crime has been committed.

- Forms used must be 'user-friendly' in order to increase compliance—a list of specific trigger indicators is particularly useful in obstetric practice.
- Patient details, date and time of the incident, staff involved, and a brief *factual* account of the incident must be included.
- It should also be made clear that any serious outcome for a patient must be reported to appropriate persons without delay.
- Completed forms should be collated and analysed at a central point.

Over a period of time it is possible to identify common factors and trends that may result in real risks to patients though they would be considered trivial when viewed in isolation.

Should a legal claim be likely to result from an adverse outcome, formal statements can be collected from the staff involved in order that legal advisors can make early decisions on potential liability and prepare a defence when appropriate.

Communication with patients following adverse events

An efficient system of risk reporting also aids good communication. A senior member of the obstetric/midwifery team must be informed of adverse outcomes in order that the family are counselled appropriately and arrangements made for referral or follow-up dependent on clinical need and the patient's wishes.

Analysis of complaints/legal claims/user views

Retrospective analysis of complaints and legal claims can be used to highlight areas where improvements in care/treatment can be made. Ongoing audit of claims and complaints is an important part of clinical governance in that Trusts must be able to demonstrate changes in practice by learning from previous mistakes. This aspect of risk management has recently been highlighted in a Department of Health Report.

It is essential also to involve consumers in the planning and development of maternity services. In the UK this can be achieved by involving representatives from the Maternity Services Liaison Committee in local clinical governance initiatives.

Confidential enquiries and audit

Invaluable information on clinical risk can be gained from the UK Department of Health's Confidential Enquires into Maternal Deaths and into Stillbirths and Infant Deaths. These national reports also recommend changes to practice in order to reduce risk.

Local clinical audit processes may also highlight areas of clinical risk and can be used to monitor areas of high risk, e.g. the 'decision to delivery' interval in emergency Caesarean section.

Risk assessments

All reported risk or near-miss situations should be formally assessed as to their frequency of occurrence and severity in order that necessary actions can be centrally prioritized. Control measures can then be identified and put into place.

Some NHS Trusts employ specialists in risk analysis to carry out formal risk assessments whilst others use their own staff. During the process of carrying out proactive risk assessments widespread consultation with all grades and disciplines of staff is necessary. This encourages local ownership of problems and may well identify latent failures within the organization, i.e. the factors that contribute indirectly to medical accident and near-miss situations. Decisions can then be made on what precautions or controls are needed. These measures can be maintained whilst monitoring future risk recurrence.

Risk analysis

The risk assessment process must include analysis of the severity of effect and the likelihood of recurrence. This will include consideration of effects on the patient, on service provision, and on the likelihood of future legal claim. A cost:benefit analysis should also be carried out at this stage. Because of the nature of health care it is not possible to create an environment that is free of risk.

Risk control

Clinical risks can be controlled by:
- Avoidance—by using alternative working practices or equipment.
- Making risks less likely—e.g. by improving staff training or a review of clinical guidelines.
- Elimination—by ceasing to provide the service.
- Insuring against those the risks that cannot be reduced or eliminated so that litigation costs are reduced. In the UK this can be achieved by membership of the Clinical Negligence Scheme for Trusts (CNST).

789

The Clinical Negligence Scheme for Trusts

The CNST is administered by the NHS Litigation Authority and acts as a form of indemnity insurance against clinical negligence claims. The aim is to promote high standards of care, to increase knowledge of clinical risk management principles, and to provide financial settlement of claims over an agreed financial excess. Comprehensive risk management standards are produced with Standard 10 providing criteria for management and communication systems in maternity care.

Risk reduction in obstetric/midwifery practice

Communication

Effective communication between health professionals and between staff and women and their families is essential to the provision of quality care. Poor communication is one of the main causes of complaint that may lead to a legal claim. Women should be encouraged to participate in decision-making and in making informed choices about the care and treatments available. Written information should be available to support verbal information given to women. Provision of information in the form of audio and video tapes should also be considered.

There should be a personal hand-over of care at shift changes for both medical and midwifery staff in order to ensure accurate sharing of information.

Policies, procedures, guidelines

These should be based on the best available evidence and reviewed and updated regularly. Clinical audit may help clarify that guidelines are suitable and are used by clinical staff. It is also important that out-of-date documents are correctly archived if required for future legal claims.

Valid consent arrangements

Ideally, consent for operative procedures should be obtained by a health professional capable of carrying out the procedure. If this is not possible, the health professional obtaining consent must have sufficient knowledge to inform the woman of the material risks, benefits, and alternatives to the proposed treatment. It is also essential to warn of any consequences of refusal of treatment and give the woman an opportunity to ask questions if she wishes.

Staffing levels

Attention should be given to provision of safe levels of both obstetric and midwifery staffing levels in all areas of practice. For labour wards this should include the recommendations of the recent report *Towards safer childbirth*:

1 Minimum consultant or equivalent cover for labour wards of 40 hours per week.
2 Midwifery staffing levels of 1.15 midwives per woman in labour.
3 Junior medical staffing will depend on available training opportunities.

Wherever possible, the use of locum or agency clinical staff should be minimal. When this group of staff are employed close supervision is necessary. Handover of patient care should be by a senior member of the obstetric/midwifery team. Written information on local procedures and guidelines should also be made freely available.

Professional competence

Statutory supervision in midwifery provides an enabling and supportive framework in order that the midwife can fulfil her responsibilities. Professional guidance and advice on assessment and management of risk is also available via the supervisory relationship.

- Induction programmes for all staff should be mandatory at commencement of employment.
- All clinical staff must receive 6 monthly training in cardiotocograph (CTG) interpretation and the management of high-risk labour (CNST standard 10).

- Regular training of all staff in neonatal and adult basic life support should also be considered as mandatory. 'Fire drills' in the management of obstetric emergencies such as major haemorrhage and shoulder dystocia are excellent methods of maintaining professional competence.
- All staff must be familiar with equipment used in their area of work and ensure it is maintained regularly.

Complaint management

All clinical staff should have a basic knowledge of local complaint procedures and have the necessary skills to deal with verbal complaints before a formal complaint becomes necessary.

Record-keeping

Keeping and maintaining a record of care given are essential, both to aid continuity of care and to provide a defence to legal claims.

- Records must be clear, unambiguous, legible, and contemporaneous.
- It is essential that all entries are readily identifiable.
- All decisions about clinical care should be recorded.
- Local arrangements must be in place for follow-up of all clinical investigations performed.
- All test and imaging results, electrocardiographs (ECGs), and CTG tracings must be stored securely within the casenotes.
- Maternity records must be stored securely for a minimum 25-year period.
- Regular audit of record-keeping standards is necessary with appropriate feedback to individuals in order that standards can be improved.

Recommendations for further reading

1 Brennan, T.A., Leape, L.L., and Laird. N. (1991). Incidence of adverse events and negligence in hospitalised patients: results of the Harvard medical study: part 1. *New England Journal of Medicine* **324**, 370–7.

2 Wilson, R.M., Runciman, W.B., and Gibber, R.W. (1995). The Quality in Australian Healthcare Study. *Medical Journal of Australia* **163**, 458–71.

3 Department of Health (1997). *The new NHS: modern, dependable*, White Paper. Department of Health, London.

4 Donaldson, L. (2000). *Organisations with memory*. Department of Health, London.

5 NHS Litigation Authority (NHSLA) (2000). *Clinical Negligence Scheme for Trusts clinical risk management standards*, Version 01. NHSLA, London.

6 Royal College of Obstetricians (RCOG) and Gynaecologists and Royal College of Midwives (1999). *Towards safer childbirth—minimum standards for the organisation of labour wards*, report of a joint working party. RCOG Press, London.

Index

Index

Index

Index

801

Index